The Frith Prescribing Guidelines for People with Intellectual Disability

'The Frith guidelines are now in their fourth edition, demonstrating their internationally important contribution. The expert editors have integrated the latest information from leaders in the field – essential reading for anyone serious about understanding and improving pharmacotherapy and pharmacovigilance for people with intellectual disabilities.'

Sally-Ann Cooper,
Professor of Learning Disabilities,
University of Glasgow

The Frith Prescribing Guidelines for People with Intellectual Disability

Fourth Edition

Edited by
David M. L. Branford
Independent Pharmacy Consultant

Satheesh K. Gangadharan
Leicestershire Partnership NHS Trust, University of Leicester, and Loughborough University

Mary Barrett
Leicestershire Partnership NHS Trust

Regi T. Alexander
Hertfordshire Partnership University NHS Foundation Trust and University of Hertfordshire

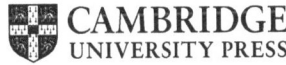

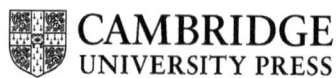
CAMBRIDGE
UNIVERSITY PRESS

Shaftesbury Road, Cambridge CB2 8EA, United Kingdom

One Liberty Plaza, 20th Floor, New York, NY 10006, USA

477 Williamstown Road, Port Melbourne, VIC 3207, Australia

314–321, 3rd Floor, Plot 3, Splendor Forum, Jasola District Centre, New Delhi – 110025, India

103 Penang Road, #05–06/07, Visioncrest Commercial, Singapore 238467

Cambridge University Press is part of Cambridge University Press & Assessment, a department of the University of Cambridge.

We share the University's mission to contribute to society through the pursuit of education, learning and research at the highest international levels of excellence.

www.cambridge.org
Information on this title: www.cambridge.org/9781009430722
DOI: 10.1017/9781009430715

First edition © Leicestershire Partnership NHS Trust 2005
Second edition © Leicestershire Partnership NHS Trust 2008
Third edition © John Wiley & Sons, Ltd 2015
Fourth edition © Royal College of Psychiatrists 2025

This publication is in copyright. Subject to statutory exception and to the provisions of relevant collective licensing agreements, no reproduction of any part may take place without the written permission of Cambridge University Press & Assessment.

First published 2005
Second edition 2008
Third edition 2015
Fourth edition 2025

A catalogue record for this publication is available from the British Library

A Cataloging-in-Publication data record for this book is available from the Library of Congress

ISBN 9781009430722 Paperback

Cambridge University Press & Assessment has no responsibility for the persistence or accuracy of URLs for external or third-party internet websites referred to in this publication and does not guarantee that any content on such websites is, or will remain, accurate or appropriate.

....

Every effort has been made in preparing this book to provide accurate and up-to-date information that is in accord with accepted standards and practice at the time of publication. Although case histories are drawn from actual cases, every effort has been made to disguise the identities of the individuals involved. Nevertheless, the authors, editors, and publishers can make no warranties that the information contained herein is totally free from error, not least because clinical standards are constantly changing through research and regulation. The authors, editors, and publishers therefore disclaim all liability for direct or consequential damages resulting from the use of material contained in this book. Readers are strongly advised to pay careful attention to information provided by the manufacturer of any drugs or equipment that they plan to use.

Contents

List of Contributors vii
Foreword xi
Lade Smith
Preface xiii
Acknowledgements xiv

1 **Intellectual Disability** 1
Ken Courtenay, Tadhgh Lane, and Indermeet Sawhney

2 **Prescribing Practice** 13
Gyles Glover, David Gerrard, and David M. L. Branford

3 **Physical Health Monitoring** 31
Mariam Omokanye, Nazurah Wahid, Praveena Peddireddi, Reena Tharian, David M. L. Branford, and Archana Anandaram

4 **Mental Health Conditions in People with Intellectual Disability** 51
Meghana Rayala, Ayomipo J. Amiola, Reena Tharian, Tadhgh Lane, and Regi T. Alexander

5 **Trauma in People with Intellectual Disability: Recognition and Intervention** 61
Elspeth Bradley and Marika Korossy

6 **Anxiety Disorders** 74
Ayomipo J. Amiola, Reena Tharian, and Regi T. Alexander

7 **Depression** 87
Adelola Idowu and David M. L. Branford

8 **Bipolar Disorders** 102
Prabhleen Jaggi, David M. L. Branford, and Regi T. Alexander

9 **Schizophrenia** 118
Dasari Michael, Amir Javaid, Muzammil Hayat, Ilyas Ali, Ayomipo J. Amiola, and Reena Tharian

10 **Aggression and Self-Injurious Behaviour** 131
Peter E. Langdon, Kris Roberts, Danielle Adams, Farshad Shaddel, and Mary Barrett

11 **Personality Disorders** 155
Ayomipo J. Amiola, Sreeja Sahadevan, Reena Tharian, Sadie Clarke, and Regi T. Alexander

12 **Sexual Offences and Paraphilias** 169
Stuart Banham, Gemma Lewin, and John Devapriam

13 **Substance Use Disorders** 180
Ayomipo J. Amiola, Sreeja Sahadevan, Saher Binnat Rafiq, and Regi T. Alexander

14 **Attention Deficit Hyperactivity Disorder** 199
Bhathika Perera

15 **Autism** 209
Dolly Sud, Danielle Adams, Rohit Shankar, and Samuel Tromans

16 **Sleep Disorders** 223
Rebecca Dodds and Laura Korb

17 **Epilepsy** 238
Lance Watkins, Márie O'Dwyer, Reza Kiani, and Rohit Shankar

18 **Dementia** 254
Shweta Gangavati, Elizabeta Mukaetova-Ladinska, Satheesh K. Gangadharan, and Remon Mosaad

19 **Eating and Drinking Difficulties** 275
Jennifer Worsfold, Jennifer Roberts, Nicky Calow, and David M. L. Branford

20 **Children and Adolescents** 297
Mark Lovell, Ashley Liew, and Keir Jones

21 **Prescribing for Health Issues in Women with Intellectual Disability** 309
Sowmy Murickal, Nnenna Kalu-Nsi, and Amala Jesu

22 **Older People** 321
Gemma Lewin, Elizabeta Mukaetova-Ladinska, Rohit Gumber, and Satheesh K. Gangadharan

Index 338

Contributors

Danielle Adams
Centre for Research in Intellectual and Developmental Disabilities (CIDD), University of Warwick, UK

Regi T. Alexander
Hertfordshire Partnership University NHS Foundation Trust and University of Hertfordshire, UK

Ilyas Ali
Nottinghamshire Healthcare NHS Foundation Trust, UK

Ayomipo J. Amiola
Hertfordshire Partnership University NHS Foundation Trust, UK

Archana Anandaram
Leicester, Leicestershire and Rutland Integrated Care Board, UK

Stuart Banham
Herefordshire and Worcestershire Health and Care NHS Trust, UK

Mary Barrett
Leicestershire Partnership NHS Trust, UK

Elspeth Bradley
University of Toronto, Canada

David M. L. Branford
Independent pharmacy consultant, Leicestershire, UK

Nicky Calow
Leicestershire Partnership NHS Trust, UK

Sadie Clarke
Hertfordshire Partnership University NHS Foundation Trust, UK

Ken Courtenay
Barnet Enfield and Haringey Mental Health NHS Trust, London, UK

John Devapriam
Herefordshire and Worcestershire Health and Care NHS Trust, UK

Rebecca Dodds
Nottinghamshire Healthcare NHS Foundation Trust, UK

Satheesh K. Gangadharan
Leicestershire Partnership NHS Trust, University of Leicester, and Loughborough University, UK

Shweta Gangavati
Leicestershire Partnership NHS Trust, UK

David Gerrard
Health Improvement Pharmacy lead, Learning Disability and Autism, NHS England

Gyles Glover
National Autism Programme, NHS England and NHS Improvement, UK

Rohit Gumber
Leicestershire Partnership NHS Trust, UK

Muzammil Hayat
Humber Teaching NHS Foundation Trust, UK

Adelola Idowu
Leicestershire Partnership NHS Trust, UK

Prabhleen Jaggi
Leicestershire Partnership NHS Trust, UK

Amir Javaid
Humber Teaching NHS Foundation Trust, UK

Amala Jesu
Leicestershire Partnership NHS Trust, UK

Keir Jones
Midlands Partnership NHS Foundation Trust, UK

Nnenna Kalu-Nsi
Core Trainee (CT3), Leicestershire Partnership NHS Trust, UK

Reza Kiani
Leicestershire Partnership NHS Trust and University of Leicester, UK

Laura Korb
Haringey Learning Disability Partnership, North London Mental Health Partnership, UK

Marika Korossy
Surrey Place Centre, Toronto, Canada

Tadhgh Lane
RADiANT, Hertfordshire Partnership University Foundation NHS Trust, UK

Peter E. Langdon
Centre for Research in Intellectual and Developmental Disabilities (CIDD), University of Warwick and Coventry and Warwickshire Partnership NHS Trust, UK

Gemma Lewin
Leicestershire Partnership NHS Trust, UK

Ashley Liew
South London and Maudsley NHS Foundation Trust, UK

Mark Lovell
Tees Esk and Wear Valleys NHS Foundation Trust, UK

Dasari Michael
Humber Teaching NHS Foundation Trust, UK

Remon Mosaad
Leicestershire Partnership NHS Trust, UK

Elizabeta Mukaetova-Ladinska
University of Leicester and Leicestershire Partnership NHS Trust, UK

Sowmy Murickal
Nottinghamshire Healthcare NHS Foundation Trust, UK

Máire O'Dwyer
School of Pharmacy and Pharmaceutical Sciences, Trinity College Dublin, Ireland

Mariam Omokanye
Nottinghamshire Healthcare NHS Foundation Trust, UK

Praveena Peddireddi
Derbyshire Healthcare NHS Foundation Trust, UK

Bhathika Perera
University College London and North East London NHS Foundation Trust, UK

Saher Binnat Rafiq
Cambridgeshire and Peterborough NHS Foundation Trust, UK

Meghana Rayala
Norfolk and Suffolk Foundation NHS Trust, UK

Jennifer Roberts
Leicestershire Partnership NHS Trust, UK

Kris Roberts
Nottinghamshire Healthcare NHS Foundation Trust, UK

Sreeja Sahadevan
Hertfordshire Partnership University NHS Foundation Trust, UK

Indermeet Sawhney
Hertfordshire Partnership University NHS Foundation Trust, UK

Farshad Shaddel
University of Oxford, UK

Rohit Shankar
Plymouth University Peninsula Schools of Medicine and Dentistry, CIDER; Cornwall Partnership NHS Foundation Trust, UK

Dolly Sud
Leicestershire Partnership NHS Trust, UK

Reena Tharian
Hertfordshire Partnership University NHS Foundation Trust, UK

Samuel Tromans
SAPPHIRE Group, Department of Population Health Sciences, University of Leicester, and Leicestershire Partnership NHS Trust, UK

Nazurah Wahid
Derbyshire Healthcare NHS Foundation Trust, UK

Lance Watkins
Swansea Bay University Health Board, UK

Jennifer Worsfold
Derbyshire Healthcare NHS Foundation Trust, UK

Foreword

Report after report has found that people with learning disability are more likely to die early of an avoidable physical disorder. In addition to the failure to recognise symptoms, diagnostic overshadowing, and even frank neglect, iatrogenic harms through poor prescribing, especially inappropriate polypharmacy, result in an unacceptable level of risk.

Changing systems in healthcare, not unlike an ocean-going liner turning around, takes a long time. However, in the meantime, as individual practitioners, we can improve our knowledge and understanding, and, above all, our prescribing, such that our individual patients will be less likely to be harmed by inadequate practice.

To guide us in this, the editors of the fourth edition of this book have brought together doctors and pharmacists, clinicians and researchers, and even librarians from different specialist areas and with differing types of experience – from trainees to the most senior consultants. Most importantly, they have brought people with lived experience together with health professionals from all across the UK to provide thoroughly comprehensive, evidence-based, up-to-date, and thoughtful guidance about how best to support our patients with intellectual disability to get drug treatments, which are tailored to their individual needs and aimed at providing health benefits with minimal adverse effects, and this of course, is the best way to prescribe.

The book covers different psychiatric disorders, but also focuses on different groups of people across the lifespan – from children and adolescents to older people – and there is a special chapter on prescribing for women. Importantly, they include a chapter on prescribing practice and physical health at the start of the book.

The *Frith Prescribing Guidelines* are now in their fourth edition. This is the ultimate reference guide for anyone working with people with intellectual disability. As that is all of us, every clinician should have a copy of this book on our shelves. I thank David Branford, Mary Barrett, Satheesh Kumar, Regi Alexander, and all the contributors for giving me and other practitioners the tools and guidance to support our patients to have better lives and achieve their potential.

Dr Lade Smith CBE, President of the Royal College of Psychiatrists

Preface

The fourth edition of the *Frith Prescribing Guidelines* is dedicated to the founding editor of this book: the late Professor Sabyasachi (Sab) Bhaumik OBE. Professor Bhaumik had been the chair of the psychiatry of intellectual disability faculty at the Royal College of Psychiatrists, London, between 2006 and 2010, and of the Royal College of Psychiatrists' Trent division before that. In 2007, he established an international links group that brought together all the activities related to intellectual disability undertaken internationally by Royal College of Psychiatrists members. At the time of his sudden and unexpected death in 2019, Sab was truly the prototype of the accomplished clinician-researcher: an inspirational role model for many of his trainees, peers, patients, and families, and a leading authority in the psychiatry of people with intellectual disability.

Recognising the lack of evidence to support the prescribing of psychotropic medication in this group, alongside Dr David Branford he created the first edition of the *Frith Prescribing Guidelines* in 2005. Over the last 18 years, the book has remained, arguably, the best-known prescribing guideline for psychotropic medication for people with intellectual disability. While its first edition was developed almost entirely based on the clinical consensus of a range of professionals in the field, the second and third editions drew on a growing scientific evidence base, while still retaining consensus clinical opinion for those areas where the evidence remained limited. This dual approach addressed, to a substantial degree, the complexity perpetually encountered by clinicians in this field.

Although the format remains largely similar with case studies and, where appropriate, algorithms, this fourth edition has many new features:

- Involvement of service users and/or their families in the planned structure and authorship of the chapters. We would particularly like to thank Tadhgh Lane and Michelle O'Reilly for their valued contributions in this regard.
- A greater reference to the evidence base.
- An expert group 'statements of confidence', provided for treatment guidelines in each of the diagnostic categories. Divided into the categories of high, medium, and low, they attempt to combine the strength of the evidence base with the experience of clinical practice.
- A strong focus on STOMP (Stopping the Over-Medication of People with a learning disability and autistic people) and STAMP (Supporting Treatment and Appropriate Medication use in Paediatrics). These programmes have spurred the development of many initiatives in England and resulted in the generation of many resources to assist both professionals and non-professionals involved with intellectual disability.
- A greater emphasis on how to reduce psychotropic medication and/or consider non-medication alternatives, as appropriate.
- Links to key documents and resources.

We hope that this format proves useful and would welcome feedback on this, and indeed any other aspects of the book, from readers to inform future editions.

Acknowledgements

The editors would like to thank all those who have given their time and expertise to help produce this fourth edition of the *Frith Prescribing Guidelines*.

A particular mention goes to Dr Lade Smith CBE, President of the Royal College of Psychiatrists, for kindly providing the Foreword.

In addition, the editors wish to formally acknowledge the valuable input the of experts by experience who have contributed to and significantly enhanced the quality of this edition, namely Dr Michelle O'Reilly, Associate Professor of Communication in Mental Health, University of Leicester and Chartered Psychologist in Health, and Mr Tadhgh Lane, member of RADiANT, Hertfordshire Partnership University foundation NHS Trust.

The editors wish to express their sincere gratitude to all the chapter authors of this fourth edition, who have freely given of their time and considerable expertise; without them, this book could not have been produced. In addition, thanks go again to all the contributors to the previous three editions, on which this edition has been built.

Finally, the editors wish to acknowledge the vital role of the late Professor Sabyasachi Bhaumik in the development of the *Frith Prescribing Guidelines*. His input as a founding editor and chapter author over the first three editions provided the bedrock for this ongoing work. We are profoundly grateful for his enthusiasm, drive, and academic rigour, which we have sought to continue as part of his legacy. He remains greatly missed and fondly remembered.

Chapter 1

Intellectual Disability

Ken Courtenay, Tadhgh Lane, and Indermeet Sawhney

Introduction

People with intellectual disability experience greater health inequalities and a disproportionate number of comorbid physical health disorders when compared with the general population (Emerson & Hatton 2013). They often have complex medication regimens to support them in managing their health (Eady et al. 2015). For these reasons, it is important that clinicians, people with intellectual disability, and their carers are well informed about the medication that they are likely to use throughout their lives.

The focus of this edition of the *Frith Prescribing Guideline*s is to guide clinicians in how to approach the treatment of people with an intellectual disability and ensure that they and their carers are at the centre of the decision-making process. This is to achieve the best possible clinical outcomes for the person while ensuring they are empowered as much as possible, and with due respect being paid to their autonomy and dignity.

Definitions

The Centre for Disease Control (CDC) defines developmental disorders as 'a group of conditions which cause an impairment in physical, learning, language or behavioural development. These conditions begin during the developmental period and may impact on day-to-day functions, and usually last throughout a person's lifetime' (Centre for Disease Control and Prevention 2022). The important aspect of the definition of developmental disorders is their origins in childhood, as compared with cognitive disorders that may occur in adults because of disease or head injury where the adult did not have signs of a developmental disorder prior to the event causing the current impairment.

Disorders of intellectual development is a term used to describe developmental disorders that includes intellectual disability (Simpson et al. 2020; Salvador-Carulla et al. 2011). The World Health Organization describes disorders of intellectual development as ' a group of etiologically diverse conditions originating during the developmental period characterised by significantly below average intellectual functioning and adaptive behaviour that are approximately two or more standard deviations below the mean (approximately less than the 2.3rd percentile), based on appropriately normed, individually administered standardized tests' (ICD-11; https://icd.who.int/browse/2024-01/mms/en#605267007).

Developmental disorders are graded according to severity, which can be helpful in clinical practice in communicating the level of functioning of a person. The categories are mild (50–70), moderate (35–49), severe (20–34), and profound (<20), graded according to scores derived from cognitive testing. Categorisations should not obscure the strengths and abilities innate to each person (American Psychiatric Association 2013).

> **Box 1.1** The American Psychiatric Association (APA) Diagnostic Criteria for Intellectual Disability (DSM-5 Criteria)
>
> 1. Deficits in general mental abilities.
> 2. Impairment in adaptive functioning for individual's age and sociocultural background which may include communication, social skills, person independence and school or work functioning.
> 3. All symptoms must have an onset during the developmental period.
> 4. The condition may be subcategorised according to severity based on adaptive functioning as mild, moderate, or severe.
>
> (American Psychiatric Association 2013)

Causes of Intellectual Disability

The causes of intellectual disability are varied and in many cases are unknown. Genetic disorders such as Fragile X syndrome (Sitzmann et al. 2018), chromosomal disorders such as Down syndrome, disorders due to structural abnormalities such as cerebral palsy, and perinatal effects such as hypoxia at birth or prematurity have all been mentioned (Karam et al. 2015) (see Table 1.1).

The Health of People with Intellectual Disability

The health outcomes for people with intellectual disability are poor, with men and women dying more than 22 years earlier than people in the general population (Glover et al. 2017; Heslop & Hoghton 2018). People with intellectual disability experience more comorbid disorders throughout their lifetime, with estimates of a mean of 11 comorbid disorders per person (Kinnear et al. 2018). Specific examples include epilepsy that is more prevalent, especially in autistic people (Lukmanji et al. 2019). Diseases associated with lifestyle are more common: for example, obesity, which can lead to metabolic disorders such as diabetes (Hsieh et al. 2014). As a result, people with intellectual disability use more medications for physical and mental health disorders across their lifetimes, exposing them to unwanted effects of medication (McMahon et al. 2020). For these reasons, it is important to be aware of the potential impact of prescribing practice on the person and their well-being when considering drug interventions, and when assessing the overall benefit to the person of using medication.

Psychiatric Disorders and Behaviours That Challenge

The diagnosis and treatment of psychiatric disorders and behaviours that challenge in people with intellectual disability may require a different approach to that in the general population. Such conditions often present differently in people with intellectual disability compared to people in the general population. The signs and symptoms may be misattributed to the person's developmental disorder – this is described as diagnostic overshadowing (Reiss & Szyszko 1983). In addition, symptoms of an underlying physical condition, or a reaction to environmental changes, may mask an underlying psychiatric disturbance (Bertelli et al. 2015). Difficulties in diagnosis may be further compounded by a person's communication challenges.

Table 1.1 Causes of intellectual disability

Period of origin	Nature of disorder	Common examples
Prenatal period	**Genetic disorders** Chromosome aberrations Single gene mutations Microdeletions	Down syndrome (trisomy 21) Tuberous sclerosis, phenylketonuria, mucopolysaccharidoses, Fragile X syndrome, Prader–Willi syndrome, Williams syndrome, Smith–Magenis syndrome
	Congenital malformations Central nervous system malformations Multiple malformation syndromes	Neural tube defects Cornelia de Lange syndrome
	Exposure Maternal infections Teratogens Pre-eclampsia, placental insufficiency Severe malnutrition Trauma Iatrogenic	Congenital rubella, HIV Foetal alcohol spectrum disorder Prematurity Intra-uterine growth retardation Physical injury Radiation, medications
Perinatal period	Infections Delivery Other causes	TORCH infections: toxoplasmosis, hepatitis B, syphilis, herpes zoster, rubella, cytomegalovirus, herpes simplex, Anoxic brain damage Hyperbilirubinaemia
Postnatal period	Infections Metabolic Endocrine Cerebrovascular Toxins Trauma Neoplasms Psychosocial factors	Encephalitis Hypoglycaemia Hypothyroidism Thrombo-embolic phenomena Lead poisoning Head injury Meningioma, craniopharyngioma Under-stimulation
Any	Untraceable or unknown	

Psychotropic medication is used to support people who have psychiatric disorders and behaviours that challenge. The use of antipsychotics has come under scrutiny in recent years because they have been used to manage behavioural challenges rather than to treat psychiatric disorders (O'Dwyer et al. 2019). Prescribing medication for reasons not connected to its recognised indications should not be part of good clinical care.

Evidence-Based Practice

The evidence base for the use of psychotropic medications is limited. Consequently, a wide range of psychotropic medications are used outside their licenced indications to manage behaviours that challenge, which may or may not be associated with an underlying psychiatric disorder (Bowring et al. 2017). In a Dutch study, 32% of the study group were prescribed antipsychotics for behavioural disturbances (de Kuijper et al. 2010). The reasons for this are many, including:

- Pressure from professionals/carers for immediate resolution of a problem
- Limited resources available for changing the environment
- Lack of appropriately trained staff in residential homes
- Shortfall in the number of psychiatrists
- Lack of input from clinical psychologists, specialist clinical pharmacists, and speech therapists.

Even with optimum resources and good professional input, some behavioural problems remain unchanged, causing serious risk to the person and others. In some cases, the use of psychotropic medication brings welcome relief: for example, using low doses of risperidone in those with autism may reduce stereotypies and disturbed behaviour (Jesner et al. 2007; Rajapakse & Pringsheim 2010).

In some cases, medications can reduce elevated levels of arousal, allowing the person to then participate in other therapeutic approaches (Ali et al. 2014). Nevertheless, clinicians who prescribe psychotropic medications outside their licenced indications may feel professionally vulnerable and open to criticism for 'unethical practice' (Bhaumik et al. 2015). Strong views exist about 'chemical straitjacketing' for behavioural disorders in the absence of adequate resources (Moncrieff 2013).

Prescribing Medication

The clinical activity of prescribing medication is part of the professional role of medical and non-medical prescribers. Clinicians have a professional responsibility to prescribe medication judiciously by taking in to account the benefits to the person of using medication and to be aware of their potential adverse consequences (General Medical Council 2021). It is essential to understand the purpose of prescribing medication and the desired impact that is required. Prescribing without a focused and defined purpose is irresponsible and potentially dangerous.

It is important to understand and to focus on the therapeutic benefit of medication for the person. What may work for one person may not be effective for another. When prescribing, the benefits to the person should be to arrest disease progression or alleviate suffering. Medications often have associated side effects that could have adverse consequences for the individual. Common effects such as tremor or weight gain can have important and distressing impacts on the person's health and, ultimately, their quality of life (Gründer et al. 2016). Excessive weight gain due to using medication predisposes to development of metabolic disorders such as diabetes mellitus that can have major consequences for a person's health and their lifespan (Raben et al. 2017).

Movement disorders may affect a person's ability to engage in activities and have psychological impacts affecting their participation in life (Sheehan et al. 2017). Additionally, the experience of undesirable effects may affect carers and family members supporting the person where a change in behaviour or physical health may be attributable to using medication (Hall & Deb 2008). For these reasons, prescribing is an important skill in clinical practice that clinicians must consider carefully and strive to achieve high standards in prescribing practice for the benefits of the person.

Prescribers have a duty to inform those using medication about the actions and impacts of medication on them, to enhance their understanding when gaining their consent to treatment (Adams et al. 2018). To achieve this, it is important to engage with people to support them in using drug regimens appropriately. For people who lack mental capacity or have fluctuating capacity, gaining their consent to treatment can be challenging, but appropriate processes are available that clinicians should abide by (Social Care Institute for Excellence 2009).

The Body and Medication

Considering the therapeutic indications for using medication, clinicians should be aware of the physical impacts of medication on the body and how the organs metabolise medication. When initiating medication, it is prudent for prescribers to be aware of potential adverse impacts due to drug interactions and to act accordingly to avoid untoward effects that could affect the overall efficacy of the medication (English et al. 2012).

Pharmacokinetics is the process of absorption, distribution, and elimination of medication by the body's organs, which affects the availability of the active components of drugs (Loucks et al. 2015). For a person using multiple medications, the potential for drug interactions is greater and can affect the bioavailability (pharmacokinetics) of the agent and therefore the impact (pharmacodynamics) of it on the body (Daniel et al. 2022). An understanding by the prescriber of the disease states of a person helps to inform how drugs will be metabolised: for example, lithium salts in a person with impaired renal function.

Pharmacodynamics is the study of the impact of the active component of drugs on the body, including the brain (Rowland 2010). Prescribers will be aware of the desired impacts of medication, but such impacts may not be uniform for everyone, especially people with intellectual disability and other developmental disorders. For example, standard doses of a medication may be over-sedating for one person but stimulating for another, or therapeutic for some but sub-therapeutic for others.

Pharmacogenomics

An emerging area of great interest is how a person's genes determine how they metabolise the active ingredients of medications. Knowledge about individual responses to how drugs are absorbed, metabolised, and impact on disease could unlock the prospect of clinicians designing drug regimens to optimise the therapeutic effects in a personalised approach (Carvalho Henriques et al. 2020). Such knowledge and skill could have impressive impacts and benefits for people with developmental disorders using complex drug regimens (Perera et al. 2022).

Polypharmacy

Given that people with developmental disorders experience greater rates of comorbid disorders, it is not surprising that they will use a variety of medications together to treat physical and mental health conditions (McMahon et al. 2020). Such complicated drug regimens may lead to drug interactions and compounding adverse effects that may negatively affect a person's quality of life (Valenza et al. 2017). Polypharmacy in clinical practice is not advised, but for many it is inevitable. Regardless, it is important that there is clarity for the person on the indications of using all medications and their potential consequences.

Prescribing Practice

When commencing medication, it is advisable that prescribers consider the maxim of 'start low and go slow', whereby lower doses than standard ones are suggested because of the sensitivity of people with intellectual disability to medication and the greater likelihood of developing adverse effects (Osugo & Cooper 2016). A slower approach to increasing doses is desirable to avoid adverse effects. Therefore, gaining an impression of the therapeutic effect may take longer than would be expected in the general population. For this reason, it is prudent not to abandon potentially beneficial medication where the impact is not immediately apparent but to agree a timescale for a therapeutic trial. This allows for a more informed evaluation of a drug's effectiveness.

In the absence of benefit, it is important to consider withdrawing medication and how this should be undertaken (Deb et al. 2020). With some agents – for example, antidepressants and antipsychotics – abrupt or rapid withdrawal is not advised because of withdrawal effects that can adversely affect a person's well-being and level of functioning (Davies & Read 2019; Hengartner et al. 2020). A programme of withdrawal can minimise the effects the person could experience (Shankar et al. 2019). For this reason, regular review of medication, especially psychotropic medication, is essential to avoid the unnecessary long-term use of agents that do not have discernible benefits to the person and may affect their quality of life because of adverse effects.

Overuse of Medication

An issue of great importance and concern is the overuse of medication in people with intellectual disability (Sheehan et al. 2015). Formal inquiries into incidents of poor care in inpatient services revealed that psychotropic medication was prescribed to excess and often without clinical indications, especially where it was used to control behaviour (Flynn 2012). In England, this issue has resulted in a review of the culture of prescribing psychotropic medication, in particular antipsychotics, leading to a public campaign to stop the overuse of medication in people with intellectual disability. The objective is to reduce reliance on psychotropic medication and to implement non-pharmacological approaches to support behaviours that may challenge services. The impact has been to highlight the inappropriate use of medication in people who often cannot advocate for themselves and to develop alternatives to medication. As a result, there have been changes in the attitudes of prescribers, carers, and families to a reliance on medication. Such an approach, and a change in clinical practice, could have beneficial effects on a person's quality of life and respect of their human rights.

Issues Affecting Prescribing in People with Intellectual Disability

Communication

Difficulties with communication are frequently encountered by clinicians treating people with intellectual disability; in addition, associated hearing or vision loss can often create physiological challenges (Smith et al. 2020). For the person, cognitive impairments can make attending to and processing information more difficult, while the prescriber may struggle to communicate effectively with the person (Martin et al. 2010). It is essential to involve the person at all stages of the decision-making process when prescribing new treatments, or when altering or withdrawing existing treatments. Consulting a family member or carer on their knowledge of the person is advisable when a person cannot express their personal views. Such an approach helps to inform the decision-making process and should ensure the person's best interests remain central (Bigby et al. 2019). It is important to involve the person if they plan to manage their own medication regimen. Where a person is supported by a carer to use medication, it is essential that carers understand the importance of the medication, its functions, and any side effects. They need advice on observing for adverse reactions and how to seek medical attention.

There are many methods and aids available to assist the clinician with communicating with a person with intellectual disability. Makaton signing is an effective method of communication for people with intellectual disability which utilises sign language, symbols, and speech to provide multiple avenues for communication (Grove & Walker 1990). Visual communication aids such as the Picture Exchange Communication System (PECS) and Talking Mats may be beneficial when supporting people who do not use spoken language (Murphy & Cameron 2008; Sulzer-Azaroff et al. 2009). Processing visual information may be easier than processing auditory information (Hollins 1996). Asking for the assistance of a family member or carer to advise on the best communication methods for the person is important.

Shared Decision-Making

While it is medically and ethically right to withdraw medications that people do not require, it is important to balance this with the positive medical benefits the person may receive from using them. An open dialogue with the person and, where necessary and appropriate, their family, carer, or advocate about the potential positives and negatives of continued use of medication is important to create a collaborative decision-making process (Sullivan & Heng 2018). Such an approach should ensure that the person's views and concerns are expressed and addressed while allowing the clinician to fully explain their concerns or views regarding medication regimens. This should help to achieve better clinical outcomes for the person.

Mental Capacity and Incapacity

Mental incapacity is where a person is unable, by the reason of impaired mental ability, to make a decision for themselves on the matter in question, or unable to communicate that decision. No one can give consent on behalf of an incompetent adult. The assessment of an adult's capacity to make a decision about their own medical treatment is a matter of clinical judgement guided by the Mental Capacity Act (Social Care Institute for Excellence 2009). It is the personal responsibility of the professional proposing to treat a person to judge whether the patient has the capacity to give valid consent. The clinician has a duty to give the patient an account in simple terms of the nature of the treatment, the benefits versus risks of the proposed treatment, and the alternative options.

Determining mental capacity can be a complex issue when supporting people with intellectual disability. A person may have capacity to make decisions in certain areas of their lives (e.g., which clothes to wear), but lack capacity in other areas (such as personal care or finances). Capacity is not fixed but can fluctuate over time: for example, a person may lose capacity while unwell (either physically or mentally), then regain capacity on recovery. Due to these complexities, it is essential that clinicians have a solid foundation in understanding mental capacity.

To demonstrate capacity in relation to treatment, a person should be able to:
- understand in simple language what the medical treatment is, its purpose and nature, and why it is proposed;
- understand its principal benefits and risks, and any alternative options;
- understand, in broad terms, what the consequences of not receiving the proposed treatment may be;
- retain the information for long enough to make an effective decision;
- weigh that information on balance and arrive at a free choice;
- communicate their decision.

In day-to-day clinical practice, decisions regarding treatments are often taken for adults who lack capacity using 'best interest' principles. There is clear guidance on formulating best interest decisions within the Mental Capacity Act of England and Wales (Social Care Institute for Excellence 2009). The key principles are:
- The person remains at the centre of the decision-making process and participates as much as they are able.
- Parents, carers, and other people close to the patient need to be consulted for information about the person's preferences, choices, and best interests.
- Consideration must be given to the least restrictive option for the person's rights and freedom.
- For decisions regarding serious medical treatment or a change in accommodation when the person is classed as 'un-befriended' (i.e., has no one to speak for them aside from paid carers), then involvement of an Independent Mental Capacity Advocate (IMCA) is required.
- Intervention from the Court of Protection should be sought for treatment decisions that are more serious or contentious.

Consent to Treatment

Guidelines for medical practitioners registered with the General Medical Council in the UK state that, wherever possible, express consent should be obtained from the person, and/or where appropriate their family/guardians if they do not have mental capacity (General Medical Council 2020). Express consent is provided either verbally or in writing, but other communication methods are acceptable if it enables the person to participate in the decision-making process. Documentation of all decisions on mental capacity is essential in clinical practice.

For a person's consent to be legally valid and professionally acceptable, they must be:
- Capable of taking the specific decision (competent)
- Acting voluntarily (free from coercion)
- Be provided with enough information (in a form they can understand) to enable them to take the decision (informed)

For adults with intellectual disability, this is often a process over time, rather than a 'one-off' effort, and particular attention should be paid to:
- The mode of communication (particularly the use of communication aids)
- The environment in which information is provided
- The person's familiarity with whoever provides the information
- The pace at which the information is provided

Person-Centred Care

Adopting a person-centred approach in care is fundamental to providing high-quality healthcare to people. The person and their family/carers should be consulted on all aspects of planning and decisions concerning their healthcare. Historically, people with intellectual disability have not been involved in decisions about their health (Sullivan & Heng 2018). Person-centred care is considered good clinical practice (van der Meer et al. 2018). Guidance on developing person-centred plans is available that should help to create holistic long-term plans for the person that recognise their needs, values, and goals in life and how to achieve them.

The six guiding principles of patient-centred care are:
- Care and support are person-centred (personalised, co-ordinated, and empowering)
- Services are created in partnership with the public and communities
- A focus on equality and the narrowing of inequalities
- Carers are identified, supported, and involved in the person's care and decision-making process
- Voluntary, community, social enterprise, and housing sectors to be involved as key partners and enablers of people
- Volunteering and social action are seen as key enablers

Conclusion

People with intellectual disability experience comorbid disorders that require complex medication regimens that can affect their quality of life. They are especially sensitive to the effects of medication. They are at risk of over-medication especially where medication is not monitored regularly, and they may not be able to advocate for themselves. Understanding mental capacity and communication styles is essential for prescribers to effectively support people with intellectual disability. Prescribing clinicians need to strive to involve people in their care with the support of families and carers.

References

Adams, D., Carr, C., Marsden, D., & Senior, K. (2018). An update on informed consent and the effect on the clinical practice of those working with people with a learning disability. *Learning Disability Practice*, **21**(4), 36–40.

Ali, A., Blickwedel, J., & Hassiotis, A. (2014). Interventions for challenging behaviour in intellectual disability. *Advances in Psychiatric Treatment*, **20**(3), 184–92.

American Psychiatric Association. (2013). DSM 5 Intellectual Disability. www.psychiatry.org/File%20Library/Psychiatrists/Practice/DSM/APA_DSM-5-Intellectual-Disability.pdf.

Bertelli, M. O., Rossi, M., Scuticchio, D., & Bianco, A. (2015). Diagnosing psychiatric disorders in people with intellectual disabilities: Issues and achievements.

Advances in Mental Health and Intellectual Disabilities, 9(5), 230–42.

Bhaumik, S., Gangadharan, S. K., Branford, D., & Barrett, M. (Eds.). (2015) *The Frith Prescribing Guidelines for People with Intellectual Disability*. John Wiley & Sons.

Bigby, C., Whiteside, M., & Douglas, J. (2019). Providing support for decision making to adults with intellectual disability: Perspectives of family members and workers in disability support services. *Journal of Intellectual & Developmental Disability*, **44**(4), 396–409.

Bowring, D. L., Totsika, V., Hastings, R. P., Toogood, S., & McMahon, M. (2017). Prevalence of psychotropic medication use and association with challenging behaviour in adults with an intellectual disability: A total population study. *Journal of Intellectual Disability Research*, **61**(6), 604–17.

Carulla, L. S., Reed, G. M., Vaez-Azizi, L. M., et al. (2011). Intellectual developmental disorders: Towards a new name, definition and framework for 'mental retardation/intellectual disability' in ICD-11. *World Psychiatry*, **10**(3), 175–80.

Carvalho Henriques, B., Yang, E. H., Lapetina, D., et al. (2020). How can drug metabolism and transporter genetics inform psychotropic prescribing? *Frontiers in Genetics*, **11**, 491895. https://doi.org/10.3389/fgene.2020.491895.

Centre for Disease Control and Prevention. (2022, April). Developmental disabilities. www.cdc.gov/ncbddd/developmental disabilities/index.html.

Daniel, W. A., Bromek, E., Danek, P. J., & Haduch, A. (2022). The mechanisms of interactions of psychotropic drugs with liver and brain cytochrome P450 and their significance for drug effect and drug-drug interactions. *Biochemical Pharmacology*, **199**, 115006.

Davies, J., & Read, J. (2019). A systematic review into the incidence, severity and duration of antidepressant withdrawal effects: Are guidelines evidence-based? *Addictive Behaviors*, **97**, 111–21.

de Kuijper, G., Hoekstra, P., Visser, F., et al. (2010). Use of antipsychotic drugs in individuals with intellectual disability (ID) in the Netherlands: Prevalence and reasons for prescription. *Journal of Intellectual Disability Research*, **54**(7), 659–67.

Deb, S., Nancarrow, T., Limbu, B., et al. (2020). UK psychiatrists' experience of withdrawal of antipsychotics prescribed for challenging behaviours in adults with intellectual disabilities and/or autism. *BJPsych Open*, **6**(5), e112.

Eady, N., Courtenay, K., & Strydom, A. (2015). Pharmacological management of behavioral and psychiatric symptoms in older adults with intellectual disability. *Drugs & Aging*, **32**(2), 95–102.

Emerson, E., & Hatton, C. (2013). *Health Inequalities and People with Intellectual Disabilities*. Cambridge University Press. https://doi.org/10.1017/CBO9781139192484.

English, B. A., Dortch, M., Ereshefsky, L., & Jhee, S. (2012). Clinically significant psychotropic drug-drug interactions in the primary care setting. *Current Psychiatry Reports*, **14**(4), 376–90.

Flynn, M. (2012). *Winterbourne View Hospital: A Serious Case Review*. South Gloucestershire Council. www.southglos.gov.uk/news/serious-case-review-winterbourne-view/.

General Medical Council. (2020). Decision making and consent. www.gmc-uk.org/-/media/documents/gmc-guidance-for-doctors-decision-making-and-consent-english_pdf-84191055.pdf.

General Medical Council. (2021). Good practice in prescribing and managing medicines and devices. www.gmc-uk.org/-/media/documents/prescribing-guidance-updated-english-20210405_pdf-85260533.pdf.

Glover, G., Williams, R., Heslop, P., Oyinlola, J., & Grey, J. (2017). Mortality in people with intellectual disabilities in England. *Journal of Intellectual Disability Research*, **61**(1), 62–74.

Grove, N., & Walker, M. (1990). The Makaton vocabulary: Using manual signs and graphic symbols to develop interpersonal communication. *Augmentative and Alternative Communication*, **6**(1), 15–28.

Gründer, G., Heinze, M., Cordes, J., et al. (2016). Effects of first-generation antipsychotics versus second-generation antipsychotics on quality of life in schizophrenia: A double-blind, randomised study. *The Lancet Psychiatry*, **3**(8), 717–29.

Hall, S., & Deb, S. (2008). A qualitative study on the knowledge and views that people with learning disabilities and their carers have of psychotropic medication prescribed for behaviour problems. *Advances in Mental Health and Learning Disabilities*, **2**(1), 29–37.

Hengartner, M. P., Davies, J., & Read, J. (2020). Antidepressant withdrawal: The tide is finally turning. *Epidemiology and Psychiatric Sciences*, **29**, e52.

Heslop, P., & Hoghton, M. (2018). The Learning Disabilities Mortality Review (LeDeR) programme. *British Journal of General Practice*, **68**(suppl 1), bjgp18X697313.

Hollins, S., Bernal, J., & Slowie, D. (1996). *Going to the Doctor*. Books Beyond Words. https://booksbeyondwords.co.uk/bookshop/paperbacks/going-doctor.

Hsieh, K., Rimmer, J. H., & Heller, T. (2014). Obesity and associated factors in adults with intellectual disability. *Journal of Intellectual Disability Research*, **58**(9), 851–63.

Jesner, O., Aref-Adib, M., & Coren, E. (2007). Risperidone for autism spectrum disorder. *Cochrane Database of Systematic Reviews*, **2007**(1), CD005040. https://doi.org/10.1002/14651858.CD005040.

Karam, S. M., Riegel, M., Segal, S. L., et al. (2015). Genetic causes of intellectual disability in a birth cohort: A population-based study. *American Journal of Medical Genetics Part A*, **167**(6), 1204–14.

Kinnear, D., Morrison, J., Allan, L., et al. (2018). Prevalence of physical conditions and multimorbidity in a cohort of adults with intellectual disabilities with and without Down syndrome: Cross-sectional study. *BMJ Open*, **8**(2), e018292.

Loucks, J., Yost, S., & Kaplan, B. (2015). An introduction to basic pharmacokinetics. *Transplantation*, **99**(5), 903–7.

Lukmanji, S., Manji, S. A., Kadhim, S., et al. (2019). The co-occurrence of epilepsy and autism: A systematic review. *Epilepsy & Behavior*, **98**, 238–48.

Martin, A.-M., O'Connor-Fenelon, M., & Lyons, R. (2010). Non-verbal communication between nurses and people with an intellectual disability: A review of the literature. *Journal of Intellectual Disabilities*, **14**(4), 303–14.

McMahon, M., Hatton, C., & Bowring, D. L. (2020). Polypharmacy and psychotropic polypharmacy in adults with intellectual disability: A cross-sectional total population study. *Journal of Intellectual Disability Research*, **64**(11), 834–51.

Moncrieff, J. (2013). Chemical cosh: Antipsychotics and chemical restraint. In *The Bitterest Pills*. London: Palgrave Macmillan, pp. 132–51.

Murphy, J., & Cameron, L. (2008). The effectiveness of Talking Mats® with people with intellectual disability. *British Journal of Learning Disabilities*, **36**(4), 232–41.

O'Dwyer, C., McCallion, P., Henman, M., et al. (2019). Prevalence and patterns of antipsychotic use and their associations with mental health and problem behaviours among older adults with intellectual disabilities. *Journal of Applied Research in Intellectual Disabilities*, **32**(4), 981–93.

Osugo, M., & Cooper, S.-A. (2016). Interventions for adults with mild intellectual disabilities and mental ill-health: A systematic review. *Journal of Intellectual Disability Research*, **60**(6), 615–22.

Perera, B., Steward, C., Courtenay, K., Andrews, T., & Shankar, R. (2022). Pharmacogenomics: An opportunity for personalised psychotropic prescribing in adults with intellectual disabilities. *BJPsych Open*, **8**(5), e157.

Raben, A. T., Marshe, V. S., Chintoh, A., et al. (2017). The complex relationship between antipsychotic-induced weight gain and therapeutic benefits: A systematic review and implications for treatment. *Frontiers in Neuroscience*, **11**, 741.

Rajapakse, T., & Pringsheim, T. (2010). Pharmacotherapeutics of Tourette syndrome and stereotypies in Autism. *Seminars in Pediatric Neurology*, **17**(4), 254–60.

Reiss, S., & Szyszko, J. (1983). Diagnostic overshadowing and professional experience with mentally retarded persons. *American Journal of Mental Deficiency*, **87**(4), 396–402.

Rowland, M. T. T. N. (2010). *Clinical Pharmacokinetics and Pharmacodynamics: Concepts and Applications*, 4th rev. ed. Lippincott Williams and Wilkins.

Shankar, R., Wilcock, M., Deb, S., et al. (2019). A structured programme to withdraw antipsychotics among adults with intellectual disabilities: The Cornwall experience. *Journal of Applied Research in Intellectual Disabilities*, **32**(6), 1389–400.

Sheehan, R., Hassiotis, A., Walters, K., et al. (2015). Mental illness, challenging behaviour, and psychotropic drug prescribing in people with intellectual disability: UK population based cohort study. *BMJ*, h4326.

Sheehan, R., Horsfall, L., Strydom, A., et al. (2017). Movement side effects of antipsychotic drugs in adults with and without intellectual disability: UK population-based cohort study. *BMJ Open*, **7**(8), e017406.

Simpson, N., Mizen, L., & Cooper, S.-A. (2020). Intellectual disabilities. *Medicine*, **48**(11), 732–6.

Sitzmann, A. F., Hagelstrom, R. T., Tassone, F., Hagerman, R. J., & Butler, M. G. (2018). Rare *FMR1* gene mutations causing fragile X syndrome: A review. *American Journal of Medical Genetics Part A*, **176**(1), 11–18.

Smith, M., Manduchi, B., Burke, É., et al. (2020). Communication difficulties in adults with Intellectual Disability: Results from a national cross-sectional study. *Research in Developmental Disabilities*, **97**, 103557.

Social Care Institute for Excellence. (2009). Mental Capacity Act 2005 at a glance. www.scie.org.uk/mca/introduction/mental-capacity-act-2005-at-a-glance.

Sullivan, W. F., & Heng, J. (2018). Supporting adults with intellectual and developmental disabilities to participate in health care decision making. *Canadian Family Physician Medecin de Famille Canadien*, **64**(Suppl 2), S32–S36.

Sulzer-Azaroff, B., Hoffman, A. O., Horton, C. B., Bondy, A., & Frost, L. (2009). The Picture Exchange Communication System (PECS). *Focus on Autism and Other Developmental Disabilities*, **24**(2), 89–103.

Valenza, P. L., McGinley, T. C., Feldman, J., et al. (2017). Dangers of polypharmacy. In *Vignettes in Patient Safety – Volume 1*, InTech. https://doi.org/10.5772/intechopen.69169.

van der Meer, L., Nieboer, A. P., Finkenflügel, H., & Cramm, J. M. (2018). The importance of person-centred care and co-creation of care for the well-being and job satisfaction of professionals working with people with intellectual disabilities. *Scandinavian Journal of Caring Sciences*, **32**(1), 76–81.

Chapter 2

Prescribing Practice

Gyles Glover, David Gerrard, and David M. L. Branford

Introduction

There are many studies of the prescribing of psychotropic medications for people with intellectual disability. This chapter provides information about that prescribing, issues associated with the data, and trends in medication usage. Excessive or unnecessary prescribing of psychotropic medication that exposes individuals to unwanted side effects and imposes unwarranted costs on services has been the focus of many medication review programmes. This chapter will review outcomes data from medication reduction programmes for individuals with intellectual disability and present practitioner guidelines. The NHS England programme STOMP (Stopping the Over-Medication of People with a learning disability and autistic people) and STAMP (Supporting Treatment and Appropriate Medication use in Paediatrics) has been the focus for many initiatives in England, resulting in the generation of numerous resources to assist both professionals and non-professionals working with people with intellectual disability.

Prevalence of Psychotropic Medication Prescribing

The English governmental inquiry into the care of people with intellectual disability, following the scandal of abuse and neglect in the largely NHS-funded, private hospital Winterbourne View (Department of Health 2012), noted that the inquiry team had 'heard deep concerns about over-use of antipsychotic and antidepressant medicines'. The concern was that these, and other psychotropic medications, were being used to manage behaviour seen as problematic or challenging by staff – a use for which they are not licenced and for which there is little, if any, good-quality evidence of their efficacy. In response, the government commissioned studies into the extent of use and the development of guidance on its appropriateness in this context.

In their guidance NG11(NICE 2015), the National Institute for Health and Care Excellence reviewed the evidence of effectiveness of a range of pharmaceutical treatments to prevent and intervene for people whose behaviour is seen as challenging. They concluded that almost all the research in this area was of low or very low quality. While there was some evidence indicating short-term (less than three months) benefit in managing behaviours, there was very little information on the long-term benefits. On the other hand, there was evidence of long-term physical health consequences, including weight gain, raised prolactin levels, and sedation.

The National Learning Disability Observatory (at that time a part of Public Health England) collaborated with the Medicines and Healthcare Products Regulatory Agency to study general practitioners' (GP) prescribing of psychotropic medication to people identified as having intellectual disability (Glover et al. 2014). The study used data for the period April 2009 to March 2012 from one of the large-scale general practice research datasets, the Clinical Practice Research Datalink. Although the use of psychotropics in this group is usually initiated at the suggestion of secondary-care consultants, most long-term prescribing, other than for current in-patients, is done by patients' GPs. The study found that, on average, 17% of adults with intellectual disability were currently being prescribed an antipsychotic (one-fifth of this group were prescribed more than one antipsychotic) and 16.9% an antidepressant (11% of this group were prescribed more than one medication from this class). The study also noted that 22.9% of adults with intellectual disability were currently prescribed an antiseizure medication, 7.1% a medication used for the management of mania or hypomania, 4.2% an anxiolytic, and 2.7% a hypnotic. Prescribing rates for antipsychotics and antidepressants rose with age, with more than a quarter of those aged 65 or older prescribed an antipsychotic, and more than 20% an antidepressant. Antipsychotics and antidepressants were commonly prescribed together, with 40% of those prescribed an antipsychotic also prescribed an antidepressant, and vice-versa. The prescribing rates for these two latter medication classes far exceeded the prevalence of the mental illnesses for which they are indicated in people with intellectual disability, as documented by Cooper et al. (2007).

In response to this and other investigations, NHS England's Chief Pharmacist initiated the STOMP programme in 2016 (Covered in more detail later in this chapter).

Four years later, Public Health England explored the practicality of using data from another general practice research dataset – The Healthcare Intelligence Network (THIN) – to monitor progress of STOMP and STAMP (Mehta and Glover 2019). This study looked at trends in quarter-year prescribing rates, comparing the six and a quarter years from January 2010 to March 2016 to the subsequent seven quarter years, following the launch of the STOMP programme, to the end of 2017. For both antipsychotics and antidepressants, in the pre-STOMP period there was a small rising trend in prescribing prevalence. After the STOMP launch, a slight falling trend appeared for antipsychotics, while for antidepressants the rising trend flattened to no trend. Before the launch, prescribing prevalence had been steady for anxiolytics and rising for antiseizure medications. After the launch, there was a decreasing trend for anxiolytics, but no change for antiseizure medications.

The findings of this study need to be seen as preliminary. Rolling out programmes such as STOMP and STAMP across the whole of England takes significant time. Major impacts would be expected to appear mainly in years two to four, thus the data window for the study closed much too early. Additionally, the utility of the findings was limited by only using data from a sample of the English population; thus it was only possible to report on England as a whole. Monitoring the roll-out of a remedial programme requires data capable of showing differences between local areas.

To provide this, NHS England added a number of items to the data collected through the system called the Health and Care of People with Learning Disabilities (NHS Digital 2022). These data are intended to be collected annually from all NHS General Practices. The data are read in an automated way from practice clinical information systems and, to secure confidentiality, provide a large series of counts of individuals meeting sets of multiple criteria. Hence, as a result of commercial difficulties with one of the suppliers of the general practice information systems, they are collected from practices covering roughly 55% of the English population, with collection more complete from the west of the country than the east.

The data reported here were collected in the summer of 2022. They give counts of the numbers of adults registered with general practitioners, where the GP had or had not recorded the presence of an intellectual disability, by age group and sex, overall and where the individual was currently prescribed four classes of medications. For three of the medication classes, these counts were further subdivided by whether specific indications for use of the medications were recorded. Using these data, it is possible to document the recent prevalence of treatment with these medication classes by age and sex. Figure 2.1 shows the results.

For all four medication groups, prescribing rates for people with intellectual disability of both genders rise during young adulthood, reaching a peak usually around the 55–64-year age band, and then show some reduction in older age groups. For people without recorded intellectual disability, this pattern was seen for antidepressants and antipsychotics, although with a second peak in the oldest age group for antipsychotics. For antiseizure medications and benzodiazepines prescribing rates rose continuously with age.

The biggest differences were in the overall rates of prescribing. Prescribing of antipsychotics was much more common in people with intellectual disability than those without: prescription with a recorded indication was 10.9 times as frequent and without a recorded indication 19.1 times. Prescribing of antidepressants was also more common but by a much smaller margin: prescription with a recorded indication was 1.4 times as common and without 2.5 times.

Antiseizure medication was, not surprisingly, much more frequently prescribed for people with intellectual disability, reflecting the much greater frequency of epilepsy. Prescriptions with a recorded epilepsy diagnosis were 27.4 times as frequent in people with intellectual disability as those without. However, some medications in this group also have indications in the treatment of affective disorders, and the figures collected do not show how commonly these wider indications were present. People with intellectual disability were prescribed antiseizure medications in the absence of epilepsy 1.9 times as frequently as people without intellectual disability. For benzodiazepines, only overall prescribing rates were reported. These were 3.7 times as frequent in people with intellectual disability as in those without.

The setting up of the STOMP programme raises the question of long-term trends in prescribing rates. Unfortunately, some of the counts shown in Figure 2.1 have not been collected more than twice. Figure 2.2 shows the time trends as far as these are available. The rate for all antipsychotic prescribing for people with intellectual disability fell by 4%. For people without intellectual disability, over the same period the rate rose by 4%. Prescribing of antidepressants without a depression diagnosis rose by 10% in people with intellectual disability, while for people without intellectual disability it rose by only 3%. Prescribing of antiseizure medications without an epilepsy diagnosis fell by 9% in people with intellectual disability while remaining unchanged at 3% for those without intellectual disability. Overall use of benzodiazepines fell in both groups.

These data give the best available indication of the profile and trends in prescribing of these medication groups in England in recent years. They go some way towards giving a national picture, but with two qualifications. First, the data source does not include people with or without intellectual disability who are currently in hospital. This is important, as there is a significant group of people with intellectual disability who have been in hospital for several years and who currently show little sign of being discharged. The second issue – non-availability of data from general practices using one commercial note system – has already been mentioned.

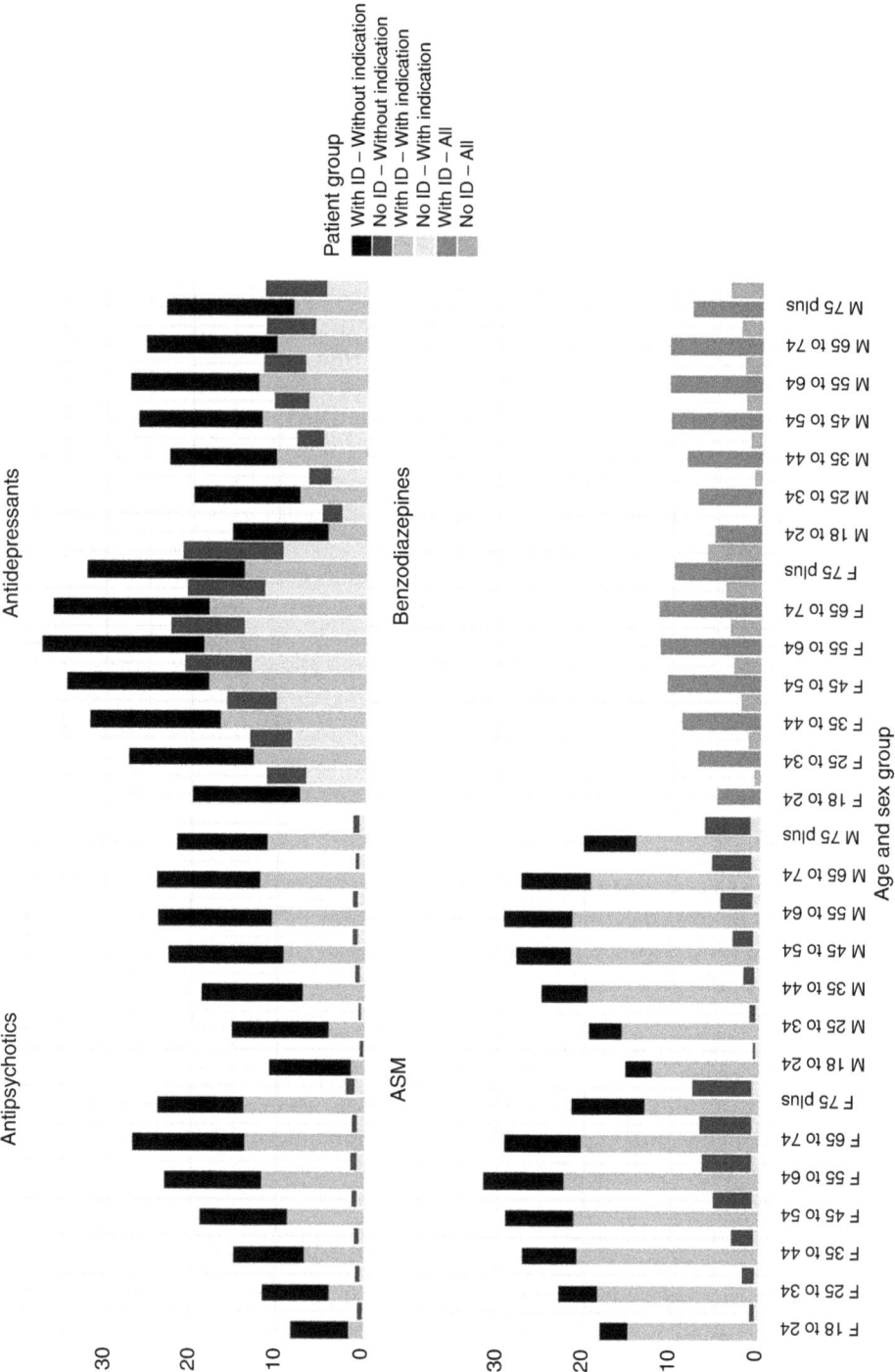

Figure 2.1 Prescribing prevalence for antipsychotics, antidepressants, antiseizure medication, and benzodiazepines, with and without key indications, by age group, for adults with and without intellectual disability, end March 2022. Created with information from NHS Digital: Health and Care of People with Learning Disabilities 2021–2.
Key: Percentage of people with intellectual disability prescribed either an antipsychotic, antiseizure medication or antidepressant but with no indication on GP record

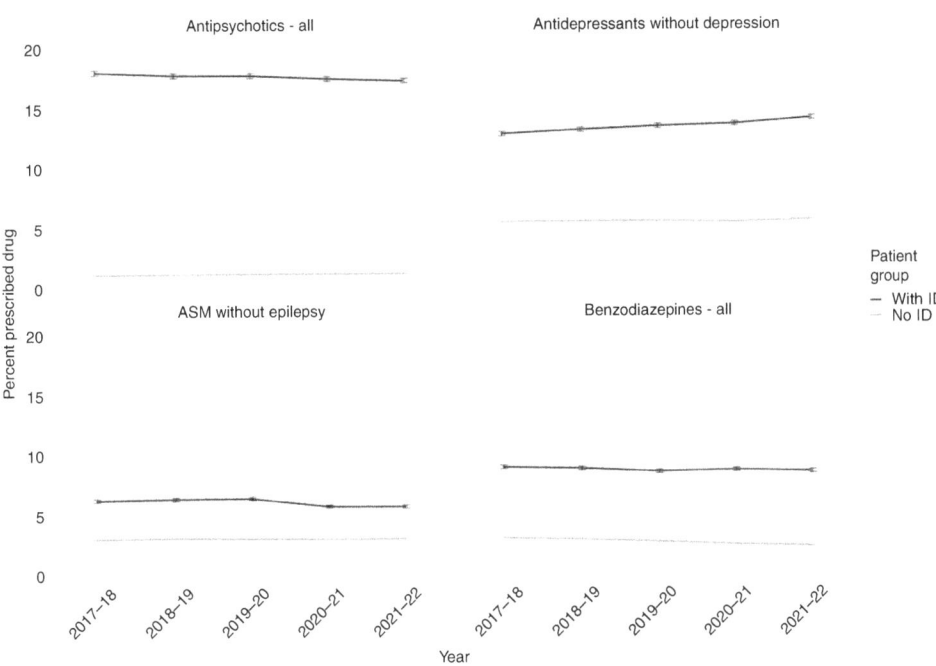

Figure 2.2 Changes from 2017/18 to 2021/2 in prescribing prevalence of antipsychotics, benzodiazepines, and antiseizure medication in the absence of an epilepsy diagnosis and antidepressants in the absence of a depression diagnosis for people with and without intellectual disability. Source: NHS Digital. Open Government Licence
Key: Dark Line – People with intellectual disability. Light Line – People without intellectual disability

Medication Review Programmes

There are many publications about psychotropic medications prescribed for people with intellectual disability. Their primary focus has been antipsychotics to manage behaviours, although some have focused on antiseizure medications for the management of epilepsy.

Other chapters of this guideline provide advice about how best to prescribe and maximise the benefits of psychotropic medication for the various conditions affecting people with intellectual disability. These chapters will also provide guidance on how to withdraw the medication when no longer required or where their use is thought to be poor practice.

There are also many publications comparing the prescribing patterns before and after an active medication review programme; however, there are few that were designed with any robust research methodology. Most are reports of programmes, have focused primarily on antipsychotics, and are dominated by American-based programmes.

The primary method used in the reported American studies was the establishment of a multidisciplinary review process. This followed the recommendation of the Accreditation Council for Services for Mentally Retarded and Other Developmentally Disabled Persons (1977).

> **Example of USA Institutional Medication Review Programme**
>
> Of the US studies, the one showing the greatest change was a seven-year programme using rigidly mandated guidelines. It demonstrated a reduction in and maintenance of antipsychotic use from 41% of an institutional population to 12% (Findholt and Emmett 1990). The study used a drug review committee with the specific remit to manage the use of psychotropic medication. The committee involved a team of psychologists, pharmacists, nurses, and physicians.

Although most such review committees operated within institutions, Lepler et al. (1993) established a similar process with community-based facilities. This process led to a low psychotropic medication use of 17% and a reduction in dose for 75% of the individuals.

Attempts to develop randomised controlled trials (RCT) of discontinuation or reduction of antipsychotics have found recruitment to be a major hurdle. Studies include:

- Ahmed et al. (2000), with additional reporting by Smith et al. (2002), managed to recruit 56 participants, of which 36 were in the intervention group. Their finding was that there was no difference between those that discontinued, those that achieved a greater than 50% reduction, and controls.
- A further attempt at an RCT, AndreaLD (McNamara et al. 2017) named AndreaLD reported on 22 randomised participants (intervention, n = 11; control, n = 11); 13 (59%) achieved progression through all four stages of reduction. Follow-up data at 6 and 9 months were obtained for 17 participants (intervention, n = 10; and control, n = 7; 77% of those randomised). There were no clinically important changes in participants' levels of aggression or challenging behaviour at the end of the study. Recruitment was challenging, which was largely a result of difficulty in identifying appropriate persons to consent and carer concerns regarding re-emergence of challenging behaviour.

Non-RCT medication review programmes from countries outside of America include:

- Jauernig and Hudson (1995) reported on a small programme located at an institution in Australia (12% achieved total withdrawal and 86% some dose reduction)
- Branford (1996a) reported on a study based in Leicestershire (UK) involving 123 people living in hospital and community settings (25% discontinued, 46% achieved a reduced dose)
- de Kuijper et al. (2014), from the Netherlands, investigated the effects of controlled discontinuation of antipsychotics prescribed for behaviours that challenge. Of 98 participants, 43 achieved complete discontinuation; at follow-up 7 had resumed use of antipsychotics. There were no significant differences in improvement of behavioural ratings between two discontinuation schedules. Higher baseline problem-behaviour rating predicted higher odds of incomplete discontinuation
- Gerrard et al. (2019) reported on the use of positive behavioural support to assist medication reduction at a Sunderland Clinic (see Case Study 2.1)

Systematic Reviews of Medication Programmes in Intellectual Disability

Two very different systematic reviews of the effectiveness of medication reviews have been published.

Sheehan and Hassiotis (2017) undertook a systematic review of programmes of reduction or discontinuation of antipsychotics for challenging behaviour in adults with intellectual disability. They included all studies published in peer review journals and all study designs. Of the 45 studies identified for full text review only 21 met the criteria for inclusion. They excluded studies that had no individual outcomes, observational studies, and studies where most individuals were taking antipsychotics for mental illnesses. All but 6 of the studies were based in institutional settings, while the remainder were in community or mixed settings.

They attempted to quantify the relative success of the various programmes; the effect of reduction or discontinuation on behaviour, physical health, mental health and cognitive functioning; and predictors of successful antipsychotic reduction or discontinuation.

They found ten studies that describe the outcome of reduction or discontinuation of antipsychotic medication, but due to the study designs they were unable to obtain a summary measure of the successful reduction or discontinuation of antipsychotics.

A similar methodology was used by a team from the Netherlands (Nabhanizadeh et al. 2019). However, they focused on studies that included the effect of medication reviews on identifying and/or reducing medication-related problems in people with intellectual disability with no restriction of type of medication, age, and level of intellectual disability. Literature databases were searched up to August 2017.

Like Sheehan and Hassiotis, they found that reviews differed in methodology, composition of the teams, institution types, study time, and the nature of the pharmacy input. Six of the included studies reviewed all medications while two studies only reviewed psychotropics and antiepileptics. All studies were performed in multidisciplinary settings by a team that consisted of a pharmacist and medical staff or caregivers. Medication reviews (a combination of medication monitoring, patient education, and patient follow-up) were mostly undertaken by pharmacists. Four of the studies described how medication reviews were performed and which steps were involved. One study (Zaal et al., 2016) used the Systematic Tool to Reduce Inappropriate Prescribing (STRIP). There are no known clinical randomised controlled or controlled prospective trial studies for this review to include.

Factors Associated with Successful or Unsuccessful Withdrawal of Antipsychotic Medications

Several factors can influence the outcome of a review programme. These include: legal requirements supported by court rulings (mostly in the USA); national guidance; financial and other incentives; the availability of a multidisciplinary team dedicated to the programme; and the availability of alternative approaches to the challenging behaviour. The chapter section on STOMP and STAMP describes the impact of a social movement approach.

Sheehan and Hassiotis (2017), in their systematic review of reduction and discontinuation programmes, concluded that predictors of poor response could not be reliably identified and that the limitations of the data were such that they could not inform a population-level approach to the issue.

Nabhanizadeh et al. (2019) concluded that there is insufficient evidence to determine whether the use of medication reviews significantly leads to a reduction of medication-related problems and prescribing errors.

STOMP and STAMP

STOMP (NHS England, 2016; Branford et al., 2019a, Branford et al. 2019b) was launched in 2016 as a 'call to action' in response to the deep concern, expressed in the Winterbourne View report (Department of Health 2012), about the overprescribing of psychotropic medication in the absence of a formal mental health diagnosis. STAMP (NHS England, 2019) followed and focused on similar prescribing principles in children and young people.

Prescribing in this way was often linked to the construct of behaviour experienced as challenging – an unlicenced indication. In 2015, the National Institute for Health and Care Excellence (NICE) guidance NG11 (NICE 2015) focused on the appropriate pathway for preventing and intervening with behaviour experienced as challenging. This included using non-pharmacological intervention as first-line, with antipsychotic medication being considered as add-on therapy only if the situation had not adequately resolved. The guidance requires adherence to strict review and monitoring timescales, as well as a written discontinuation plan produced at the point of initiation. This is to ensure that medication use is appropriate and for the shortest time.

Pledges for STOMP and STAMP

From the launch in 2016 until 2019, the social movement approach, or 'call to action', invited health and social care providers to pledge to demonstrate commitment to the principles of STOMP and STAMP: a focus on quality-of-life improvement; education for the person, family, carer team, and professionals; alternative strategies to medication; and a commitment to work in collaboration. The pledge commitments are still valid, and in 2019 were enshrined within the NHS Long-Term Plan, placing emphasis on providers to deliver meaningful STOMP and STAMP interventions.

Examples of STOMP Pledge Commitments

- We will actively explore alternatives to medication
- We will ensure people with intellectual disability, autism or both, of any age, and their circle of support, are fully informed about their medication and involved in decisions about their care
- We will ensure all staff within the organisation have an understanding of psychotropic medication, including why it is being used and its potential side effects
- We will ensure all people are able to speak up if they have a concern that someone is receiving inappropriate medication
- We will maintain accurate records about a person's health, well-being, and behaviour
- We will ensure that medication, if needed, is started, reviewed and monitored in line with relevant NICE guidance
- We will work in partnership with people with intellectual disability, autism or both, their families, care teams, healthcare professionals, commissioners and others to stop over-medication

(NHS England 2016)

Guidance for STOMP and STAMP

The Royal College of Psychiatrists published a position statement in 2021 (Royal College of Psychiatry Position Statement PS05/21, 2021) highlighting the principles of STOMP for its members. NICE has also produced a list of standards to enable organisations to audit prescribing performance.

1. **Royal College of Psychiatrists Position Statement principles include:**

    Utilise effective multidisciplinary working

    Prescribing psychotropic medication for the right indication, for the right reason at the right time

    Ensuring full adherence to mental capacity legislation

    Ensuring robust monitoring of psychotropic medication

2. **NICE NG11 Standards describe:**

    Consideration of antipsychotic medication after non-pharmacological interventions do not fully work, if there is a risk of severe harm to self or others, and always in combination with non-pharmacological intervention

    Medication choice to be dictated by the person's (or family's) preference, side effects, response to previous medication, and interaction potential

    When initiating, identify target behaviour, decide on a monitoring method, start with lowest dose, formally review side effects

    - Review benefit and side effects after 3–4 weeks
    - Stop after 6 weeks if no benefit

    If continued beyond 6 weeks:

    Review after 3 months and then 6 monthly thereafter

    When prescribing is transferred to primary care, document:

    - The behaviours of concern
    - How to monitor benefit and side-effect burden
    - The anticipated length of treatment
    - A written plan of how to reduce and withdraw medication

Deprescribing Guidance

There is limited evidence to guide deprescribing of psychotropic medication being used for behaviour seen as challenging. A range of considerations is needed to guide the process (Branford 1996b; de Kuijper et al., 2014). The reviews must be person-centred and holistic (Sheehan and Hassiotis 2017) and may benefit from ongoing intervention from behavioural specialists (Lee et al. 2018; Gerrard et al. 2019). NHS England produced a general guide to undertaking STOMP and STAMP reviews in 2019 (see Figure 2.3).

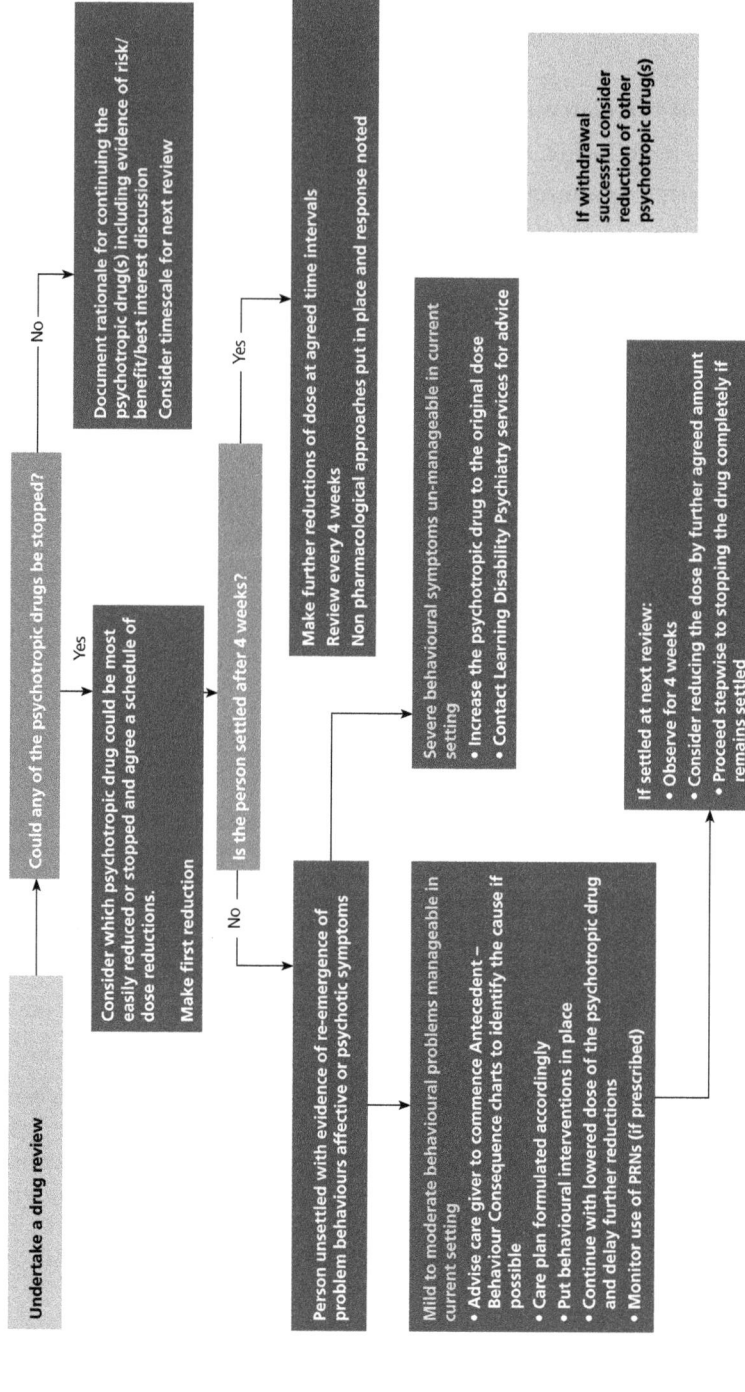

Figure 2.3 A general guide to undertaking STOMP and STAMP reviews, produced by NHS England. Open Government Licence.

Case Study 2.1: The Sunderland Clinic: Impact of Multidisciplinary Team Working (Gerrard et al. 2019)

A positive behavioural support (PBS)-led clinic was developed as a model for delivering STOMP medication reviews. It involved a full multidisciplinary team (MDT) including nursing, psychology, pharmacy, occupational therapy, speech and language therapy (SALT), and physiotherapy.

This ensured a holistic review of the person, with full assessment of behaviour experienced as challenging, sensory and environmental issues, physical health (via GP), and a full medication history.

The team identified people thought to be inappropriately prescribed psychotropic medication with no formal mental health diagnosis. They worked with the person and care team, with family input, to decide if medication could be challenged. In line with the NICE NG 11 principles, a behavioural support plan was devised and implemented before the medication work began. This was agreed with all relevant parties, including the person, before deprescribing was commenced. The PBS nurse would train care teams and families to produce monitoring data to help inform prescribing decisions as well as implementing a range of supportive interventions such as active support and intensive intervention.

Reductions were flexible and based on data and the ongoing opinion of the person and carers. In the first two years of the clinic 18 medications were stopped, with a further 35 being reduced.

Case Study 2.2: Practical Deprescribing Example

Elsie is 40 and has a severe intellectual disability with no verbal communication. She presents with behaviour experienced as challenging in the form of grabbing others and moaning. Her GP highlighted a raised prolactin level above 3,000, although she shows no symptoms of hyperprolactinaemia. She has taken risperidone 2mg daily for more than 10 years without having a formal diagnosis of a mental health condition and no records of efficacy or benefit.

Elsie had a STOMP medication review including an intensive behavioural assessment, physical health check, and environmental analysis. It was agreed with family members and her care team to challenge the risperidone. Targets for measuring the impact of change were agreed and positive behavioural support interventions were implemented to support the medication reduction.

Over six months the medication was reduced and stopped, guided by behavioural data and interpretation. The schedule was flexible, allowing each reduction to reach steady state plus at least four weeks to monitor impact.

Case Study 2.3: Consequence of Over-Medication

Priya is 36, is autistic, and has a moderate intellectual disability. Priya has gained 5 stones in weight over the last 10 years and has been pre-diabetic for the last two years. The GP has highlighted concern about her medications, as reviewed at her recent annual health check (AHC).

- Olanzapine 20mg daily – thought to be for challenging behaviour as there is no record of a serious mental health diagnosis
- Valproate 200mg twice a day – unclear if Priya ever received an epilepsy diagnosis
- Paroxetine 40mg each day – depressive episode 8 years ago
- Lorazepam 1mg up to three times a day when required for aggression. This had been misinterpreted as to be given once a day.

Priya's case highlights the potential problems posed by inappropriate or poorly reviewed medication

Olanzapine has been prescribed at the same dose for more than 10 years without a specialist review. There is no clear indication and no plan for how it should be reviewed. The medication has a significant impact on weight gain and may have driven Priya's increased weight and diabetic risk.

Valproate is being prescribed to a woman of childbearing age without consideration for enrolment in the pregnancy prevention programme. The indication is unclear and has not been reassessed or challenged.

Paroxetine, an antidepressant with a short half-life (approx. 1 day), making deprescribing more complex, has been left in place despite the depressive episode happening several years ago.

Lorazepam has been prescribed for crisis situations but has been utilised as a daily dose for several years, without indication or challenge. Dependency is a significant issue making deprescribing more complex.

A STOMP review is key to ensuring medications are used appropriately with a clear plan for review, monitoring, and removal if felt to be no longer beneficial.

Withdrawal Problems with Psychotropic Medication

Evidence of Withdrawal Problems

There is a confusing terminology associated with withdrawal problems. Classically, medications such as opioids and benzodiazepines are regarded as 'addictive' in that the person suffers a degree of craving when they stop the medication, and that the withdrawal is associated with a range of symptoms that they did not suffer before. It was many years before there was general agreement of a benzodiazepine withdrawal syndrome because it was widely thought that the symptoms suffered were just a return of pre-existing anxiety or insomnia.

There is a similar debate underway regarding selective serotonin reuptake inhibitors (SSRIs), where difficulties in withdrawing the medications are frequently experienced. This has been called a 'discontinuation syndrome', rather than withdrawal.

Finally, there is the issue of relapse. Does the withdrawal of the psychotropic precipitate relapse, or is it just that many mental health illnesses are periodic in nature and the protective nature of the medication leaves the person exposed to such a relapse? Table 2.1 provides further information on withdrawal problems associated with psychotropic medications.

Table 2.1 Withdrawal problems associated with psychotropic medications

Psychotropic medication being withdrawn	Reported presentations	Guidance if occurring
All antipsychotics	Dopaminergic syndrome Withdrawal dyskinesia, akathisia, dystonia, tardive dyskinesia	Slow down the rate of withdrawal
Chlorpromazine, clozapine, olanzapine, quetiapine	Cholinergic syndrome Nausea, vomiting, headache, restlessness, anxiety, insomnia, fatigue, malaise, myalgia, diaphoresis, rhinitis, paraesthesia, loose bowels	Generally occur within first week or two of dose reduction. No specific recommendations
Clozapine	Rebound psychosis	Represcribe clozapine
Antimuscarinics used to manage extrapyramidal side effects of older antipsychotics	Cholinergic syndrome	Withdraw slowly. May take up to 3 months to withdraw successfully
Benzodiazepines	Benzodiazepine withdrawal syndrome: Many symptoms have been reported including physical symptoms of anxiety, depression, difficulty sleeping, dizziness, face and neck pain, headaches, inability to concentrate, increased sensitivity to light, noise, touch and smell. Severe withdrawal symptoms can include: derealisation (feeling out of touch with reality), hallucinations, memory loss, muscle twitching, paranoia and delusions, seizures.	British National Formulary recommends transfer to diazepam and slowly withdraw (Ashton Manual)
Z drug hypnotics	insomnia, anxiety, euphoria irritability, tremor, inner restlessness, speech difficulties, abdominal pain, hypertension, tonic-clonic seizures, and confusion/disorientation/delirium	Slow taper and introduce sleep hygiene
Tricyclic antidepressants	Anxiety, fast or irregular heartbeat, flu-like symptoms, insomnia, low blood pressure, problems with movement, restlessness, spontaneous orgasm, strange dreams	Slow withdrawal

Table 2.1 (cont.)

Psychotropic medication being withdrawn	Reported presentations	Guidance if occurring
SSRI and related antidepressants	Dizziness or vertigo, electric shock sensations in head, flu-like symptoms, problems with movement, sensory disturbance (such as smelling something that isn't there), stomach cramps, strange dreams, tinnitus	Most sources suggest that withdrawal effects are short lived; however, recent concerns suggest much slower withdrawal may be needed
Melatonin	None reported	
Methylphenidate	Fatigue and disturbed sleep patterns are common signs of methylphenidate withdrawal. Users undergoing detoxification also report cravings for methylphenidate. Some users develop depression after halting methylphenidate use.	Treat sleep disturbance with short-term hypnotic
Lithium	Unclear if a specific withdrawal syndrome but concerns about withdrawal precipitating relapse	Slow withdrawal

Recognising Relapse and Recurrence

One of the biggest fears of all concerned with deprescribing is the fear of relapse. It is important to understand the terminology:

- Relapse is the return to a full syndrome once remission has occurred

Many mental illnesses are of a relapsing/remitting nature. Most also have discontinuation studies that demonstrate that stopping the psychotropic will increase the likelihood of relapse. Relapse is often measured by hospitalisation and, in the modern era of limited bed availability, is to be avoided at all costs. Such a relapse is usually associated with a marked change in the severity of the illness and a deterioration in the social functioning of the patient.

A full relapse will not only affect the patient but is also likely to impact on family, friends, and relationships.

Many authors identify sleep disturbance to be one of the key initial signs of a relapse.

- Recurrence is a further episode occurring following some degree of recovery or reduction in impact

Many mental illnesses comprise a galaxy of behaviours and experiences that may worsen in the short or long term with the reduction of the psychotropic. Part of the development of a deprescribing plan is an understanding of these behaviours and experiences and whether the person, carers, and family have strategies in place to manage them.

The Frith Prescribing Guidelines Editors' Expert Group Consensus Statements

Statements of High Confidence

People with intellectual disability are commonly prescribed psychotropic medications. This is occurring more in the intellectual disability population than the general population and increases with age.

For much of the last 50 years, antipsychotics have remained the most prescribed psychotropic medication, followed by antiseizure medications.

More recent studies have shown a very gradual decline in antipsychotic use (static in general population) and benzodiazepine use (decline in both), a significant increase in antidepressants, a gradual increase in antiseizure medications independent of epilepsy (same in general population), and an increase in multiple psychotropic medication prescribing (more than 1 psychotropic medication group) (same in general population)

Overall, 95% of NHS provider Trusts signed up to the pledges of STOMP and STAMP.

Statements of Medium Confidence

Multidisciplinary review programmes are useful for psychotropic medication reduction. However there is no robust evidence on any particular methodology or whether the use of medication reviews significantly leads to a reduction of medication-related problems and prescribing errors.

Statements of Low Confidence

How to deprescribe psychotropic medication as a process or pathway:

Although there is a series of position statements and general guidance are available for prescribers, these are generally based on consensus guidance or extrapolated from guidance on opiate withdrawal.

Resource Box

TITLE	LINK
	STOMP Awareness
NHSE STOMP	NHS England » Stopping over-medication of people with a learning disability, autism or both (STOMP): www.england.nhs.uk/learning-disabilities/improving-health/stomp/
NHSE STAMP	NHS England » Supporting Treatment and Appropriate Medication in Paediatrics (STAMP): www.england.nhs.uk/learning-disabilities/improving-health/stamp/
MindEd STOMP modules	**Stopping over-medication of people with a learning disability and autistic people: www.minded.org.uk/Component/Details/742766** • Inappropriate medication prescribing: www.minded.org.uk/Component/Details/742762 • Psychotropic medication 1: www.minded.org.uk/Component/Details/755706

(cont.)

TITLE	LINK
	- Psychotropic medication 2: www.minded.org.uk/Component/Details/755709 - Psychotropic medication 3: www.minded.org.uk/Component/Details/755712 - How to challenge inappropriate medication 1: www.minded.org.uk/Component/Details/755715 - How to challenge inappropriate medication 2: www.minded.org.uk/Component/Details/744479
	Alternatives to medication
Positive Behavioural Support	An Introduction to PBS: www.youtube.com/watch?v=epjud2Of6I0 Positive Behaviour Support (PBS) | bild: www.bild.org.uk/positive-behaviour-support-pbs/
	Guidance for Healthcare Professionals
NICE Guidance Challenging behaviour NG11	Overview | Challenging behaviour and learning disabilities: prevention and interventions for people with learning disabilities whose behaviour challenges | Guidance | NICE: www.nice.org.uk/guidance/ng11
RCPsych Position Statement 2021	position-statement-ps0521-stomp-stamp.pdf (rcpsych.ac.uk): www.rcpsych.ac.uk/docs/default-source/improving-care/better-mh-policy/position-statements/position-statement-ps0521-stomp-stamp.pdf?sfvrsn=684d09b3_6
FuturesNHS Collaboration platform STOMP and STAMP	STOMP and STAMP – FutureNHS Collaboration Platform (registration required): https://future.nhs.uk/NationalSTOMPSTAMP Community of Practice – additional resources
	Medication Information
Medication Information	Easy read medication leaflets | Project (spectrom.wixsite.com): https://spectrom.wixsite.com/project/easy-read-medication-leaflets Easy Health: www.easyhealth.org.uk
	Regulation
CQC Guidance	Care Quality Commission: Brief guide: psychotropic medication in intellectual and developmental disability: www.cqc.org.uk/sites/default/files/Brief_guide_psychotropic_medication_in_intellectual_and_developmental_disability.pdf

References

Accreditation Council for Services for Mentally Retarded and Other Developmental Persons (1977). *Standards for Services for Developmentally Disabled Individuals.* Chicago: Joint Commission on Accreditation of Hospitals.

Ahmed, Z., Fraser, W., Kerr, M. P., et al. (2000). Reducing antipsychotic medication in people with a learning disability. *British Journal of Psychiatry*, **178**, 42–6.

Ashton Manual (n.d.). Benzodiazepines: How They Work and How to Withdraw. www.benzo.org.uk/manual/bzsched.htm.

Branford, D. (1996a). A review of antipsychotic drugs prescribed for people with learning disability who live in Leicestershire. *Journal of Intellectual Disability Research*, **40**, 4 358–68.

Branford, D. (1996b). Factors associated with the successful or unsuccessful withdrawal of antipsychotic drug therapy prescribed for people with learning disabilities. *Journal of Intellectual Disability Research*; **40**, 322–9.

Branford, D., Gerrard, D., Saleem, N., Shaw, C., & Webster, A. (2019a). Stopping over-medication of people with intellectual disability, Autism or both (STOMP) in England part 1 – history and background of STOMP. *Advances in Mental Health and Intellectual Disabilities*, **13**(1), pp. 31–40. https://doi.org/10.1108/AMHID-02-2018-0004.

Branford, D., Gerrard, D., Saleem, N., Shaw, C., & Webster, A. (2019b). Stopping over-medication of people with an intellectual disability, autism or both (STOMP) in England part 2 – the story so far. *Advances in Mental Health and Intellectual Disabilities*, **13**(1), 41–51. https://doi.org/10.1108/AMHID-02-2018-0005.

Cooper, S. A., Smiley, E., Morrison, J., Williamson, A. & Allan, L. (2007). Mental ill-health in adults with intellectual disabilities: prevalence and associated factors. *British Journal of Psychiatry*, **190**, 27–35.

de Kuijper, G. M., Evenhuis, H., Minderaa, R., & Hoekstra, P. J. (2014). Effects of controlled discontinuation of long-term used antipsychotics for behavioural symptoms in individuals with intellectual disability. *Journal of Intellectual Disability Research*, **58**, 71–83.

Department of Health (2012), Transforming care: A national response to Winterbourne View Hospital. Department of Health Review: Final report, Department of Health, London. www.gov.uk/government/publications/winterbourne-view-hospital-department-of-health-review-and-response.

Findholt, N. E., & Emmett, C. G. (1990). Impact of interdisciplinary team review on psychotropic drug use with persons who have mental retardation. *Mental Retardation*, **28**(1), 41–6.

Gerrard, D., Rhodes, J., Lee, R., & Ling, J. (2019), Using positive behavioural support for STOMP challenge. *Advances in Mental Health and Intellectual Disabilities*, **13**(¾), 102–12.

Glover, G., Williams, R., Branford, D., Holland, A., & Strydom, A. (2014). Use of medication for challenging behaviour in people with intellectual disability. *British Journal of Psychiatry*, **2054**(1), 6–7. https://doi.org/10.1192/bjp.bp.113.141267.

Jauernig, R., & Hudson, A. (1995) Evaluation of an Interdisciplinary Review Committee managing the use of psychotropic medication with people with intellectual disabilities. *Australia and New Zealand Journal of Developmental Disabilities*, **20**, 51–61.

Lee, R. M, Rhodes, J. A., & Gerrard, D. (2018). Positive Behavioural Support as an alternative to medication. *Tizard Learning Disability Review*, **24**(1), 1–8. https://doi.org/10.1108/TLDR-06-2018-0018.

Lepler, S., Hodas, A., & Cotter-Mack, A. (1993). Implementation of an interdisciplinary psychotropic drug review process for community based facilities. *Mental Retardation*, **31**(5), 307–15.

McNamara, R., Randell, E., Gillespie, D., et al. (2017). A pilot randomised controlled trial of community-led ANtipsychotic Drug REduction for adults with learning disabilities. *Health Technology Assessment*, **21**(47), 1–92. https://doi.org/10.3310/hta21470.

Mehta, H., & Glover, G. (2019) Psychotropic drugs and people with learning disabilities or autism, 2019. Public Health England. www.gov.uk/government/publications/psychotropic-drugs-and-people-with-learning-disabilities-or-autism/psychotropic-drugs-and-people-with-learning-disabilities-or-autism-executive-summary.

Nabhanizadeh, A., Oppewal, A., Boot, F. H., & Maes-Festen, D. (2019). Effectiveness of medication reviews in identifying and reducing medication-related problems among people with intellectual disabilities: A systematic review. *Journal of Applied Research in Intellectual Disabilities*, 32, 750–761. https://doi.org/10.1111/jar.12580.

NHS Digital (2022) Health and Care of People with Learning Disabilities. Data series/Collection. https://digital.nhs.uk/data-and-information/publications/statistical/health-and-care-of-people-with-learning-disabilities.

National Institute for Health and Care Excellence (NICE) (2015). Challenging behaviour and learning disabilities: Prevention and interventions for people with learning disabilities whose behaviour challenges. National Institute for Health and Care Excellence. www.nice.org.uk/guidance/ng11.

National Institute for Health and Care Excellence (NICE) (2016). Mental health problems in people with learning disabilities: prevention, assessment and management NG54. www.nice.org.uk/guidance/ng54.

NHS (2019). Long term plan. www.longtermplan.nhs.uk/.

NHS England (2016). Doctors urged to help stop 'chemical restraint' as leading health professionals sign joint pledge. www.england.nhs.uk/2016/06/over-medication-pledge/.

NHS England (2019). Stopping the overmedication of children and young people with a learning disability, autism or both (STOMP) and supporting treatment and appropriate medication in paediatrics (STAMP). www.england.nhs.uk/learning-disabilities/improving-health/stamp/.

NHS England (2016a). Stopping Over-Medication of People with a Learning Disability (STOMPLD) Pledge. www.england.nhs.uk/2016/06/over-medication-pledge/.

NHS England (2016b). Stopping Over-Medication of People with a Learning Disability (STOMPLD). www.england.nhs.uk/learning-disabilities/improving-health/stomp/?UID=4643034442024219163158.

Public Health England (2019). Psychotropic drugs and people with learning disabilities or autism. www.gov.uk/government/publications/psychotropic-drugs-and-people-with-learning-disabilities-or-autism.

Royal College of Psychiatrists: Faculty of Psychiatry of Intellectual Disability Report (2016). Psychotropic drug prescribing for people with intellectual disabilities, mental health problems and/or behaviours that challenge: practice guidelines. FR/ID/09 http://www.rcpsych.ac.uk/pdf/FR_ID_09_for_website.pdf.

Royal College of Psychiatry Position Statement PS05/21 (2021). Stopping the overmedication of people with intellectual disability, autism or both (STOMP) and supporting treatment and appropriate medication in paediatrics (STAMP). www.rcpsych.ac.uk/docs/default-source/improving-care/better-mh-policy/position-statements/position-statement-ps0521-stomp-stamp.pdf?sfvrsn=684d09b3_6.

Sheehan, R., & Hassiotis, A. (2017). Reduction or discontinuation of antipsychotics for challenging behaviour in adults with intellectual disability: A systematic review. *The Lancet Psychiatry*, 4(3), 238–56.

Smith, C., Felce, D., Ahmed, Z., et al. (2002). Sedative effects on responsiveness: Evaluating the reduction of antipsychotic medication in people with intellectual disabilities using a conditional probability approach. *Journal of Intellectual Disability Research*, 46, 464–71.

Zaal, R. J., Ebbers, S., Borms, M., et al. (2016). Medication review using a Systematic Tool to Reduce Inappropriate Prescribing (STRIP) in adults with an intellectual disability: A pilot study. *Research in Developmental Disabilities*, 55, 132–42. https://doi.org/10.1016/j.ridd.2016.03.014.

Chapter 3

Physical Health Monitoring

Mariam Omokanye, Nazurah Wahid, Praveena Peddireddi, Reena Tharian, David M. L. Branford, and Archana Anandaram

Introduction

There is a high incidence of physical health problems in people with intellectual disability, most of which require monitoring of some kind. In addition to the monitoring recommended for people with intellectual disability on psychotropic medications, this chapter focuses on two specific problems associated with psychotropic medication: obesity and constipation.

General Physical Health in People with Intellectual Disability and the Annual Health Check

Prevalence

A 2021 systematic review sought to better understand the prevalence and incidence of physical health conditions in people with an intellectual disability (Liao et al. 2021). The results revealed that, for high-income countries, epilepsy, eye and ear disorders, cerebral palsy, obesity, osteoporosis, congenital health defects and thyroid disorders, had the highest prevalence among people with an intellectual disability. The importance of targeted health initiatives was emphasised further by findings suggesting that conditions such as asthma and diabetes are more prevalent among people with intellectual disability compared to the general population. This systematic review joins the LeDeR programme (Learning Disability Mortality Review (LeDeR) 2019) in England in highlighting the under-detection of cancer among people with intellectual disability.

The Annual Health Check

Anyone over the age of 14 who is on the learning disability primary care register in England can have an annual health check (https://www.england.nhs.uk/learning-disabilities/improving-health/annual-health-checks/) (doa 21/06/24). Health checks have resulted in improved detection of both major (e.g., cancer) and minor (e.g., excessive ear wax) health conditions (Robertson et al. 2014). Furthermore, a study published in 2022 concluded that 'health checks are associated with a trend to improved survival for people with intellectual disability' (Kennedy et al. 2022, p. 6).

Reasonable Adjustments

The Equality Act 2010 places a duty on all public bodies to make reasonable adjustments to allow effective participation of people with disabilities. Reasonable adjustments act to remove barriers that people with disabilities may face when accessing services.

Between 2016 and 2020 a series of guides were developed to share information, ideas, and good practice in making reasonable adjustments for people with an intellectual disability in specific health service areas. The guides are aimed at health and social care professionals and family members who provide support for these individuals. There is also an easy-read summary for each service area. A key link for further information is available here: https://www.england.nhs.uk/learning-disabilities/improving-health/reasonable-adjustments/ (doa 21/06/24).

In 2018, The LeDeR programme highlighted dysphagia as 'one of the most common long-term conditions experienced by people with a learning disability' (LeDeR Programme: Action from Learning NHS England and NHS Improvement, 2019). Dysphagia is covered in more detail in Chapter 21.

Physical Health Monitoring Recommended when Prescribing Specific Medications

Where psychotropic medication is prescribed for people with an intellectual disability, monitoring for adverse effects has often been found to be inadequate (Tyrer et al. 2014). Tables 3.1–3.8 contain the recommendations for monitoring associated with various psychotropic medications. Effective monitoring often has a requirement for blood or other tests. This may present several logistical problems. For further advice about blood testing in people with intellectual disability, the following webpage gives information about reasonable adjustments: https://www.gov.uk/government/publications/blood-tests-and-people-with-learning-disabilities/blood-tests-for-people-with-learning-disabilities-making-reasonable-adjustments-guidance (doa 21/06/24).

Table 3.1 Antidepressants: minimum required monitoring for the relevant antidepressants (South West London & St George's Mental Health NHS Trust guideline, Leth-Møller et al. 2016)

Parameter	Frequency	When to consider increased or reduced monitoring
Electrocardiogram (ECG)	Baseline ECG required for citalopram, escitalopram and tricyclic antidepressants	Annual ECG in the elderly and those with cardiac disease Additional ECG if signs of cardiac arrythmia during treatment
Blood pressure	Baseline and annually for venlafaxine, phenelzine and tricyclic antidepressants	
Liver function tests	Baseline and annually for isocarboxazid	
Sodium	To be checked in all patients who develop drowsiness, confusion or convulsions particularly within the first 2 weeks of treatment	Increased index of suspicion in those taking SSRIs, particularly citalopram

Table 3.2 Antipsychotics (National Institute of Health and Care Excellent Guideline CG 178 (2014), The Maudsley Prescribing Guidelines 14th edition (2021))

Parameter	Frequency	When to consider increased or reduced monitoring
Body mass index	Baseline, weekly for the first 6 weeks, at 3 months, and then annually	More frequent monitoring if the person is gaining weight
Full blood count	Baseline and then annually	Increased monitoring for clozapine as per summary of product characteristics
Urea and electrolytes	Baseline and then annually	
Blood lipids	Baseline, 3 months after treatment and then annually	
Plasma glucose or haemoglobin A1c (HbA1c) test	Baseline, 3 months after treatment, and then annually	
Prolactin	Baseline, 6 months after starting treatment, and then annually	May not be required for aripiprazole, clozapine, quetiapine, or olanzapine if dose is 20 mg/day or less
Liver function tests	Baseline, annually	
Creatinine kinase	If neuroleptic malignant syndrome is suspected	
Pulse and blood pressure	Baseline, during dose titration and at each dose change	May not be required for amisulpride, aripiprazole, trifluoperazine, and sulpride
Electrocardiogram (ECG)	Baseline, after each medication change and then annually	May not be required for antipsychotics with no effect or a low-to-moderate effect on the QT interval and where there are no other risk factors for arrythmia

High-dose antipsychotic therapy (HDAT) may require additional monitoring depending on local policies (Rajan and Clarke 2013). High dose may occur when the total daily dose of a single antipsychotic exceeds the upper limit stated in the summary of product characteristics (SPC) or British National Formulary with respect to the age of the patient and the indication being treated or where the total daily dose of two or more antipsychotics exceeds the SPC or British National Formulary maximum using the percentage method. The consensus statement on HDAT from the Royal College of Psychiatrists is available here: www.rcpsych.ac.uk/docs/default-source/improving-care/better-mh-policy/college-reports/college-report-cr190.pdf?sfvrsn=54f5d9a2_11.

Table 3.3 Mood stabilisers (South West London & St George's Mental Health NHS Trust guideline; n.d)

Parameter	Frequency	When to consider increased or reduced monitoring
Body mass index	Baseline, after 6 months, and then annually for valproate. Baseline and then 6-monthly for lithium	Increased if evidence of weight gain
Full blood count	Baseline, after 6 months, and then annually for Valproate and Carbamazepine	
Liver function tests	Baseline, after 6 months and then annually for valproate and carbamazepine	
Urea and electrolytes	Baseline and 6-monthly for lithium	Increased if evidence of impairment
Thyroid function test	Baseline and 6-monthly for lithium	Increased if evidence of impairment
Lithium levels (12-hour post-dose)	One week after starting treatment, one week after every dose change, and weekly until levels are stable; 3-monthly thereafter	Increased if evidence of renal impairment or if evidence of toxicity
Electrocardiogram (ECG)	Baseline for lithium where there is a risk factor for existing cardiovascular disease	

Table 3.4 Medication used for ADHD (NICE guideline NG87, 2018; South West London & St George's Mental Health NHS Trust guideline, n.d)

Parameter	Frequency	When to consider increased or reduced monitoring
Body mass index	Baseline, 3 months after initiation, 6 months after initiation, and 6-monthly thereafter	
Blood pressure and heart rate	Baseline, before and after each dose change, and 6-monthly thereafter	
Electrocardiogram (ECG)	Baseline and 6-monthly where there is a family history, past medical history or risk factor for cardiovascular disease	

Table 3.5 Anti-dementia medication
Cardiac status should be assessed before prescribing Acetyl Cholinesterase Inhibitors for dementia (Rowland et al. 2007)

Parameter	Frequency	When to consider increased or reduced monitoring:
Electrocardiogram	Baseline (for high-risk groups)	Not indicated for memantine
Pulse	1 month, 2 months, and 6 months after initiation, annually thereafter	Not indicated for memantine

More information on monitoring needed for anti-dementia medications is available in Chapter 18 ('Dementia') in this volume.

Table 3.6 Anxiolytics and hypnotics (South West London & St George's Mental Health NHS Trust guideline)

Parameter/Frequency

No routine monitoring may be required for zopiclone, benzodiazepines, promethazine, melatonin and pregabalin.

The precise monitoring requirements may vary depending on local policies, but Tables 3.7 and 3.8 provide an overarching view on the monitoring requirements.

Table 3.7 Summary of recommended routine physical health monitoring for patients on antipsychotics (Hertfordshire Partnership University NHS Foundation Trust, 2020)
To be read in conjunction with Table 3.2

		Baseline	3 months	6 months	Annual Review/ Health check
a	Personal and Family History	✓			
b	Smoking	✓	✓	✓	✓
c	Alcohol and drug use	✓	✓	✓	✓
d	Allergies/drug sensitivities	✓	✓	✓	✓
e	Exercise and dietary habits*	✓	✓	✓	✓
f	Dental health	✓			✓
g	Weight (BMI/waist circumference), ideally plotted on a chart	✓	✓	✓	✓
h	Blood pressure	✓	✓	✓	✓
i	Blood lipid profile and fasting plasma glucose /HbA1c; consider other relevant blood tests or investigations required	✓	✓	✓	✓
j	ECG (the need for a baseline ECG should be considered). An ECG should be performed if there are cardiovascular risk factors, including a strong family history	✓			✓

Table 3.7 (cont.)

		Baseline	3 months	6 months	Annual Review/ Health check
	of heart disease or if medication which cause ECG abnormalities such as haloperidol are being prescribed. Referral to cardiology should be considered in service users with persistent tachycardia (heart rate raised above 100 bpm on 3 occasions) for investigations to rule out myocarditis and cardiomyopathy.				
k	Sexual health and contraception. Consider the need for a pregnancy test	✓			✓
l	Check engagement with primary care	✓			✓
n	Screen for side effects (including sexual)		✓	✓	✓
o	Offer information about medication	✓	✓	✓	✓
p	Health promotion and signposting where appropriate	✓			✓

Table 3.8 Psychotropic medication requiring specific tests and monitoring for serious mental health illness (Hertfordshire Partnership University NHS Foundation Trust, 2020)
To be read in conjunction with Tables 3.1, 3.2 and 3.3

Serious mental illness	Baseline and initial	Maintenance
Psychosis/bipolar disorder)	Full blood count (FBC) Urea and electrolytes (U&Es) Renal function (serum creatinine or e-GFR) Liver function tests (LFTs) Fasting blood glucose (if possible), HbA_{1c} (average blood glucose level) Blood lipid profile (fasting if possible) Prolactin level Electrocardiogram (ECG) if clinically indicated Blood pressure, weight, waist circumference	Annual health check FBC annually U&Es annually Renal function (serum creatinine or e-GFR) annually LFTs annually Fasting (if possible) blood glucose, HbA_{1c} annually Blood lipid profile (fasting if possible) annually

Table 3.8 (cont.)

Serious mental illness	Baseline and initial	Maintenance
MEDICATION		
Mood stabilisers	**BASELINE and INITIAL**	**MAINTENANCE**
Lithium	U&Es e-GFR (estimated glomerular filtration rate) Thyroid function tests Serum calcium levels Cardiac function: ECG if clinically indicated Blood pressure Weight and height (BMI) Lithium level weekly until therapeutic level & one week after each dose change, then 3-monthly for first 12 months	Annual health check Lithium level – 3-monthly for first 12 months and then every 6 months thereafter if stable, or every 3 months for people in any of the following groups: • older adults • people taking other medicines that interact with lithium • people who are at risk of renal or thyroid dysfunction, raised calcium levels, or other complications • people who have poor symptom control • people with poor adherence • people whose last lithium plasma level was 0.8 mmol/L or higher e-GFR (estimated glomerular filtration rate) 6-monthly Thyroid function tests – 6-monthly Serum calcium levels – annually Fasting (if possible) blood glucose, HbA_{1c} (average blood glucose level) annually Blood lipid profile (fasting if possible) annually
Sodium valproate valproic acid	LFTs at baseline and periodically during first 6 months Clotting screen FBC at baseline and at 6 months Blood pressure at baseline and at 6 months Weight and height at baseline, weight at 3 and 6 months Blood lipid profile (fasting if possible)	Annual health check LFTs annually Clotting screen annually FBC annually Blood pressure annually Weight/BMI annually Fasting (if possible) blood glucose, HbA_{1c} annually Blood lipid profile (fasting if possible) annually

Table 3.8 (cont.)

Serious mental illness	Baseline and initial	Maintenance
	Fasting (if possible) blood glucose, HbA_{1c} (average blood glucose level) Valproate is contraindicated in girls and women of childbearing potential, unless the conditions of the pregnancy prevention programme are met Pregnancy must be ruled out and highly effective contraception in place for girls and women of childbearing potential	Plasma levels if required to detect non-compliance or toxicity (plasma levels to ensure adequate dosing are of limited use) For girls and women of childbearing potential, review the need for treatment with sodium valproate and complete
Carbamazepine	Plasma level 2 weeks after initiation FBC baseline and at 6 months LFTs baseline and at 6 months U&Es baseline and at 6 months Blood pressure Weight and height, monitor weight periodically thereafter	Annual health check U&Es 6-monthly Plasma levels can be used to ensure adequate dosing and treatment compliance Plasma level 2 weeks after dose change, then every 6 months Fasting (if possible) blood glucose, HbA_{1c} (average blood glucose level) annually Blood lipid profile (fasting if possible) annually
Lamotrigine	See clinical notes section for advice and counselling regarding blood disorders, skin reactions, and hypersensitivity syndrome	Annual health check
Antidepressants	**BASELINE and INITIAL**	**MAINTENANCE**
Venlafaxine	Blood pressure and pulse at baseline and regularly after initiation	Blood pressure and pulse – review periodically and after dose changes
Agomelatine	LFTs at baseline and weeks 3, 6, 12, 24	LFTs regularly as clinically indicated and at increase of dose
SSRIs and others	No specific monitoring required	No specific monitoring required
Antipsychotics	**BASELINE and INITIAL**	**MAINTENANCE**
Amisulpride Aripiprazole Olanzapine Quetiapine Risperidone	FBC Blood glucose (fasting if possible), baseline then at 3 months and 1 year (olanzapine also at 1 month and 6 month)	Annual health check FBC annually Blood glucose (fasting if possible) annually HbA_{1c} annually

Table 3.8 (cont.)

Serious mental illness	Baseline and initial	Maintenance
First-generation antipsychotics Clozapine (see below) Refer to High Dose Antipsychotic Therapy (HDAT) policy for monitoring those on high dose antipsychotics.	HbA$_{1c}$ (average blood glucose level) baseline and 3 months Blood lipid profile baseline then at 3 months and 1 year (olanzapine 3-monthly for first year then annually) LFTs U&Es Prolactin ECG if clinically indicated (and after target dose is reached during in-patient admission and before discharge if medication regimen has changed) (mandatory prior to haloperidol) Blood pressure/pulse baseline and frequently during dose titration then at 12 weeks and 1 year Weight baseline, weekly for 6 weeks (if possible) then at 12 weeks, 6 months and 1 year (plotted on a chart) (olanzapine, weekly for 6 weeks then at 12 weeks and every 3 months for first year, then annually) Waist circumference (plotted on a chart)	Blood lipid profile – annually LFTs – annually U&Es – annually Prolactin level annually for antipsychotics likely to cause a rise in prolactin or if signs or symptoms of raised prolactin. ECG if clinically indicated e.g., high-dose antipsychotic or presence of cardiovascular risk Blood pressure/pulse annually Weight annually (plotted on a chart) Waist circumference annually (plotted on a chart) Glasgow Antipsychotic Side effects Scale (GASS-C)/LUNSERs/ Barnes Akathisia Rating Scale for side-effect monitoring
Clozapine	FBC Blood glucose (fasting if possible) baseline then at 1, 3, 6, and 12 months HbA$_{1c}$ (average blood glucose level) baseline and at 3 months Blood lipid profile baseline, then at 3, 6, and 12 months LFTs at baseline and then at 6 months U&Es at baseline ECG Blood pressure and pulse baseline, frequently during dose	Annual health check FBC as per monitoring guidelines Fasting blood glucose (if possible) and HbA$_{1c}$ (average blood glucose level) every 6 months U&Es – annually LFTs – annually Blood lipid profile – annually ECG annually if high dose >600mg/day or otherwise indicated. Blood pressure and pulse – minimum 6-monthly

Table 3.8 (cont.)

Serious mental illness	Baseline and initial	Maintenance
	titration then at 3 months and 12 months Weight at baseline, weekly for 6 weeks (if possible) then at 12 weeks, 6 months, and 1 year (plotted on a chart) Waist circumference baseline then at 12 weeks and 1 year (plotted on a chart) Assessment of bowel movements	Weight minimum 6-monthly (plotted on a chart) or at each review. Waist circumference annually (plotted on a chart) Glasgow Antipsychotic Side effects Scale (GASS-C) – 6-monthly Bowel movements at each review

The next two sections consider the clinical guidance around two specific issues: overweight/obesity and constipation.

Weight Gain and Obesity

Definitions and Categories

Overweight and obese are defined as abnormal or excessive fat accumulation that presents a risk to health (World Health Organization 2022). The NICE guidelines on the identification, assessment, and management of obesity (NICE Clinical Guideline 189, 2014; updated September 2022) set out clinically useful categories based on body mass index (BMI), central adiposity and waist circumference.

Traditionally, BMI was used as the basis for diagnosing obesity and was calculated by dividing the weight in kilogrammes by the square of the height in metres. A BMI of less than 18.5 was considered within the underweight range, 18.5 to <25 within the healthy weight range, 25.0 to <30 within the overweight range, and 30.0+ within the obese range. The updated National Institute of Health and Care guideline suggested that for those from Black, Asian, and Minority Ethnic (BAME) backgrounds, the BMI cut offs for being overweight and obese should be lower by about 2.5 (i.e., BMI 23 to 27.4 overweight and above 27.5 obese). Further, this highlighted the limitations of relying on BMI alone and emphasised the need to monitor central adiposity by recording the waist to height ratio, if the BMI was 35 or less. Ideally, the waist measurement should be half your height or less. Waist circumference by itself can be used as an indicator for increased or significant risk of physical health complications. A waist circumference in men of 94–101 centimetres indicates increased risk and over 102 centimetres indicates significant risk, while in women it is 80–7 centimetres and over 88 centimetres respectively.

Obesity has a greater prevalence among people with intellectual disability. The most recent data from primary care in England showed a prevalence of 37%, compared to 30% in those without an intellectual disability (Public Health England 2020). This overrepresentation has been a consistent finding over the years, among both men and women

(Samele et al. 2006, Melville et al. 2008, Biswas et al. 2016). Contributory factors may include proportionately higher calorie intake, lower levels of physical activity and exercise, limited availability of appropriate community leisure facilities, lack of skilled staff, day services, dietary advice and lifestyle changes, a genetic predisposition in some cases, and the greater use of psychotropic medication (Biswas et al. 2016). The consequences of obesity, which include hypertension, type 2 diabetes mellitus, cardiac disease, and cancers, can be significant contributors to the increased mortality rates that are reported in people with an intellectual disability (Public Health England 2020).

Psychotropic Medication and Obesity

Weight gain is a long recognised and common problem in psychiatric practice. While there are several illness-related and environmental factors that contribute to this, the side effects of psychotropic medication, and particularly of atypical antipsychotics, cannot be overemphasised. Being overweight/obese is 2–3 times more common in those treated with antipsychotics than in the general population (Holt & Peveler 2009).

Mental health or intellectual disability in-patient wards have been described as potentially obesogenic environments (Russell et al. 2018) and the cascade iatrogenesis concept may be particularly relevant in such settings (Holt 2019). The latter refers to how a series of multiple medical complications can be set in motion by a seemingly innocuous first event. Antipsychotic or other psychotropic medication, limited exercise, a sedentary lifestyle, increased calorie intake, weight gain, obesity, type 2 diabetes, hypertension, and dyslipidaemias can become the cascade that leads on to more serious cardiac events or other complications. Although robust monitoring standards for psychotropic medication are now available (NICE Clinical Guideline NG11, 2015; NICE Evidence Summary, 2017; Royal College of Psychiatrists 2016; Alexander et al. 2017), there is evidence to suggest scope for further improvement in monitoring for side effects, particularly obesity and metabolic syndrome, to facilitate early interventions.

Interventions: General Principles

The NICE guidelines on the identification, assessment, and management of obesity (NICE Clinical Guideline 189, 2014; updated September 2022) set out the general principles for intervention. These include discussion with the patient, agreement on a course of action, tailoring interventions to individual needs and recognising that 'one approach will not fit all' as far as interventions go.

Interventions: Lifestyle Changes, Diet, Exercise, and Behavioural Approaches

Outside of mental health settings, there is good evidence for lifestyle changes being effective. The Diabetes Remission Clinical trial (DiRECT) used a low-calorie total diet replacement followed by stepped food reintroduction and support in people with type 2 diabetes. A quarter of participants lost more than 15 kilogrammes in year 1 and maintained an average weight loss of 10 kilogrammes in year 2 (Lean et al. 2019). Comparably impressive evidence, however, has not been identified in the case of antipsychotic- or psychotropic-induced weight gain.

A wide range of behavioural approaches have been developed, including counselling, cognitive behavioural therapy (CBT), self-monitoring, stimulus control, goal setting, slowing rate of eating, social supports, problem solving, assertiveness training, cognitive restructuring, relapse prevention, and mindfulness. Although there is evidence that mindfulness as a technique is useful in addressing obesity and unhealthy eating habits (Carrière et al. 2018), it has not been widely used in mental health or intellectual disabilities settings. A feasibility study to test its applicability in an in-patient forensic intellectual disability setting has recently been reported (Amiola et al. 2022). For further details on lifestyle measures, please refer to the NICE clinical guidelines 189: www.nice.org.uk/guidance/cg189.

Interventions: Switching of Psychotropics

Psychotropic medication has different propensities to cause weight gain and obesity (see Table 3.9).

Table 3.9 Obesogenic risk of antipsychotics and antidepressants

Grade of risk of obesity	Antipsychotics	Antidepressants
High	Clozapine Olanzapine	Mirtazapine All tricyclics (within this group, lofepramine has the least potential to cause weight gain) Paroxetine Citalopram
Moderate	Quetiapine Risperidone Paliperidone Chlorpromazine Flupenthixol Promazine Pipotiazine Iloperidone	SSRIs excluding paroxetine and citalopram
Low	Aripiprazole Amisulpiride Lurasidone Sulpiride Haloperidol Trifluoperazine Sertindole Pimozide Perphenazine Loxapine Fluphenazine Cariprazine Brexipiprazole Benperidol Asenapine	Agomelatine

The general principle would be to either try to lower the dose of the currently prescribed antipsychotic or switch to one which has a lower degree of risk of weight gain or obesity (The Maudsley Prescribing Guidelines 2021; The Maudsley Practice Guidelines for Physical Health Conditions in Psychiatry 2021; Choice and Medication n.d.). Earlier studies showed some promise in switching from Olanzapine to Aripiprazole (Newcomer et al. 2003). This promise, however, has not been sustained. The evidence of efficacy of this approach has been well summarised by Holt (2019), and unfortunately there isn't much robust evidence that switching is effective. There is also little evidence of an antipsychotic dose-response regarding weight gain, and hence lowering the antipsychotic dose rarely achieves weight loss.

Interventions: Medication

Orlistat, metformin, liraglutide, and semaglutide offer pharmacological options for the management of obesity. Recommendations for their use are summarised in Table 3.10. (NICE Clinical Guideline CG 189, 2014, updated 2022; NICE Evidence summary 14, 2017; The Maudsley Prescribing Guidelines 2021; The Maudsley Practice Guidelines for Physical Health Conditions in Psychiatry 2021).

Table 3.10 Advantages, disadvantages, monitoring, and length of treatment

	Orlistat	Metformin	Liraglutide	Semaglutide
Advantages	Evidence for use in clozapine- and olanzapine-induced weight gain	Does not stimulate insulin production and hence little risk of hypoglycaemia, if used alone. Low cost	Effective in patients treated with olanzapine or clozapine	Can be given once weekly
Disadvantages	Should follow a low-fat diet	Off-label use Risk of lactic acidosis, Vitamin B12 deficiency	High monthly cost Daily injections	Injections, although weekly
Monitoring	Side effects: diarrhoea, gas, stomach pain, oily stools. A fatty diet can cause steatorrhea and potential malabsorption of oral medication	Monitor renal functions 3–6 monthly; intermittent vitamin B12 level monitoring	Side effects: nausea, vomiting, abdominal pain, headache, increased heart rate, increased risk of pancreatitis, hypoglycaemia, diarrhoea, constipation, fatigue	Side effects: nausea, diarrhoea, vomiting, constipation, abdominal pain, headache, fatigue, hypoglycaemia

Table 3.10 (cont.)

	Orlistat	Metformin	Liraglutide	Semaglutide
How long to continue	Continue beyond 3 months only if there is a 5% weight loss	Deprescribing: discussion of pros and cons at 6-month mark	Should be discontinued after 12 weeks if patients have not lost at least 5% of their initial body weight	2 years maximum

Interventions: Bariatric Surgery

In England (NICE Clinical Guideline 189, 2014), bariatric surgery for obesity may be indicated if the following conditions are met:

- The person has
  - a BMI of 40 or more, or
  - a BMI between 35 and 40 and other significant disease (e.g., type 2 diabetes or high blood pressure) that could be improved if they lost weight.
- All appropriate non-surgical measures have been tried but the person has not achieved or maintained adequate, clinically beneficial weight loss
- The person has been receiving or will receive intensive management in a tier 3 obesity service
- The person is generally fit for anaesthesia and surgery
- The person commits to the need for long-term follow-up

The types of bariatric surgery may include gastric bypass or sleeve gastrectomy (The Maudsley Practice Guidelines for Physical Health Conditions in Psychiatry 2021). There are no published reports about its use in people with intellectual disabilities and obesity. There is one systematic review (Kouidrat et al. 2017) on the use of bariatric surgery in people with severe mental illness; it concludes that while there are few studies in this area, psychosis should not be a contraindication where an individual has severe obesity and where surgery would otherwise be recommended. The same should apply to people with intellectual disability.

A general algorithm for the management of obesity in people with an intellectual disability is provided in Figure 3.1.

Constipation

Up to 40% of people with intellectual disability experience constipation (Mathew et al. 2021). Constipation, where missed or inadequately treated, can result in behavioural disturbance, faecal impaction, intestinal obstruction, and death (Mathew et al. 2021). Despite being described as 'both preventable and amenable to treatment', the number of people with an intellectual disability who have died because of constipation remains concerning (Learning Disability Mortality Review (LeDeR) Programme: Action from Learning NHS England and NHS Improvement, n.d.).

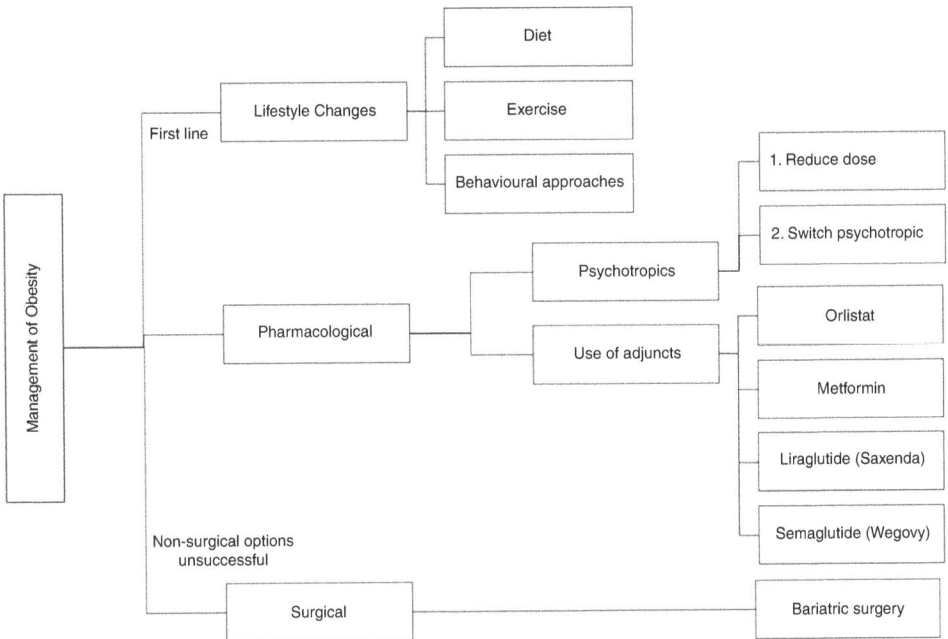

Figure 3.1 Algorithm for the management of obesity

Among people with intellectual disability, constipation is 'most commonly secondary to neuromuscular abnormalities, immobility, diet and medication side effects' (Morad et al. 2007). Antipsychotic medication can be associated with constipation, with the risk being three times greater with clozapine (Shirazi et al. 2016). Despite its potential for fatal consequences, constipation is a frequently overlooked side effect of clozapine treatment (Shirazi et al. 2016). The risk of constipation with clozapine is associated with its anticholinergic activity (Talley et al. 2003), peripheral clozapine serotonergic antagonism (Crowell 2004), strong histamine H1 receptor antagonism (Shirazi et al. 2016), and, specific to the norclozapine metabolite, potent agonist activity at delta opioid receptors (Olianas et al. 2009). The risk of constipation with clozapine is compounded further by the reduced intestinal sensitivity to distention resulting in patients often not complaining of feeling any pain or discomfort (MyPsych, NHS Greater Glasgow and Clyde web site, n.d.).

Signs and Symptoms
- Reduced bowel movement
- Excessive straining
- Lower abdominal pain, discomfort, distension, or bloating
- Hard stools
- Rectal bleeding
- Severe cases: confusion, nausea, reduced appetite, overflow diarrhoea, urinary retention

Conservative Treatment

- Healthy, balanced diet (e.g., high sorbitol fruits, daily fibre content of 30g)
- Regular meals
- Drinking water adequately (e.g., 2 litres for men and 1.6 litres for women)
- Increasing activity levels
- Optimising toilet routines (e.g., taking into account any physical or sensory difficulties)

Treatment with Medication

- Note that laxatives may not be suitable in all circumstances. Check British National Formulary for contraindications (e.g., fluid and electrolyte disturbance, dehydration, faecal impaction)
- Bulk-forming laxatives (e.g., ispaghula husk) act by retaining fluid within the stool and increasing faecal mass, stimulating peristalsis; also have stool-softening properties
- Osmotic laxatives (e.g., lactulose) act by increasing the amount of fluid in the large bowel, producing distension, which leads to stimulation of peristalsis
- Stimulant laxatives (e.g., senna, bisacodyl, docusate, sodium pico-sulfate) cause peristalsis by stimulating colonic and/or rectal nerves
- Prokinetic laxatives (e.g., prucalopride) stimulate intestinal motility.

Treatment of Clozapine Induced Constipation

Specialist Pharmacy Service (2022) developed the following guidance:

- Start stimulant laxatives and review after 24 hours
- Add an osmotic laxative or stool softener (e.g., docusate sodium) if necessary and review after 48 hours
- Increase laxative doses (up to the maximum licenced dose) every 48 hours until resolution of symptoms
- Avoid bulk-forming laxatives due to clozapine induced gastric hypomotility
- Consider high-dose macrogol or repeated doses of suppositories in cases of faecal impaction
- In severe cases of constipation, liaise with a gastroenterologist for advice
- Care plans to be developed to prevent future episodes of constipation

The Frith Prescribing Guidelines Editors' Expert Group Consensus Statements

Statements of High Confidence

Being overweight or obese is 2–3 times higher in people with intellectual disability treated with antipsychotics than in the general population.

In the general population, metformin is associated with a mean reduction in body weight over 3–6 months.

In the general population, liraglutide helps to induce and sustain clinically significant weight loss in patients with obesity.

The risk of constipation is three times greater with clozapine compared to other antipsychotics.

Statements of Medium Confidence

Annual health checks are associated with a trend towards improved survival for people with intellectual disability

Health checks have resulted in improved detection of both major (e.g., cancer) and minor (e.g., excessive ear wax) health conditions

Statements of Low Confidence

There is limited evidence that diet control or exercise is effective for antipsychotic- or psychotropic-induced weight gain for people with intellectual disability.

Behavioural approaches (including mindfulness) are effective among people with intellectual disability who are overweight or obese.

Resource Box

- The Easy Health website (www.easyhealth.org.uk) holds 390 resources about 120 health conditions or topics in their library, including easy-read leaflets and accessible patient information videos. The site also signposts to links for other useful resources.
- Beyond Words (booksbeyondwords.co.uk) is an online resource which offers a variety of paid resources to support communication through pictures.

References

Alexander, R. T., Shankar, R., Cooper, S. A., et al. (2017). Challenges and pitfalls of antipsychotic prescribing in people with learning disability. *British Journal of General Practice*, **67**(661), 372–3.

Amiola, A., Temple, P., Dickerson, H., et al. (2022). A pilot project to introduce the Compassionate Approach to Living Mindfully for Prevention of Disease (Calmpod) in weight management in a forensic intellectual disability unit. *BJPsych Open*, **8**(S1), S82–S83.

Beyond Words. (n.d.). *Beyond Words*. https://booksbeyondwords.co.uk.

Biswas, A., Shaherbano, S., & Hiremath, A. (2024). Obesity in people with intellectual disabilities. University of Herfordshire. www.intellectualdisability.info/physical-health/obesity-in-people-with-intellectual-disabilities.

Carrière, K., Khoury, B., Günak, M. M., & Knäuper, B. (2018) Mindfulness-based interventions for weight loss: A systematic review and meta-analysis. *Obesity Reviews*, Feb; **19**(2), 164–77. https://doi.org/10.1111/obr.12623. Epub 2017 Oct 27. PMID: 29076610.

Choice and Medication. (n.d.). Website. www.choiceandmedication.org.

Crowell, M. D. (2004). Role of serotonin in the pathophysiology of the irritable bowel syndrome. *British Journal of Pharmacology*, **141**(8), 1285–93. https://doi.org/10.1038/sj.bjp.0705762.

Holt, R. I. and Peveler, R. C. (2009). Obesity, serious mental illness and antipsychotic drugs. *Diabetes, Obesity and Metabolism*, **11**(7), 665–79.

Holt, R. I. (2019). The management of obesity in people with severe mental illness: an unresolved conundrum. *Psychotherapy and Psychosomatics*, **88**(6), 327–32.

Hertfordshire Partnership University NHS Foundation Trust (2020). Physical Health Policy Procedure for the Assessment, Examination and Physical Wellbeing

Support of Service Users. www.hpft.nhs.uk/media/1842/item-13a-physical-health-strategy-final-board-paper.pdf.

Kennedy, N., Kennedy, J., Kerr, M., Dredge, S., & Brophy, S. (2022). Health checks for adults with intellectual disability and association with survival rates: A linked electronic records matched cohort study in Wales, UK. *BMJ Open*, **12**(4), p.e049441. https://doi.org/10.1136/bmjopen-2021-049441.

Kouidrat Y, Amad A, Stubbs B, Moore S, & Gaughran F. (2017) Surgical management of obesity among people with schizophrenia and bipolar disorder: A systematic review of outcomes and recommendations for future research. *Obesity Surgery*, Jul; 27(7), 1889–95.

Lean, M. E., Leslie, W. S., Barnes, A. C., et al. (2019). Durability of a primary care-led weight-management intervention for remission of type 2 diabetes: 2-year results of the DiRECT open-label, cluster-randomised trial. *The Lancet Diabetes & Endocrinology*, 7(5), 344–55.

Learning Disability Mortality Review (LeDeR) Programme Annual Report. (2020). www.bristol.ac.uk/media-library/sites/sps/leder/LeDeR_2019_annual_report_FINAL2.pdf.

Learning Disability Mortality Review (LeDeR) Programme: Action from Learning NHS England and NHS Improvement. (n.d.). www.england.nhs.uk/wp-content/uploads/2019/05/action-from-learning.pdf.

Leth-Møller, K. B., Hansen, A. H., Torstensson, M., et al. (2016). Antidepressants and the risk of hyponatremia: A Danish register-based population study. *BMJ Open*, 6(5). https://doi.org/10.1136/bmjopen-2016-011200.

Liao, P., Vajdic, C., Trollor, J., & Reppermund, S. (2021). Prevalence and incidence of physical health conditions in people with intellectual disability – a systematic review. *PLOS ONE*, **16**(8), p.e0256294. https://doi.org/10.1371/journal.pone.0256294.

Mathew, R., Attarha, B.O., Kallumkal, G., et al. (2021). A primary care approach to constipation in adults with intellectual and developmental disabilities. *Advances in Medicine*, **2021**, p.3248052. https://doi.org/10.1155/2021/3248052.

Melville, C. A., Cooper, S. A., Morrison, J., et al. (2008). The prevalence and determinants of obesity in adults with intellectual disabilities. *Journal of Applied Research in Intellectual Disabilities*, **21**(5), 425–37.

Morad, M., Nelson, N. P., Merrick, J., Davidson, P. W., & Carmeli, E. (2007). Prevalence and risk factors of constipation in adults with intellectual disability in residential care centres in Israel. *Research in Developmental Disabilities*, **28**(6), 580–6. https://doi.org/10.1016/j.ridd.2006.08.002.

MyPsych, NHS Greater Glasgow and Clyde web site (n.d.). Clozapine and Constipation. https://rightdecisions.scot.nhs.uk/mypsych-app/working-in-greater-glasgow-clyde/medicines-companion/clozapine/clozapine-and-constipation/.

National Institute of Health and Care Excellence (NICE) (2014). Psychosis and schizophrenia in adults: prevention and management. Guideline CG178. www.nice.org.uk/guidance/cg178.

National Institute of Health and Care Excellence (NICE) (2014). Obesity: Identification, Assessment and Management. Clinical Guideline CG 189, updated September 2022. www.nice.org.uk/guidance/cg189.

National Institute for Health and Care Excellence (NICE) (2015). Challenging behaviour and learning disabilities: prevention and interventions for people with learning disabilities whose behaviour challenges, NG 11. www.nice.org.uk/guidance/ng11.

National Institute for Health and Care Excellence (NICE) (2016). Mental health problems in people with learning disabilities: prevention, assessment and management NG54. www.nice.org.uk/guidance/ng54.

National Institute for Health and Care Excellence (NICE) (2017). Obese, Overweight with risk factors: Liraglutide (Saxenda) Evidence Summary. www.nice.org.uk/guidance/ta875.

National Institute for Health and Care Excellence (NICE) (2018). Clinical Guideline 87; www.nice.org.uk/guidance/ng87/chap

ter/Recommendations#maintenance-and-monitoring.

National Institute for Health and Care Excellence (NICE) (2020). Liraglutide for managing overweight and obesity, Technology appraisal guidance [TA664.] Published 9 December 2020. www.nice.org.uk/guidance/ta664.

National Institute for Health and Care Excellence (NICE) (2012). Semaglutide for obesity, published February 2022. www.nice.org.uk/news/article/nice-recommends-new-drug-for-people-living-with-obesity.

NHS England (n.d.). Annual health checks. www.england.nhs.uk/learning-disabilities/improving-health/annual-health-checks/.

Olianas, M.C., Dedoni, S., Ambu, R., & Onali, P. (2009). Agonist activity of N-desmethylclozapine at δ-opioid receptors of human frontal cortex. *European Journal of Pharmacology*, **607**(1–3), 96–101. https://doi.org/10.1016/j.ejphar.2009.02.025.

Prajapathi, A. R. (2014). Role of metformin in the management of antipsychotic-induced weight gain. *Progress in Neurology and Psychiatry*, Nov–Dec, 33–8. https://wchh.onlinelibrary.wiley.com/doi/pdf/10.1002/pnp.358.

Rajan, L., & Clarke, I. (2013). Audit of combination and high-dose antipsychotic treatment in the community. *The Psychiatrist*, **37**(9), 302–7. https://doi.org/10.1192/pb.bp.112.039750.

Robertson, J., Hatton, C., Emerson, E., & Baines, S. (2014). The impact of health checks for people with intellectual disabilities: An updated systematic review of evidence. *Research in Developmental Disabilities*, **35**(10), 2450–62. https://doi.org/10.1016/j.ridd.2014.06.007.

Rowland, J. P., Rigby, J., Harper, A. C., & Rowland, R. (2007). Cardiovascular monitoring with acetylcholinesterase inhibitors: A clinical protocol. *Advances in Psychiatric Treatment*, **13**(3), 178–84. https://doi.org/10.1192/apt.bp.106.002725.

Royal College of Psychiatrists (2016) Psychotropic drug prescribing for people with intellectual disability, mental health problems and/or behaviours that challenge: practice guidelines. www.rcpsych.ac.uk/docs/default-source/members/faculties/intellectual-disability/id-faculty-report-id-09.pdf?sfvrsn=55b66f2c_6.

Royal College of Psychiatrists (2014; January 2023 revision) Report CR190: The risks and benefits of high-dose antipsychotic medication. www.rcpsych.ac.uk/docs/default-source/improving-care/better-mh-policy/college-reports/college-report-cr190.pdf?sfvrsn=54f5d9a2_11.

Russell, R., Chester, V., Watson, J., et al. (2018). The prevalence of overweight and obesity levels among forensic inpatients with learning disability. *British Journal of Learning Disabilities*, **46**(2), 101–108.

Samele, C., Seymour, L., Morris, B., et al. (2006) A formal investigation into health inequalities experienced by people with learning difficulties and people with mental health problems – Area Studies Report. Report to the Disability Rights Commission (DRC). The Sainsbury Centre for Mental Health.

Shirazi, A., Stubbs, B., Gomez, L., et al. (2016). Prevalence and predictors of clozapine-associated constipation: A systematic review and meta-analysis. *International Journal of Molecular Sciences*, **17**(6), 863. https://doi.org/10.3390/ijms17060863.

SPS – Specialist Pharmacy Service (2022). Managing constipation in people taking clozapine. www.sps.nhs.uk/articles/managing-constipation-in-people-taking-clozapine/.

South West London & St George's Mental Health NHS Trust guideline. Guidance for recommended on going physical monitoring of psychotropic medication in primary care. https://swlstg.nhs.uk/download.cfm?ver=1101.

Talley, N. J., Jones, M., Nuyts, G., & Dubois, D. (2003). Risk factors for chronic constipation based on a general practice sample. *The American Journal of Gastroenterology*, **98**(5), 1107–11. https://doi.org/10.1111/j.1572-0241.2003.07465.x.

Taylor, D. M., Gaughran, F. & Pillinger, T. (2020) (Eds.), *The Maudsley Practice Guidelines for physical health conditions in psychiatry.* Wiley Blackwell.

Taylor, D. M., Barnes, T. R. and Young, A. H., et al. (2021) *The Maudsley Prescribing Guidelines in Psychiatry.* Wiley Blackwell.

Mencap (2018). Treat me well: Reasonable adjustments for people with a learning disability in hospital. www.mencap.org.uk/sites/default/files/2018-06/Treat%20me%20well%20top%2010%20reasonable%20adjustments.pdf.

Tyrer, P., Cooper, S.-A., & Hassiotis, A. (2014). Drug treatments in people with intellectual disability and challenging behaviour. *British Medical Journal*, **349**(jul04 1), g4323–g4323. https://doi.org/10.1136/bmj.g4323.

World Health Organization. Health topics: obesity. www.who.int/health-topics/obesity/#tab=tab_1.

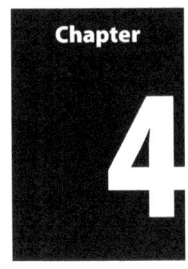

Chapter 4

Mental Health Conditions in People with Intellectual Disability

Meghana Rayala, Ayomipo J. Amiola, Reena Tharian, Tadhgh Lane, and Regi T. Alexander

Introduction

Intellectual disability refers to conditions characterised by significant impairment of both intellectual and adaptive functioning, with onset during the developmental period (i.e., before the age of 18). A retrospective diagnosis, when presenting to services after the age of 18, can also be made. Based on the extent of this impairment as measured using standardised tests and clinical judgement, the condition can vary in severity as mild, moderate, severe, or profound. (International Classification Diseases (ICD) 11 (WHO, 2022); Diagnostic and Statistical Manual (DSM) 5 (APA, 2013).) The worldwide prevalence of intellectual disability is estimated to be around 1–2% (Emerson & Baines, 2011). Among individuals with intellectual disability, approximately 85% have mild intellectual disability, 10% have moderate intellectual disability, 4% have severe intellectual disability, and 2% have profound intellectual disability (King et al., 2009).

How Common Is Co-Existing Mental Health Morbidity in Intellectual Disability?

Mental Health Conditions

Intellectual disability is associated with high mental health, behavioural, and neurodevelopmental disorder comorbidity (Matson and Cervantes 2013). People with intellectual disability develop psychiatric conditions at rates similar to or higher than the general population (Buckles, Luckasson & Keefe 2013). This may not be surprising, given the complex interplay of developmental factors, psychological and social disadvantages, and physical health comorbidity that they are exposed to (Cooper 2020). The estimated prevalence of mental health problems in people with intellectual disability is 15–20%, depending on the diagnostic criteria used. Some epidemiological studies suggest a prevalence rate as high as 31–41%, and this extensive comorbidity can lead to severe debilitation in many people (Matson and Cervantes 2013; Morgan et al. 2008). This in turn causes increased contact with health and social care services, including admissions to in-patient psychiatric units and secure hospital settings. Prevalence rates for specific mental health disorders derived from population-based studies are not without inherent bias due to inadequate methods of identification. As a result, they may not always be generalisable, but nevertheless give an idea about the disease burden in people with intellectual disability (Smiley et al. 2005) (see Table 4.1). The rates in hospital settings can be significantly higher due to the selected nature of the population (Chester et al. 2023).

Table 4.1 Population-based prevalence rates of mental health conditions (from Smiley 2005)

Condition	Rate
Schizophrenia	3%
Bipolar affective disorder	1.5%
Depression	4%
Generalised anxiety disorder	6%
Specific phobia	6%
Agoraphobia	1.5%
Obsessive-compulsive disorder	2.5%
Dementia at age 65 years or over	20%
Autistic spectrum disorder	7%
'Severe problem' behaviour	10–15%

Challenging Behaviour

A significant proportion of people with intellectual disability display behaviours that challenge, with prevalence increasing as the degree of disability becomes more severe. A prevalence of around 5–15% in educational, health, or social care services and 30–40% in hospital settings (NICE 2015; Devapriam and Alexander 2019) has been reported.

Challenging behaviour is defined as behaviour which is of such intensity, frequency, or duration as to threaten the quality of life and/or the physical safety of the individual or others and is likely to lead to responses that are restrictive, aversive, or result in exclusion (Royal College of Psychiatrists, British Psychological Society & Royal College of Speech and Language Therapists 2007). This definition is quite broad and can cover a range of presentations, from relatively minor acts of aggression to serious violence. Thus, the dividing line between challenging behaviour and offending behaviour can be blurred, although a range of offence, patient, and system factors have been proposed to distinguish them (Chester et al. 2023). Likewise, while many mental illnesses and disorders may present with challenging behaviour, not all challenging behaviour is the result of a mental illness or disorder. It must be recognised as a descriptive concept and not a diagnosis. It might be unrelated to, or it can be a manifestation of, an underlying mental health disorder, and the association is strongest in those with severe disorders of intellectual disability. The behaviour might be also related to physical health problems, communication difficulties, or environmental changes – and, in many cases, a combination of these (Royal College of Psychiatrists 2016). This makes it important to ascertain the underlying causes and associations before making decisions about treatment, particularly prescribing (Royal College of Psychiatrists 2013, 2016; NICE 2016). Chapter 10 in this volume provides more information on aggression and self-injurious behaviour – two common types of challenging behaviour seen in people with intellectual disability.

Approach to Assessment and Treatment

There must be a clear diagnostic assessment and formulation before any prescribing of psychotropic medication. This must be followed by regular review and monitoring of the prescribing (NICE 2016; Royal College of Psychiatrists 2016).

Diagnostic Assessment

Reaching a consensus about diagnosis in people with intellectual disability can be complex. Prior to any prescribing, a full diagnostic assessment should be completed that covers the following planes:

1. Degree of intellectual disability
2. Cause of intellectual disability
3. Autism
4. Any other neurodevelopmental disorder (e.g., attention deficit hyperactivity disorder, dyspraxias, etc.)
5. Mental illnesses (if not enough features of the full syndrome, record a narrative account of the symptoms that are present)
6. Personality disorder
7. Substance use disorders
8. Physical illnesses
9. Experience of trauma due to any cause
10. Types of challenging behaviour

Following this structure, behaviour that challenges is not treated as a diagnosis, but as a presenting symptom in the context of a range of biopsychosocial factors. The prescriber generates a multiaxial diagnosis and formulation, which becomes the target for intervention. A multidisciplinary team involvement, including family and carers, for reaching the formulation and offering interventions is recommended (NICE 2016; Royal College of Psychiatrists 2016).

Formulation and Understanding Challenging Behaviour

Challenging behaviour may serve a purpose for the person, such as drawing attention from others, stimulation, avoidance, or pain reduction, all of which can maintain the behaviour (Hastings et al. 2013). It is important to have a conceptual framework to understand challenging behaviour in relation to its social, vulnerability, and maintaining factors. The social effects include how the challenging behaviour has resulted in the individual missing out on a typical community life in some way and the risks such behaviours pose to themselves and others. The vulnerability factors include physical illness, mental illness, sensory problems, lack of communication skills, or limited life situations and inequalities experienced by people with intellectual disability which put them at risk of presenting with challenging behaviour.

The 5-P model of the **p**resenting problem, **p**redisposing, **p**recipitating, **p**erpetuating, and **p**rotective factors (Macneil et al. 2012) offers a useful structure for psychological formulation. The HELP framework of **h**ealth (physical health), **e**nvironment, **l**ived experience (trauma), and **p**sychiatric problems (Green et al. 2018) is a patient-centred way of structuring the targets for therapeutic intervention. The therapeutic approach to the experience of past trauma in people with intellectual disability is addressed in detail in Chapter 5.

Interventions Other than Psychotropic Medication

Once assessment and formulation are completed, interventions are developed to target these. Any underlying causes identified through the HELP framework must be addressed. This may mean the identification and treatment of undetected physical health causes (e.g., constipation, pain, etc.), mitigation of environmental stress factors, addressing past traumas and adverse life experiences, and treating psychiatric comorbidity. A positive behavioural support (PBS) plan is developed, which is a framework developed from functional assessment of behaviour; understanding the interplay of biological, social, psychological, and environmental factors contributing to the behaviour; and developing patient-centred, evidence-based interventions (Carr et al. 2002; Beavers et al. 2013; Langdon et al. 2017). Alongside PBS, other psychological interventions must be offered as appropriate (NICE 2016; Royal College of Psychiatrists 2016).

Criteria and Guidance for Prescribing

Any clinician prescribing for people with intellectual disability must be aware of the relevant guidelines set out by the National Institute for Health & Care Excellence (NICE), the Royal College of Psychiatrists, and other medical regulatory bodies. In people with intellectual disability who have a mental health condition or behaviour that challenges, there are three broad situations in which they might meet mental healthcare professionals (Royal College of Psychiatrists 2016). These are: the presence of behaviour that challenges but is not associated with symptoms that meet the criteria of any mental illness or any other mental disorder; the presence of behaviour that challenges and is associated with symptoms that clearly meet the diagnostic criteria for a mental illness or any other mental disorder; and the presence of behaviour that challenges and is associated with some mental health symptoms, but these do not fulfil the diagnostic criteria for a mental illness or any other mental disorder. Interventions must be offered based on which of these three categories they fall into

Challenging Behaviour and No Mental Illness/Mental Disorder

- In general, there should be no primary role for treatment with psychotropic medication in this group. As behaviour is driven by psychological factors, environmental factors, or physical health causes, treatment addressing these is paramount.
- Studies from across the world have shown psychotropic medication prescription rates of 30–60% for those with intellectual disability and challenging behaviour. This rate is very high considering the relative lack of robust evidence for effects of medications on challenging behaviours. In England, a national programme to stop over-medication of people with learning difficulties (STOMP-LD) has been developed to rationalise prescribing practice in this area (Alexander & Tharian 2021). Prescribing practice and STOMP are discussed in detail in Chapter 2.
- Prescribing for a very short period could be considered to alleviate a serious risk to the safety of the individual or others while other modalities of treatment are being implemented.
- Antipsychotics should be considered to manage behaviour that challenges only if
    - psychological or other interventions alone have not produced the desired outcome within an agreed reasonable time; or

- treatment for any co-existing mental or physical health problem has not led to a reduction in the behaviour; or
- the risk to the person or others is very severe.
  (NICE 2015; Royal College of Psychiatrists 2016)

• In this context, the prescribing would be off label, and hence prescribers should follow recommendations set out by regulatory bodies for such prescribing (GMC, 2021).

Challenging Behaviour and a Clear Mental Illness/Mental Disorder

• Where recognising mental illness among people with intellectual disability or autism is complicated because of communication difficulties, atypical presentations, diagnostic overshadowing, or difficulties accessing services, the clinician must rely on accurate descriptions and narrative account of the symptoms (Langdon & Murphy 2021).
• Treatment should follow established guidelines for the mental illness or mental disorder. Guidelines of specific mental health diagnoses are discussed in depth in other chapters.
• While prescribing, the common practice of 'start low and go slow' might be relevant, especially in those with a more severe degree of intellectual disability. This approach should be balanced against the risk of under-treating and adversely affecting the prognosis, particularly in those with serious mental illness comorbidity (NICE 2016). Medications are effective at the same doses as for those without an intellectual disability and there is no clear evidence that they have more side effects (Frighi et al. 2011; NICE 2016).

Challenging Behaviour and Some Features of a Mental Illness/Mental Disorder

• Consider whether the presentation could be described as an atypical variation of a mental illness or disorder as described in the ICD or DSM systems. Give a clear narrative account of this (Royal College of Psychiatrists 2016).
• If that is not the case, consider whether there are specific affective, psychotic, and/or behavioural symptoms or cluster of symptoms which could be areas for intervention. Give a clear, narrative account of this (Royal College of Psychiatrists 2016). Five such symptom clusters have been described (Royal College of Psychiatrists 2016; Devapriam & Alexander 2019; Langdon et al. 2017; Alexander & Tharian 2021):
  - Cognitive, perceptual symptoms (e.g., chronic, low-level features like ideas of reference, pseudo-hallucinations, persecutory or self-referential ideas, fleeting hallucinations, etc.).
  - Affective dysregulation symptoms (e.g., affective instability, mood swings, chronic dysthymia-like features, emotional detachment, etc.).
  - Anxiety symptoms (cognitive and somatic).
  - Self-injurious behaviour (e.g., repetitive stereotyped behaviour, extreme tissue damage, co-occurring self-injury and aggression, self-injury with agitation when interrupted, mixed type).
  - Aggression towards others (e.g., affective, predatory, organic, and ictal).

- This prescribing would be off licence, should be for the shortest period possible, and should be monitored and audited regularly.
- If there is no clinical improvement within three months, then stopping the medication in favour of other treatment options must be considered.

General Points for All Three Categories

- A good diagnostic clarification and psychological formulation should be completed in all cases.
- Careful attention should be paid to physical health causes, environmental causes, and experience of trauma.
- When prescribing any medication, side effects and potential medication interactions should be monitored carefully, particularly in those with more severe degrees of intellectual disability.
- Prescribers should make sure they are aware of all the medications the patient is receiving when prescribing and consider the risk of medication interactions.
- Patients and carers should be involved in discussions about treatment options (General Medical Council Good Practice 2021), particularly when psychotropic medication is prescribed.
- When prescribing, there must be regular follow ups to assess if continuing the medications is warranted.
- Standardised scales that give an objective measurement of treatment outcome must be used.
    - The Clinical Global Impression (CGI) scale is a quick and easy tool that could be used for this purpose. It offers a global improvement score and an efficacy index which balances therapeutic effects with any side effects (Guy Clinical Global Impression 1976).
    - The Health of the Nation Outcome Scale (HoNOS) is another option for monitoring change over time.
    - Measures like the Liverpool University Neuroleptic Side Effect Rating Scale (LUNSERS) (Day et al. 1995) and the Glasgow Antipsychotic Side-effect Scale (GASS) (Waddell & Taylor 2008) can be used to record side effects (Royal College of Psychiatrists 2016).
- Using both narrative accounts and standardised measures in this way will help the prescriber in determining the effectivity of the medications and guide in continuing or discontinuing them in consultation with patients and their carers (Royal College of Psychiatrists 2016).

Audit Standards and Assessment Framework

The Royal College of Psychiatrists set out four standards and six recommendations for the use of psychotropic medication in this patient group (Royal College of Psychiatrists 2016). These were developed after careful consideration of the latest NICE recommendations (NG11(2015), NG54 (2016)) in this area and remain relevant now. They are reproduced below.

Standards
1. The indication(s) and rationale for prescribing the psychotropic drug should be clearly stated, including whether the prescribing is off-label, polypharmacy, or high dose.
2. Consent-to-treatment procedures (or best-interests decision-making processes) should be followed and documented.
3. There should be regular monitoring of treatment response and side effects (preferably every 3 months or less, at a minimum every 6 months).
4. Review and evaluation of the need for continuation or discontinuation of the psychotropic drug should be undertaken on a regular basis (preferably every 3 months or less, at a minimum every 6 months) or whenever there is a request from patients, carers, or other professionals.

Recommendations
1. All psychotropic prescribing should adhere to the four prescribing standards described above.
2. All initiations of psychotropic drugs for people with intellectual disability, whether from primary or secondary care, should be by a prescriber who is competent in the care of people with intellectual disability.
3. Psychotropic drug prescribing should be seen as part of a wider multidisciplinary and holistic care plan.
4. Regular reviews of the drugs should occur either according to NICE quality standards or when requested by the patient, carer, or other professionals.
5. There should be a national audit on prescribing practice that considers all the standards mentioned above.
6. Regulators and commissioners should use these standards for quality checks on services.

The evidence base about prescribing is limited and is often related to the difficulties of conducting randomised, controlled trials in people with disorders of intellectual development (intellectual disability). The few that have been completed (National Institute for Health & Care Excellence (CG142) 2012; Tyrer et al. 2009; Ahmed et al. 2000; De Kuijper et al. 2014) are limited by the difference between patients who are enrolled in research and those who are treated in clinics. Large-scale naturalistic studies and national audits might be the best way forward in gathering an evidence base that resembles the clinical experience, as done in other branches of medicine and surgery. There have been some attempts within psychiatry for this, such as the National Prescribing Observatory for Mental Health Audits. However, even these audits rely on categorical diagnoses and do not record the narrative accounts (Royal College of Psychiatrists 2016).

Self-Assessment
The self-assessment framework tool proposed by the Royal College of Psychiatrists is useful for clinicians to audit or monitor their clinical practice in prescribing psychotropic medications for people with intellectual disability and is available here (page 15): www.rcpsych.ac.uk/docs/default-source/members/faculties/intellectual-disability/id-fr-id-095701b41885e84150b11ccc989330357c.pdf?sfvrsn=55b66f2c_4.

Resource Box

1. NICE (NG11) (2015): Challenging behaviour and learning disabilities: prevention and interventions for children with learning disabilities whose behaviour challenges. www.nice.org.uk/guidance/ng11.
2. NICE guidelines (NG54) (2016): Mental Health problems in people with learning disabilities: Prevention, assessment, and management. www.nice.org.uk/guidance/ng54.
3. Royal College of Psychiatrists: Faculty of Psychiatry of Intellectual Disability report. Psychotropic drug prescribing for people with disorders of intellectual development (Intellectual disability), mental health problems and/or behaviours that challenge: practice guidelines. 2016. FR/ID/09. www.rcpsych.ac.uk/docs/default-source/members/faculties/intellectual-disability/id-faculty-report-id-09.pdf?sfvrsn=55b66f2c_6.
4. Scheepers, M., & Kerr, M. (Eds.). (2019). Seminars in the Psychiatry of Intellectual Disability (3rd ed., College Seminars Series). Cambridge: Cambridge University Press. Chp. 15: 'Challenging behaviour and use of pharmacological interventions'. https://doi.org/10.1017/9781108617444.
5. Bhaumik, S., and Alexander, R. (Eds.), *Oxford textbook of the psychiatry of intellectual disability*, Oxford Textbooks in Psychiatry (Oxford, 2020; online edn), Oxford Academic. https://doi.org/10.1093/med/9780198794585.001.0001.
6. Langdon, P. & Murphy, G. (2021). Working in community settings with people with learning disabilities and autistic people who are at risk of coming into contact with the criminal justice system. A resource for health and social care staff. Health Education England. www.researchgate.net/publication/354089773_Working_in_community_settings_with_people_with_learning_disabilities_and_autistic_people_who_are_at_risk_of_coming_into_contact_with_the_criminal_justice_system_A_resource_for_health_and_social_care_s.

References

Ahmed, Z., Fraser, W., Kerr, M. P., et al. (2000). Reducing antipsychotic medication in people with a learning disability. *British Journal of Psychiatry*, 176, 42–6.

Alexander, R., & Tharian, R. (2021). Medication Treatments, in P. E. Langdon & G. H. Murphy (ed.) Working in community settings with people with learning disabilities and autistic people who are at risk of coming into contact with the criminal justice settings. A resource for health and social care staff. Health Education England. http://wrap.warwick.ac.uk/156472/7/WRAP-Working-community-learning-disabilities-autistic-risk-criminal-justice-system-2021.pdf, pp. 84–91.

American Psychiatric Association (2013). *Diagnostic and statistical manual of mental disorders (DSM-5 (R))*. 5th ed. American Psychiatric Association Publishing.

Beavers, G. A., Iwata, B. A., & Lerman, D. C. (2013). Thirty years of research on the functional analysis of problem behavior. *Journal of Applied Behavior Analysis*, 46(1), 1–21.

Buckles, J., Luckasson, R., & Keefe, E. (2013). A systematic review of the prevalence of psychiatric disorders in adults with intellectual disability, 2003–2010. *Journal of Mental Health Research in Intellectual Disabilities*, 6(3), 181–207.

Carr, E. G., Dunlap, G., Horner, R. H., et al. (2002). Positive behavior support: Evolution of an applied science. *Journal of Positive Behavior Interventions*, 4(1), 4–16.

Chester, V., Tharian, P., Slinger, M., Varughese, A., & Alexander, R. T. (2023). Overview of offenders with intellectual disability, in J. M. McCarthy,

R. T. Alexander, & E. Chaplin (eds.), *Forensic aspects of neurodevelopmental disorders: A clinician's guide.* Cambridge University Press, pp. 24–33.

Cooper, S. A. (2020). Types of mental disorders in people with intellectual disability. In S. Bhaumik & R. Alexander (Eds.), *Oxford textbook of the psychiatry of intellectual disability.* Oxford University Press.

Day, J. C., Wood, G., Dewey, M., & Bentall, R. P. (1995) A self-rating scale for measuring neuroleptic side-effects: Validation in a group of schizophrenic patients. *British Journal of Psychiatry,* **166**(5), 650–3.

De Kuijper, G., Evenhuis, H., Minderaa, R. B., et al. (2014) Effects of controlled discontinuation of long-term used antipsychotics for behavioural symptoms in individuals with intellectual disability. *Journal of Intellectual Disability Research,* **58**, 71–83.

Devapriam, J., & Alexander, R. (2019) Challenging behaviour and use of pharmacological interventions in *Seminars in the Psychiatry of Intellectual Disability* (3rd ed., College Seminars Series). Cambridge University Press.

Devapriam, J., Rosenbach, A., & Alexander, R. (2015). In-patient services for people with intellectual disability and mental health or behavioural difficulties. *BJPsych Advances,* **21**(2), 116–23.

Emerson, E., & Baines, S. (2011). Health inequalities and people with learning disabilities in the UK. *Tizard Learning Disability Review,* **16**(1), 42–48. https://doi.org/10.5042/tldr.2011.0008.

Frighi, E., Stephenson, M. T., Morovat, A., et al (2011). Safety of antipsychotics in people with intellectual disability. *British Journal of Psychiatry,* **199**, 289–95.

General Medical Council (2021). *Good practice in prescribing and managing medicines and devices.* https://www.gmc-uk.org/-/media/documents/prescribing-guidance-updated-english-20210405_pdf-85260533.pdf.

Glover, G., Bernard, S., Branford, D., et al. (2014). Use of medication for challenging behaviour in people with intellectual disability. *British Journal of Psychiatry,* **205**, 6–7.

Green, L., McNeil, K., Korossy, M., et al. (2018). HELP for behaviours that challenge in adults with intellectual and developmental disabilities. *Canadian Family Physician,* **64** (Suppl 2), S23–S31.

Guy, W (ed.) (1976) *Clinical Global Impression (CGI). In ECDEU Assessment Manual for Psychopharmacology.* US Department of Health, Education, and Welfare (http://www.psywellness.com.sg/docs/CGI.pdf).

Hastings, R. P., Allen, A., Baker, P. et al. (2013). A conceptual framework for understanding why challenging behaviours occur in people with developmental difficulties. *International Journal of Positive Behavioural Support,* **3**(2), 5–13.

Heyvaert, M., Maes, B., & Onghena, P. A. (2010). Meta-analysis of intervention effects on challenging behaviour among persons with intellectual disabilities. *Journal of Intellectual Disability Research,* **54** part 7, 634–49.

King, B. H. (2020). *Intellectual disability.* McGraw-Hill Education LLC.

King, B. H., Toth, K. E. Hodapp, R. M. D.E. (2009). Intellectual disability. In *Comprehensive textbook of psychiatry,* 9th ed. B. J. Sadock, V. A. Sadock, & P. Ruiz (Eds.). Lippincott, pp. 3444–74.

Langdon, P. E., Dalton, D., Brolly, K., Temple, P., Thomas, C., & Webster, T. (2017). Using positive behavioural support as a treatment for trauma symptoms with a man with intellectual disabilities. *International Journal of Positive Behavioural Support,* **7**(1), 31–7.

Matson, J. L., & Cervantes, P. E. (2013). Comorbidity among persons with intellectual disabilities. *Research in Autism Spectrum Disorders,* **7**(11), 1318–22.

Morgan, V. A., Leonard, H., Bourke, J., & Jablensky, A. (2008). Intellectual disability co-occurring with schizophrenia and other psychiatric illness: population-based study. *The British Journal of Psychiatry,* **193**(5), 364–72. https://doi.org/10.1192/bjp.bp.107.044461.

NICE guidelines (2012). (CG142) Autism spectrum disorder in adults: Diagnosis and management. NICE. www.nice.org.uk/guidance/cg142.

Royal College of Psychiatrists (2013). People with learning disability and mental health, behavioural or forensic problems: the role of in-patient services. Faculty of Psychiatry of Intellectual Disability report. www.rcpsych.ac.uk/docs/default-source/members/faculties/intellectual-disability/id-fr-id-03.pdf?sfvrsn=cbbf8b72_2.

NICE (2015) NICE guidance: Learning disability: Behaviour that challenges (QS101). www.nice.org.uk/guidance/qs101.

Royal College of Psychiatrists, British Psychological Society & Royal College of Speech and Language Therapists (2007). Challenging behaviour, a unified approach. Clinical and service guidelines for supporting people with learning disabilities who are at risk of receiving abusive or restrictive practices College Report CR14. www.rcpsych.ac.uk/docs/default-source/improving-care/better-mh-policy/college-reports/college-report-cr144.pdf?sfvrsn=73e437e8_2.

Smiley, E. (2005). Epidemiology of mental health problems in adults with learning disability: an update. *Advances in Psychiatric Treatment*, **11**(3), 214–22.

Smith, A., Petty, M., Oughton, I., & Alexander, R. T. (2010). Establishing a work-based learning programme: vocational rehabilitation in a forensic learning disability setting. *British Journal of Occupational Therapy*, **73**(9), 431–6.

Tyrer, P., Oliver-Africano, P., Romeo, R., et al. (2009). Neuroleptics in the treatment of aggressive challenging behaviour that challenges for people with intellectual disabilities: a randomised controlled trial (NACHBID). *Health Technology Assessment*, **13**: iii–iv, ix–xi, 1–54.

Waddell, L., & Taylor, M. (2008). A new self-rating scale for detecting atypical or second-generation antipsychotic side effects. *Journal of Psychopharmacology*, **22**(3), 238–43.

World Health Organization. (2022). *ICD-11: International classification of diseases* (11th revisions). https://icd.who.int/.

Chapter 5

Trauma in People with Intellectual Disability
Recognition and Intervention

Elspeth Bradley and Marika Korossy

Introduction

Well documented in the lives of people with intellectual disability are greatly increased occurrences of adverse life events, exposure to abuse (emotional, physical, sexual), neglect, exploitation, victimisation, and hate crimes, in contrast to the general population (Keesler, 2014b; McNally et al., 2021). Shockingly, abuse has been reported in developmental service systems at even higher rates (Sobsey, 1991, 1994) and in specialist treatment units such as Winterbourne View and Whorlton Hall (Richards, 2020). People with intellectual disability also experience trauma in association with physical restraint to manage behaviours that challenge services (Wilton, 2020), negative consequences of psychotropic medication for such behaviours (Scheifes et al., 2016), greater exposure to painful medical procedures consequent to health issues, particularly in early and late stages of life (e.g., syndrome-related medical conditions, seizures), and greater-than-typical discontinuities in care related to hospital admissions, respite, and staff turnover in group and institutional living. Everyday traumas also occur related to unique intellectual disability-related neurobiology: for example, hyperacusis in Williams syndrome, distress from sensory hypersensitivities, and difficulties in sensory processing as occur in autism. A two-phased approach to trauma has been proposed (Núñez-Polo et al., 2016) that acknowledges not only trauma consequent to the abuse and adversity already described, but also trauma associated with living with intellectual and developmental disability per se (see also Sinason, 1992).

Trauma and Mental Health

> Trauma is not the only cause of mental health challenges for people with intellectual disability, but it's among the most significant. Ignoring the impact of trauma on individuals with intellectual disability creates environments where challenging behaviors are often ineffectively met with physical, chemical, or mechanical restraint intended to control behaviors. These interventions are not only ineffective, but they may also retraumatise the individual causing further psychological harm. (Horton, 2016).

The sequela of trauma includes severe mental illness, with patients with mild intellectual disability and borderline intellectual functioning having significantly greater rates of all trauma categories and being more likely to have post-traumatic stress disorder (PTSD) compared to other patients with severe mental illness in an outpatient setting (Nieuwenhuis et al., 2019).

PTSD is an outcome of single-trauma experiences. Individuals who experienced chronic, repeated, and prolonged traumas (such as childhood physical, sexual, or emotional abuse; bullying; witnessing violence where they live; community or school violence; neglect; loss of a close relationship; disruptions in care; serious illness or accident) tend to experience more complex reactions extending beyond those typically observed in PTSD (National Institute for Health and Care Excellence-NICE, 2018a; Brewin, 2020; WHO, 2022). In complex trauma (complex PTSD or C-PTSD) – also referred to as developmental or relational trauma, complex trauma, and disorders of extreme stress (Luxenberg et al., 2001) – these reactions affect three key domains: emotion regulation, self-identity, and relational capacities (Cloitre, 2020). Symptoms include prolonged feelings of terror, emotional numbness, worthlessness, helplessness, distortions in identity or sense of self, and feeling on edge (hyperarousal). Symptoms and behaviours of complex PTSD overlap with PTSD and include avoidance, changes in mood, physical and emotional reactions, and hypervigilance (Mayo Clinic Staff, 2022; NHS, 2022b).

What Is Trauma?

Trauma refers to the negative impact on a person consequent to an experienced event(s). Any event that is beyond the individual's ability to cope, or from which they are unable to escape, may be traumatising. Coping must be considered in the context of personal, developmental, and emotional capacities, and any supports that may (or may not) be available. Thus, an event that is traumatising to one person may not be to another; this appreciation may be missed in standardised criteria for PTSD. Autistic people, for example, are thought to be at increased risk of developing PTSD that fulfils the *American Diagnostic and Statistical Manual* fifth edition (DSM-5) criteria even though the traumatic event per se may not meet those criteria (Rumball et al., 2020).

People with intellectual disability are reliant on others to a greater or lesser extent, and are invariably living in support situations in which they are powerless to change their circumstance or leave should they feel threatened, in danger, or unsafe. While trauma is personally experienced, its impact may be observable to others by changes in the individual's behaviour. Some individuals may be able to share in words aspects of their painful and distressing experiences. However, regardless of the capacity to self-report, trauma has increasingly become recognised as fundamentally being experienced in the body. This involves activation of the autonomic nervous system (ANS) that results in a shutting down of cortical cognitive rational processing in favour of automatic survival responses (fight-flight-freeze from sympathetic nervous system activity and shutdown from dorsal vagal parasympathetic nerve activity) (Levine, 1997; Van der Kolk, 2014; Porges, 2017; Perry & Winfrey, 2021). The behaviours associated with these survival responses overlap with behaviours that challenge services (Bradley & Korossy, 2022). Unresolved trauma leaves the individual's nervous system vulnerable to acute and chronic dysregulation related to present-day environmental and interpersonal triggers that are reminders of the past trauma event (re-experiencing). Chronic 'hijacking' of the ANS into survival mode interrupts the usual homeostatic rest and repair function of the parasympathetic/vagal component of the ANS (Porges, 2017), leading to health issues through the life span. Reviews of large population-based studies of adverse early childhood experiences link higher adverse early childhood experiences scores to greater chronic health problems, mental illness, and substance use problems in adolescence through adulthood (Lanius et al., 2010; Ontario Agency for Health Protection and Promotion [Public Health Ontario] et al., 2020; Queen's University FMGH, 2022; Porges 2022). People with intellectual disability have even higher adverse early childhood experience scores than others in the general population (Keesler, 2014a; Horton, 2016).

Trauma and Behaviours that Challenge Services

In general, behaviours that challenge services are associated with greater severity of intellectual disability and when intellectual disability and autism co-exist, demonstrating the impact of cognitive functioning and the additional impact of communication functioning. In recent years there has been a greater focus on the role of emotional functioning in behaviours that challenge services (Mazefsky, 2014; Woodcock & Blackwell, 2020). The greater prevalence of such behaviours in services for autism and intellectual disability, compared to intellectual disability alone, was found to be associated with differences in emotional regulation (Licence et al., 2020).

A meta-analysis of 69 studies found that systematic consideration of idiosyncratic emotional, as well as cognitive, factors could optimise intervention outcomes for behaviours that challenge services (Woodcock & Blackwell, 2020). Emotional outbursts, a feature of these behaviours, are associated with differences in sensory processing, masking of emotions in unsafe environments, and differences in safety perception (Chung et al., 2022). Tunnicliff et al. (2014) describe emotional arousal and temper outbursts, while Woodcock et al. (2009), comparing individuals with Prader–Willi syndrome (PWS) to those with Fragile X syndrome, describe negative emotional behaviours (temper outbursts and repetitive questions) following changes in routines or expectations. Those with Prader–Willi Syndrome engaged more in temper outbursts, while those with Fragile X more with repetitive and self-injurious behaviours.

Others have examined emotional factors more directly through ANS functioning. Manning and colleagues (2019) found that transcutaneous vagus nerve stimulation reduced temper outbursts in Prader–Willi Syndrome, while Beck et al. (2017) described new treatments for mental disorders arising from dysregulated neuro-circuitry in brain and ANS functioning involving non-invasive brain and peripheral stimulation. Porges (co-founder of the Polyvagal Institute) and colleagues (Heilman et al., 2011; Porges et al., 2014; Bulbena et al., 2017; Patriquin et al., 2019) have described atypical autonomic regulation in several syndromes associated with intellectual disabilities (Fragile X syndrome, Ehlers–Danlos syndrome, autism) and have developed an evidence-based therapeutic listening intervention that accesses the vagus nerve through the portal of the ear, which they propose helps to calm the patient's physiological and emotional state (Rosenberg, 2017). Using technology that can comfortably sense and communicate ANS arousal in daily life, Picard and colleagues at the Massachusetts Institute of Technology have been investigating emotional responses in autism while also providing personalised feedback (Picard, 2009). Technology to investigate the production, perception, and meaning of nonverbal vocalisations from nonverbal and minimally verbal individuals in natural environments is being developed (Narain et al., 2020a, 2020b). These emerging technologies to track emotional responses, along with novel treatments for emotional dysregulation, clearly have implications for both the understanding of and interventions for behaviours that challenge services, especially for those individuals with greater severity of intellectual disabilities and little or no language.

Meanwhile, Sappok and colleagues are drawing attention to different stages in emotional development and emotional functioning as predicting behaviours that challenge services. They found a greater prevalence of behaviours that challenge services in individuals with more severe intellectual disability and autism, correlated with less well-developed emotional functioning (Sappok et al., 2014). Emotional resilience is associated with the nature of early developmental attachment relationships, with emotional dysregulation being associated with insecure attachments in early life (Raju et al., 2012). Adults with intellectual disability appear to be at greater risk of experiencing difficulties in attachment relationships (Hamadi & Fletcher, 2021). More work is needed to understand these emotional vulnerabilities, the impact of trauma, and association with behaviours that challenge services.

Drawing on the similarity of behaviours that challenge services with survival responses of the ANS (fight-flight-freeze and shutdown), and reports from people with autism, it has been proposed that these behaviours may be adaptive responses by the individual to danger, threat, and feeling unsafe (Bradley & Korossy, 2022). In this context, in people with intellectual disability, they may be marker(s) of past or ongoing adversity and trauma, especially for those without language whose only way to communicate their emotional distress is through their behaviour (e.g., Howlin & Clements, 1995; Hubert & Hollins, 2006; Kildahl et al., 2020a). As such, referral for behaviours that challenge services should trigger care givers and the clinical team into an exploration through case notes and client and informant reports, of possible adversity and trauma. Of note in this regard, a study of adults with intellectual disability and autistic spectrum disorder identified trauma-related symptoms as being more easily captured in a measure of 'challenging behaviours' (Aberrant Behaviour Checklist – especially the irritability and hyperactivity scales) than on a screening measure for psychiatric disorder developed for this population (Kildahl et al., 2020a).

Trauma and Psychiatric Diagnoses

Studies consistently document increased psychopathology in people with intellectual disability compared to general population norms, with increased prevalence of mood, anxiety, and psychotic-related disorders as well as behaviours that challenge services. However, symptoms and behaviours of Trauma- and Stressor-Related Disorders, as in the American classificatory system (DSM-5), and complex PTSD, as in the International Classification of Diseases by the World Health Organization (ICD-11), overlap with criteria for these mood, anxiety, and psychotic-related psychiatric disorders. Unless the possibility of trauma is specifically investigated, it will likely remain unrecognised as contributing to mental distress (Kildahl, 2020b; Didden & Mevissen, 2022) and consequently untreated. This will lead to the individual remaining in unsafe circumstances or reliving past trauma experiences. Unrecognised, this trauma-related mental distress may end up being considered as a 'treatment resistant' psychiatric disorder or 'challenging behaviour' (Bradley et al., 2012). Exploring the experiences of mental health clinicians working with PTSD, Kildahl et al. (2020b), describe several factors that contribute to challenges identifying trauma and trauma- related symptoms in adults with intellectual disability and autism and suggest that 'if we do not look for it, we do not see it'.

In comparison to the many studies of psychopathology and psychiatric disorder in those with an intellectual disability who present with behaviours that challenge services, only a few have specifically focused on trauma (e.g., Ryan, 1994; Daveney et al., 2019; Nieuwenhuis et al., 2019; McCarthy, 2001). In a meta-analysis of seven identified studies of PTSD, Daveney et al. (2019) determined a prevalence rate of 10%, comparable to the upper limit of the condition in those without intellectual disability. They concluded that PTSD can be diagnosed in people with intellectual disability but may go unrecognised by healthcare professionals, particularly in those presenting with apparent mood disorders or challenging behavior. Given greater adverse childhood experience in those with an intellectual disability, occurrence of complex PTSD is also likely to be greater. The reported greater rates of personality disorder in intellectual disability may represent, in part, unrecognised complex PTSD (Mind for Better Mental Health, 2021, p. 10); more research in this area is urgently needed. At this stage it is not known to what extent these increased prevalence rates of major psychiatric disorders (anxiety, mood, psychotic as well as personality disorder) are unidentified trauma- and stressor-related disorders with accompanying affect dysregulation, mood, anxiety, and psychotic-related symptoms (Didden & Mevissen, 2022). The distinction is important as the focus of treatment is different.

Treatment of Trauma

The first necessary step in healing from and preventing trauma is attention to the patient's physical and emotional safety: being safe and feeling safe (Menschner & Maul, 2016). This involves organisational system changes (Keesler, 2014a; Horton, 2016) to ensure that the individual is not only living in a safe physical environment, but, crucially, feels safe where they live, work, and spend time and in any interpersonal encounters (with caregivers, peers, etc.) they may have (Larkin, 2014).

Once safely supported in daily life, individual trauma therapy involves assisting the traumatised individual, in a physically safe space and in the context of a safe therapeutic relationship, to work through the pain and fear of trauma-related thoughts, feelings, and bodily experiences so as to restore healthy autonomic nervous system (ANS) homeostatic regulation and diminished dysregulation from trauma-related triggers (Raju et al., 2012, tbls 2 & 3; Van der Kolk, 2000, 2014; Dana, 2018; Porges & Dana, 2018).

Several evidence-based psychological treatments of trauma are available: for example, cognitive behavioural therapy (CBT), eye movement desensitisation and reprocessing therapy (EMDR), body-based therapies, and several others have been shown, with appropriate developmental adaptations, to be effective with people with intellectual disability (Keeseler, 2020). It cannot be over-emphasised that, critical to any organisational change or individual therapy, the focus is on the service recipient's *felt sense of safety* where they live, work, and spend recreational time, in social and, especially, in care-giving interpersonal relationships.

Medication, Trauma, and Intellectual Disability

Being safe and feeling safe is crucial in the treatment and prevention of trauma. Medication is often considered when symptoms of anxiety, mood, and dissociation are especially troublesome; however, Luxenberg et al. (2001) caution that rapidly shifting symptoms are often not occasions for medication adjustments, but opportunities for mastery and learning how to manage and tolerate painful emotional states using, for example, cognitive behaviour therapy, relaxation exercises, imagery, etc. They note that without a good therapeutic alliance, and close collaboration between providers, it is difficult to assess such developments effectively.

In the absence of specific guidelines for trauma symptom medications for those with an intellectual disability, those prepared for the general population remain applicable. (NICE, 2018b; NHS Resources, 2022a, 2022b), with the added general caveats when prescribing for people with intellectual disability.

National Institute for Health and Care Excellence guideline (NG116) published in 2018 on PTSD recommends the following:

1. Do not offer drug treatments, including benzodiazepines, to prevent PTSD in adults.
2. NICE emphasises the primary treatment approach for PTSD being psychological, as highlighted in the earlier sections of this chapter.
3. NICE suggested the following drug treatments in addition to the use of psychological approaches if there are disabling symptoms that needs management.
4. Consider a selective serotonin reuptake inhibitor (SSRI), such as sertraline, for adults with a diagnosis of PTSD if the person has a preference for drug treatment, and review regularly.
5. Consider venlafaxine (however, the guidance points out that venlafaxine is unlicenced for use in PTSD).
6. Consider antipsychotic medications like risperidone for adults with PTSD, if there are disabling symptoms such as hyperarousal or psychotic symptoms which did not respond to other medications. Use of risperidone for PTSD is again outside the licenced indication.

As described in Chapter 4 and in this chapter, the experience of trauma is an important part of the diagnostic clarification and psychological formulation for people with intellectual disability who present either with behaviours that challenge or mental health difficulties (Rayala et al., 2023). Positive outcomes for behaviours that challenge using beta-adrenoceptor blocking medications such as propranolol have been described in clinical practice; however, to date randomised controlled trials have not been conducted to study the impact of such medication (Ward et al., 2013).

Trauma treatment and healing necessitates an understanding of the context of the patient's life and consideration of behaviours that challenge services from the patient's unique 'inside-out' perspective. One should not automatically give weight to perspectives from others who may be unfamiliar with the patient's experience of living with intellectual disability in general, or more specifically unaware of how unique biological syndromes give rise to differences in sensory experiences and perceptions and consequent actions (i.e., 'the outside-in' perspective). Verbal accounts from autistic people document how their perspective on why they are behaving in certain ways (inside-out) differs from intentions inferred in current criteria for some psychiatric diagnoses (Bradley et al., 2014).

Case Study 5.1

Stefan is a 32-year-old man diagnosed with mild intellectual disability, epilepsy, autism, and behaviours that challenge services. He lived with his family and attended a specialist college until the age of 25, at which point he moved into supported living. Since then, Stefan has been supported by a series of care providers, with most packages lasting a maximum of three years, including requiring him to move areas.

Stefan is prescribed sertraline for mood and anxiety, risperidone for agitation and anxiety, lamotrigine for epilepsy, and lorazepam 'as needed' for agitation. He receives input from a community nurse from the intellectual disability team and medication reviews from an intellectual disability psychiatrist.

Stefan's care provider contacts the intellectual disability team to report that 'he is going into crisis again'. Stefan has been displaying increasingly agitated behaviour, has assaulted several staff members, and has hit a member of the public. Stefan's care provider wants to withdraw from providing care, stating 'he will no longer engage with us' and 'he needs to be in hospital'.

The intellectual disability intensive support team are called in and work with the provider to review Stefan's support plans and adjust his medication. Input is sought from Stefan's GP to check for any physical illnesses that might be contributing to his presentation. The psychiatrist reviews Stefan to check there is no acute mental illness. Occupational therapy updates his sensory profile. An increase in support hours is requested from social services.

After the initial crisis has subsided, the intellectual disability team agree on a detailed review of Stefan's case history to look into reasons for the pattern of placement breakdown. Case notes highlight a number of factors indicating possible trauma, including frequent hospitalisations for epilepsy during childhood, physical abuse during his teenage years, multiple moves and separations, and being subject to physical restraint by some care providers. The psychiatrist makes additional diagnoses of PTSD (single and repeated trauma events, e.g., medical procedures) and complex PTSD (developmental relational trauma, e.g., associated with abuses, loss, and restraints).

The intellectual disability team psychologist works with Stefan's care provider to develop a trauma-informed care approach that includes consideration of Stefan's 'inside-out' experience of services to ensure that Stefan is safe and, importantly, feels safe where he lives, works, spends time, and in his social emotional supports and peer relationships. Staff learn to recognise and reduce the occurrence of triggers for Stefan's distress. They work with the occupational therapist to develop a sensory toolkit Stefan can use to 'self-soothe' when he shows agitation and emotional dysregulation. Working with Stefan's team, his family doctor writes a social prescription that ensures his physical environment meets his autism needs (e.g., attention to any sensory triggers) and trauma needs (e.g., opportunity to be out in the healing environment of nature and access to walks to assist emotional regulation). Individual trauma therapy is offered using tools that assist sharing and management of emotional distress (e.g., Books Beyond Words: https://booksbeyond words.co.uk/); his community nurse, whom he trusts, leads on this, supported by the psychologist.

He is also assessed to determine whether some evidence-based trauma therapies may be helpful to him (e.g., EMDR, trauma-sensitive yoga). Given emerging understanding in the neurobiology of trauma and growing recognition that trauma is stored in the physiology of the body, the team is interested in exploring body-based therapies (e.g., sensorimotor therapies, somatic experiencing, and mindfulness techniques).

With these supports in place, Stefan is able to start making more choices around his care and support – for example, interviewing for new support staff. He is better able to manage his times of anxiety and distress, and his use of 'as needed' medication is greatly reduced. His seizure control also improves, reducing the number of hospital visits needed, which has a further positive effect on his mental health. With all these supports in place it is now possible to review more systematically Stefan's previous psychiatric symptoms and prescribed psychotropic medication. In particular, consideration is given to whether his behaviours that challenge services are actually 'adaptive' responses associated with his early developmental trauma (complex PTSD); also, might his agitated states (emotional dysregulation) be addressed through ANS co-regulation therapy (Polyvagal Institute)?

Stefan and his care team recognise that he will need long-term support and there will likely always be 'ups and downs'; however, they now share a positive focus for the future that also empowers and includes Stefan at the core, offers continuity of understanding and care, and minimises any future trauma, which they plan to work towards together.

Conclusion

Much remains to be understood about trauma, behaviours that challenge services, and psychiatric disorder in intellectual disability. Greater understanding may require a shift from current categorical psychiatric diagnoses to a more dimensional approach with a formulation based on brain science and ANS functioning. Meanwhile given the evidence of adversity, negative life events, and trauma in the lives of people with intellectual disability, including when receiving health, social, and developmental services, urgent implementation of trauma-informed approaches in these services is needed both to prevent further trauma and to allow healing from trauma that has occurred (McNally et al., 2021; Keesler, 2014a; Cook & Hole, 2021). An ethical argument for engendering feeling safe and considering the perspective of people with intellectual disability in these regards, wherever they are being supported or receiving treatment, has been proposed (Bradley & Vogt, forthcoming).

The Frith Prescribing Guidelines Editors' Expert Group Consensus Statements

Statements of High Confidence

1. People with intellectual disability have greatly increased occurrences of adverse life events, exposure to abuse (emotional, physical, sexual), neglect, exploitation, victimisation, and hate crimes, in contrast to the general population.
2. Unless the possibility of trauma is specifically investigated, trauma will likely remain unrecognised as contributing to the mental distress.
3. The prevalence rate of post-traumatic stress syndrome (PTSD) of 10% is comparable to the upper limit of the condition in those without intellectual disability.

Statements of Medium Confidence

1. Unresolved trauma leaves the individual's nervous system vulnerable to acute and chronic dysregulation related to present-day environmental and interpersonal triggers that are reminders of the past trauma event (re-experiencing).
2. Atypical autonomic regulation occurs in several syndromes associated with intellectual disability.
3. Emotional resilience is associated with the nature of early developmental attachment relationships, with emotional dysregulation being associated with insecure attachments in early life.

Statements of Low Confidence

1. For adults with intellectual disability and autism, identified trauma-related symptoms are more easily captured in a measure of 'challenging behaviours'.
2. Although there are no studies in people with intellectual disability, the advice for those without intellectual disability and PTSD is to consider venlafaxine or a selective serotonin reuptake inhibitor (SSRI), such as sertraline, if there is a preference for medication treatment.

> **Resource Box**
>
> Beail, N., Frankish, P., Skelly, A. (Eds.) (2021) *Trauma and intellectual disability: Acknowledgement, identification and intervention.* Pavilion Publishing and Media.
>
> Dunn, C. (2018) *Trauma and individuals with intellectual and developmental disabilities* University of Tennessee Centre on Developmental Disabilities; Vanderbilt Kennedy Centre for Excellence in Developmental Disabilities. https://vkc.vumc.org/assets/files/tip sheets/traumatips.pdf.
>
> Frankish, P. (2019) *Trauma-informed care in intellectual disability: A self-study guide for health and social care support staff.* Pavilion Publishing and Media.
>
> Harvey, K. (2023) Trauma and healing in the lives of people with intellectual disability. AADIDE (webinar). www.aaidd.org/education/webinars/register-for-upcoming-webi nars/2023/01/12/default-calendar/trauma-and-healing-in-the-lives-of-people-with-intel lectual-disability.
>
> Kildahl, A. N., Helverschou, S. B., Bakken, T. L., & Oddli, H. W. (2020) 'If we do not look for it, we do not see it': Clinicians' experiences and understanding of identifying post-traumatic stress disorder in adults with autism and intellectual disability. *Journal of Applied Research in Intellectual Disabilities*, 33(5), 1119–32. https://onlinelibrary.wiley.com/doi/full/10.111 1/jar.12734.
>
> Marcal, S., & Trifoso, S. (2017) A trauma-informed toolkit for providers in the field of intellectual & developmental disabilities. www.pacesconnection.com/fileSendAction/fcT ype/0/fcOid/468137553002812476/filePointer/468137553002812517/fodoid/468137553 002812512/DIDE%20TOOLKIT%20%20CFDS%20HEARTS%20NETWORK%205-28%20Fina lR2.pdf.
>
> Palay, L. (2022) *The way through: Trauma responsive care in intellectual disability.* NADD Press.
>
> Wilcox, P. (2020) Trauma and developmental disabilities. Traumatic Stress Institute of Klingberg Family Centers. www.traumaticstressinstitute.org/trauma-and-developmen tal-disabilities/.

References

Beck, R. W., Laugharne, J., Laugharne, R., et al. (2017) Abnormal cortical asymmetry as a target for neuromodulation in neuropsychiatric disorders: A narrative review and concept proposal. *Neuroscience & Biobehavioral Reviews*, December 01(83), 21–31.

Bradley, E., Caldwell, P., & Underwood, L. (2014) Autism spectrum disorder. In E. Tsakanikos & J. McCarthy (Eds.). *Handbook of Psychopathology in Intellectual Disability: Research, Practice and Policy.* Springer, pp. 237–64.

Bradley, E., & Korossy, M. (2022) Are difficult behaviours described in intellectual and developmental disabilities and autism actually adaptive responses to feeling unsafe? *Journal on Developmental Disabilities*, 27(3). Online First. https://oadd.org/wp-content/u ploads/2022/09/V27-N3-JoDD-22-390-Bradl ey-and-Korossy-v3.pdf.

Bradley, E., Sinclair, L., & Greenbaum, R. (2012) Trauma and adolescents with intellectual disabilities: Interprofessional clinical and service perspectives. *Journal of Child & Adolescent Trauma*, 5(1), 33–46. https://doi .org/10.1080/19361521.2012.646412.

Bradley, E., & Vogt, J. (forthcoming) Engendering a feeling of safety for people with developmental disabilities (Intellectual Disabilities/ASD), as an ethical imperative in preventing emotional distress and behaviours that challenge services. In A. Bianchi & J. Vogt (Eds.). *Intellectual Disabilities and Autism: Ethics and Practice*. Springer.

Brewin, C. R. (2020) Complex post-traumatic stress disorder: A new diagnosis in ICD-11. *BJPsych Advances*, **26**(3):145–52. www.cambridge.org/core/services/aop-cambridge-core/content/view/2977140CBDAAF402610715BB609F688C/S2056467819000483a.pdf/complex-post-traumatic-stress-disorder-a-new-diagnosis-in-icd-11.pdf.

Bulbena, A., Baeza-Velasco, C., Bulbena-Cabre, A., et al. (2017) Psychiatric and psychological aspects in the Ehlers–Danlos syndromes. *American Journal of Medical Genetics Part C: Seminars in Medical Genetics*, March 01; **175**(1), 237–45.

Chung, J. C. Y., Mevorach, C., & Woodcock, K. A. (2022) Establishing the transdiagnostic contextual pathways of emotional outbursts. *Scientific Reports*, **12**(1), 7414–4. www.ncbi.nlm.nih.gov/pmc/articles/PMC9076826/pdf/41598_2022_Article_11474.pdf.

Cloitre, M. (2020) ICD-11 complex post-traumatic stress disorder: Simplifying diagnosis in trauma populations. *British Journal of Psychiatry*, March 01; **216**(3), 129–31. www.cambridge.org/core/services/aop-cambridge-core/content/view/E53B8CD7CF9B725FE651720EE58E93A4/S0007125020000434a.pdf/icd-11-complex-post-traumatic-stress-disorder-simplifying-diagnosis-in-trauma-populations.pdf.

Cook, S., & Hole, R. (2021) Trauma, intellectual and/or developmental disability, and multiple, complex needs: A scoping review of the literature. *Research in Developmental Disabilities*, August 01(115), 103939.

Dana, D. (2018) *The polyvagal theory in therapy: engaging the rhythm of regulation*. W. W. Norton & Company.

Daveney, J., Hassiotis, A., Katona, C., Matcham, F., & Sen, P. (2019) Ascertainment and prevalence of post-traumatic stress disorder (PTSD) in people with intellectual disabilities. *Journal of Mental Health Research in Intellectual Disabilities*, **12**(3–4), 211–33. https://discovery.ucl.ac.uk/id/eprint/10077508/1/Daveney%20et%20al%20PTSD%20prevalence%20and%20assessment%20in%20PWID_April%202019.pdf.

Didden, R., & Mevissen, L. (2022) Trauma in individuals with intellectual and developmental disabilities: Introduction to the special issue. *Research in Developmental Disabilities*, January 01(120), 104122.

Hamadi, L., & Fletcher, H. K. (2021) Are people with an intellectual disability at increased risk of attachment difficulties? A critical review. *Journal of Intellectual Disabilities*, **25**(1), 114–30

Heilman, K. J., Harden, E. R., Zageris, D. M., Berry-Kravis, E., & Porges, S. W. (2011) Autonomic regulation in Fragile X syndrome. *Developmental Psychobiology*, December 01; **53**(8), 785–95.

Horton, C. (2016) An unseen population: DIDE and trauma. *Texas Parent to Parent (Txp2p) Quarterly Newsletter*, **16**(3), 3–4. https://learn.nctsn.org/mod/resource/view.php?id=11675.

Howlin, P., & Clements, J. (1995) Is it possible to assess the impact of abuse on children with pervasive developmental disorders? *Journal of Autism and Developmental Disorders*; **25**(4), 337–53.

Hubert, J., & Hollins, S. (2006) Men with severe learning disabilities and challenging behaviour in long-stay hospital care: Qualitative study. *British Journal of Psychiatry*, Jan; **188**, 70–4.

Keesler, J. M. (2014a) A call for the integration of trauma-informed care among intellectual and developmental disability organizations. *Journal of Policy and Practice in Intellectual Disabilities*, **11**(1), 34–42.

Keesler, J. M. (2014b) Trauma through the lens of service coordinators: Exploring their awareness of adverse life events among adults with intellectual disabilities. *Advances in Mental Health and Intellectual Disabilities*, **8**(3), 151–64.

Keesler, J. M. (2020) Trauma-specific treatment for individuals with intellectual and developmental disabilities: A review of the literature from 2008 to 2018. *Journal of Policy and Practice in Intellectual Disabilities*, **17**(4), 332–45. https://doi.org/10.1111/jppi.12347.

Kildahl, A. N., Oddli, H. W., & Helverschou, S B. (2020a) Potentially traumatic experiences and behavioural symptoms in adults with autism and intellectual disability referred for psychiatric assessment. *Research in Developmental Disabilities*, December **01**(107), 103788.

Kildahl, A. N., Helverschou, S. B., Bakken, T. L., & Oddli, H. W. (2020b) 'If we do not look for it, we do not see it': Clinicians' experiences and understanding of identifying post-traumatic stress disorder in adults with autism and intellectual disability. *Journal of Applied Research in Intellectual Disabilities*, **33**, 1119–32.

Lanius, R. A., Vermetten, E., & Pain, C. (2010) *The Impact of Early Life Trauma on Health and Disease: The Hidden Epidemic*. Cambridge University Press.

Larkin, H., Felitti, V. J., & Anda, R. F. (2014) Social work and adverse childhood experiences research: Implications for practice and health policy. *Social Work in Public Health*, **29**(1), 1–16.

Levine, P. A. (1997) *Waking the Tiger: Healing Trauma : The Innate Capacity to Transform Overwhelming Experiences*. North Atlantic Books.

Licence, L., Oliver, C., Moss, J., & Richards, C. (2020) Prevalence and risk-markers of self-harm in autistic children and adults. *Journal of Autism and Developmental Disorders*, October 01; **50**(10), 3561–74.

Luxenberg, T., Spinazzola, J., & Van der Kolk, B. A. (2001) Complex trauma and disorders of extreme stress (DESNOS) diagnosis. lesson 25 – part one: Assessment; lesson 26 – part two: Treatment. *Directions in Psychiatry*, **21**(25 & 26), 373–414. file:///C:/Users/User/https://citeseerx.ist.psu.edu/document?repid=rep1&type=pdf&doi=84a82072bad93c4e7a2f2b385623e9420ef2dce8.

Manning, K. E., Beresford-Webb, J. A., Aman, L. C. S., et al. (2019) Transcutaneous vagus nerve stimulation (t-VNS): A novel effective treatment for temper outbursts in adults with Prader–Willi syndrome indicated by results from a non-blind study. *PLoS One*, December 03; **14**(12), e0223750. www.ncbi.nlm.nih.gov/pmc/articles/PMC6890246/pdf/pone.0223750.pdf.

Mayo Clinic Staff (2022) Post-traumatic stress disorder (PTSD). https://www.mayoclinic.org/diseases-conditions/post-traumatic-stress-disorder/symptoms-causes/syc–20355967.

Mazefsky, C. A., & White, S. W. Emotion regulation: Concepts & practice in autism spectrum disorder. *Child and Adolescent Psychiatric Clinics of North America*, 2014 January 01; **23**(1):15–24. www.ncbi.nlm.nih.gov/pmc/articles/PMC3830422/pdf/nihms504610.pdf.

McCarthy, J. (2001) Post-traumatic stress disorder in people with learning disability. *Advances in Psychiatric Treatment*, **7**(3), 163–9.

McNally, P., Taggart, L., & Shevlin, M. (2021) Trauma experiences of people with an intellectual disability and their implications: A scoping review. *Journal of Applied Research in Intellectual Disabilities*, **34**(4), 927–49. https://onlinelibrary.wiley.com/doi/epdf/10.1111/jar.12872.

Menschner, C., & Maul, A. (2016) *Key Ingredients for Successful Trauma-Informed Care Implementation*. Hamilton, New Jersey. www.samhsa.gov/sites/default/files/programs_campaigns/childrens_mental_health/atc-whitepaper-040616.pdf.

Mind for Better Health. (2021) Post-traumatic stress disorder (PTSD). www.mind.org.uk/media/7135/ptsd-and-complex-ptsd-2021-pdf-version.pdf.

Narain, J., & Johnson, K. (2020a) Personalized modelling of real-world vocalizations from nonverbal individuals. In *Proceedings of the 2020 International Conference on Multimodal Interaction*. Association for Computing Machinery, pp. 665–9.

Narain, J., Johnson, K. T., O'Brien, A., et al. (2020b) Nonverbal vocalizations as speech: characterizing natural-environment audio from nonverbal individuals with autism. In *Proceedings of the 2020 International Conference on Multimodal Interaction*, pp. 40–3. www.semanticscholar.org/paper/Nonverbal-Vocalizations-as-Speech%3A-Characterizing-Narain-Johnson/25a7344cef8811f797a7818a91d05cac3735460a.

National Institute for Health and Care Excellence (NICE). (2018a) Post-traumatic stress disorder [NG 116]. Guideline. NICE National Institute for Health and Care Excellence. www.nice.org.uk/guidance/ng116.

National Institute for Health and Care Excellence (NICE). (2018b) Post-traumatic stress disorder [NG 116] – guidance – recommendations. NICE National Institute for Health and Care Excellence. www.nice.org.uk/guidance/ng116.

NHS. (2022a) Complex PTSD – post-traumatic stress disorder. www.nhs.uk/mental-health/conditions/post-traumatic-stress-disorder-ptsd/complex.

NHS. (2022b) Symptoms – post-traumatic stress disorder. www.nhs.uk/mental-health/conditions/post-traumatic-stress-disorder-ptsd/symptoms/.

Nieuwenhuis, J. G., Smits, H. J.H., Noorthoorn, E. O., et al. (2019) Not recognized enough: The effects and associations of trauma and intellectual disability in severely mentally ill outpatients. *European Psychiatry*, 2019 May 01;**58**, 63–9. https://pubmed.ncbi.nlm.nih.gov/30836316/.

Núñez-Polo, M. H., Carrasco, A. A., Muñoz, I. B., Zapata, M. R., & Cafranga, A. M. (2016) Integrative therapy focused on trauma for people with intellectual disability (TIT-ID): A therapeutic answer to abuse and intellectual disability experience in the individual and the family. *Journal of Intellectual Disability: Diagnosis and Treatment*, **4**(1), 29–40.

Ontario Agency for Health Protection and Promotion (Public Health Ontario). (2020) *Interventions to prevent and mitigate the impact of adverse childhood experiences (ACEs) in Canada: A literature review*. Queen's Printer for Ontario. www.publichealthontario.ca/-/media/documents/a/2020/adverse-childhood-experiences-report.pdf?la=en.

Patriquin, M. A., Hartwig, E. M., Friedman, B. H., Porges, S. W., & Scarpa, A. (2019) Autonomic response in autism spectrum disorder: Relationship to social and cognitive functioning. *Biological Psychology*, July 01(145), 185–97.

Perry, B. D., & Winfrey, O. (2021) *What Happened to You? Conversations on Trauma, Resilience, and Healing*. Flatiron Books.

Picard, R. W. (2009) Future affective technology for autism and emotion communication. *Philosophical Transactions of the Royal Society of London. Series B, Biological Sciences*, December 12; **364**(1535), 3575–84. www.ncbi.nlm.nih.gov/pmc/articles/PMC2781888/pdf/rstb20090143.pdf.

Porges, S. W., Bazhenova, O. V., Bal, E., et al. (2014) Reducing auditory hypersensitivities in autistic spectrum disorder: Preliminary findings evaluating the listening project protocol. *Frontiers in Pediatrics*, Aug; **1**(2), 80.

Porges, S. W. (2022) Polyvagal theory: A science of safety. *Frontiers in Integrative Neuroscience*, **16**, 871227. www.frontiersin.org/articles/10.3389/fnint.2022.871227/full.

Porges, S. W. (2017) *The Pocket Guide to the Polyvagal Theory: The Transformative Power of Feeling Safe*. 1st ed. W. W. Norton & Company.

Porges, S. W., & Dana, D. (2018) *Clinical Applications of the Polyvagal Theory: The Emergence of Polyvagal-Informed Therapies*. 1st ed. W. W. Norton & Company.

Queen's University FMGH (2022). Adverse childhood experiences. *Horizons*. (Issue 2), 1–25. https://familymedicine.queensu.ca/source/Family%20Medicine/Horizons%20Fall%202022FF.pdf.

Raju, R., Corrigan, F. M., Davidson, A. J. W., & Johnson, D. (2014) Assessing and managing mild to moderate emotion dysregulation. *Advances in Psychiatric Treatment*. 2012; **18**, 82–93. www.cambridge.org/core/services/aop-cambridge-core/content/view/9FC4277C47E368BFFA800E7D8ED531D5/S1355514600016308a.pdf/assessing_and_managing_mild_to_moderate_emotion_dysregulation.pdf.

Rayala, M., Amiola, A., Tharian, R., & Alexander, R. (2023) Mental health conditions in people with intellectual disabilities (DIDe). In M. Barrett, D., Branford, S., Gangadharan, & R. Alexander (eds.), *Frith Treatment Guidelines for People with Disorders of*

Intellectual Development (DIDe). Cambridge University Press.

Richards, M. (2020) Whorlton Hall, Winterbourne ... person-centred care is long dead for people with learning disabilities and autism. *Disability & Society*, **35**(3), 500–5. www.tandfonline.com/doi/pdf/10.1080/09687599.2019.1646530?needAccess=true.

Rosenberg, S. (2017) *Accessing the Healing Power of the Vagus Nerve: Self-Help Exercises for Anxiety, Depression, Trauma, and Autism*. North Atlantic Books.

Rumball, F., Happé, F., & Grey, N. (2020) Experience of trauma and PTSD symptoms in autistic adults: Risk of PTSD development following DSM-5 and non-DSM-5 traumatic life events. *Autism Research*, **13**(12), 2122–32. https://onlinelibrary.wiley.com/doi/10.1002/aur.2306.

Ryan, R. (1994) Posttraumatic stress disorder in persons with developmental disabilities. *Community Mental Health Journal*, **30**(1), 45–54.

Sappok, T., Budczies, J., Dziobek, I., et al. (2014) The missing link: Delayed emotional development predicts challenging behavior in adults with intellectual disability. *Journal of Autism and Developmental Disorders*, April 01; **44**(4), 786–800.

Scheifes, A., Walraven, S., Stolker, J. J., et al. (2016) Adverse events and the relation with quality of life in adults with intellectual disability and challenging behaviour using psychotropic drugs. *Research in Developmental Disabilities*, March 01; **49–50**: 13–21.

Sinason, V. (1992) *Mental Handicap and the Hhuman Condition: New Approaches from the Tavistock*. Free Association Books.

Sobsey, D., & Doe, T. (1991) Patterns of sexual abuse and assault. *Sexuality and Disability*, **9**, 243–59.

Sobsey, R. (1994) *Violence and Abuse in the Lives of People with Disabilities: The End of Silent Acceptance?* P. H. Brookes Pub. Co.

Tunnicliffe, P., Woodcock, K., Bull, L., Oliver, C., & Penhallow, J. (2014) Temper outbursts in Prader–Willi syndrome: Causes, behavioural and emotional sequence and responses by carers. *Journal of Intellectual Disability Research*, February 01; **58**(2), 134–50.

Van der Kolk, B. (2000) Posttraumatic stress disorder and the nature of trauma. *Dialogues in Clinical Neuroscience*, March 01; **2**(1), 7–22.

Van der Kolk, B. A. (2014) *The Body Keeps the Score: Brain, Mind, and Body in the Healing of Trauma*. Penguin Books.

Ward, F., Tharian, P., Roy, M., Deb, S., & Unwin, G. L. (2013) Efficacy of beta blockers in the management of problem behaviours in people with intellectual disabilities: A systematic review. *Research in Developmental Disabilities*, Dec; **34**(12), 4293–303.

Wilton, J. (2020) *Briefing 54: Trauma, challenging behaviour, and restrictive interventions in schools*. Centre for Mental Health. www.centreformentalhealth.org.uk/wp-content/uploads/2020/01/Briefing_54_traumainformed-schools_0.pdf.

Woodcock, K., Oliver, C., & Humphreys, G. (2009) Associations between repetitive questioning, resistance to change, temper outbursts and anxiety in Prader–Willi and Fragile-X syndromes. *Journal of Intellectual Disability Research*, March 01; **53**(3): 265–78.

Woodcock, K. A., & Blackwell, S. (2020). Psychological treatment strategies for challenging behaviours in neurodevelopmental disorders: What lies beyond a purely behavioural approach? *Current Opinion in Psychiatry*. March 01; **33**(2), 92–109.

World Health Organization (2022). 6B41 complex post traumatic stress disorder. In: *ICD-11 International Classification of Diseases*. 11th rev. ed. Geneva, Switzerland. https://icd.who.int/browse11/l-m/en#/http://id.who.int/icd/entity/585833559.

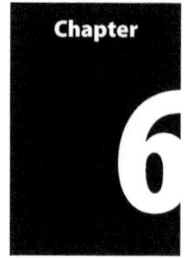

Chapter 6

Anxiety Disorders

Ayomipo J. Amiola, Reena Tharian, and Regi T. Alexander

Introduction

What Are Anxiety Disorders?

Anxiety disorders are a group of mental disorders characterised by excessive fear and anxiety and related behavioural disturbances, with symptoms that are severe enough to result in significant distress or substantial impairment in personal, family, social, educational, occupational, or other important areas of functioning. This group includes generalised anxiety disorder, panic disorder, agoraphobia, specific phobia, social anxiety disorder, separation anxiety disorder, selective mutism, and other specified anxiety or fear-related disorders (ICD-11; DSM-5). This chapter focuses on treatment approaches for generalised anxiety disorder and panic disorder.

The clinical presentation of anxiety includes cognitive, physical, and behavioural components (Harrison et al, 2017). Cognitive or psychological elements include poor concentration, worrying thoughts, fearful anticipation, and irritability. Physical symptoms include signs of autonomic arousal, such as dry mouth, difficulty in swallowing, epigastric discomfort, excessive wind, frequent or loose motions, chest constriction and discomfort, difficulty inhaling, palpitations, discomfort in the chest, awareness of missed heartbeats, frequent or urgent micturition, failure of erection, menstrual discomfort, and muscle tension. Other physiological symptoms include dizziness, tingling sensations in the extremities, feeling of breathlessness, and sleep disturbances (including insomnia and night terrors). Although all these symptoms can occur in any of the anxiety disorders, each disorder has a characteristic pattern. In generalised anxiety disorder, anxiety is continuous, and unrelated to triggers. In phobic anxiety disorders, anxiety is intermittent, arising in specific circumstances. In panic disorder, anxiety is intermittent, but its occurrence is unrelated to any circumstances.

Why Do You Develop an Anxiety Disorder?

Anxiety disorders are a result of complex interactions between genetic, neurobiological, and environmental risk factors (Bhaumik & Alexander 2020). They tend to run in families, and genetic risk factors contribute substantially to the aetiology (Tambs 2009). People with intellectual disability due to genetic syndromal causes are at increased risk of anxiety compared to those with intellectual disability of mixed aetiology and the general population (Edwards et al. 2022). From a developmental perspective, Duff (1981) and colleagues showed that adults with intellectual disability were more fearful in general and showed a more intense level of fear than their chronological-age-matched controls although they reported less overall fear than their mental-age-matched controls. People with intellectual disability also often have a history of early childhood adversity and trauma, extending into their adulthood and occurring at a rate higher than that in the general population. This increases their vulnerability to stressful life events and can precipitate anxiety disorders (Cooray & Bakala 2005).

How Are Anxiety Disorders Different in People with Intellectual Disability?

In clinical practice generally, a psychiatric illness is diagnosed only when symptoms can be clearly elicited and are consistent with criteria provided in standard diagnostic manuals. In people with intellectual disability, this unambiguous clarity may not be there. This can be due to communication difficulties, diagnostic overshadowing, atypical presentations, and the presence of other comorbid conditions. As a result, eliciting the key diagnostic criteria may not be as straightforward as in the general population. Hence behavioural phenomena such as agitation, screaming, crying, withdrawal, regressive/clingy behaviour, or freezing has been described as relevant in the diagnosis of anxiety in people with intellectual disability (Khreim &Mikkelson, 1997).

Due to cognitive and communicative difficulties, many people across the whole spectrum of intellectual disability are unlikely to be able to verbalise the key diagnostic features. There may be a particular issue with expressing complex cognitions such as derealisation, depersonalisation, fear of losing control, 'feeling of impending death', or 'going crazy'. Nevertheless, symptoms such as restlessness, being easily fatigued, irritability, and sleep disturbance should be elicitable in the clinical setting. Furthermore, as mentioned earlier, when anxiety cannot be verbally expressed, behavioural phenomena such as agitation, screaming, crying, withdrawal, regressive/clingy behaviour, or freezing may be elicitable and can be interpreted as behavioural evidence of fear. This, however, is nonspecific and may well reflect other diagnoses or a response to environmental stresses. More reliable signs may include behavioural correlates that reflect the verbal components of the relevant anxiety disorders, such as increased drinking, hyperventilation, sweating, urinary frequency, hyperactivity, irritability, vomiting, diarrhoea, tremulousness, and agitation (Cooray & Bakala 2005; Bhaumik & Alexander 2020).

Although several informant and self-rated guidelines have been developed to improve accuracy of clinical diagnoses, the reliability of these instruments is variable. The Diagnostic Criteria for psychiatric disorders for use in adults with learning disabilities DC-LD (2001) was developed by the Royal College of Psychiatrists, and the Diagnostic Manual – Intellectual Disability DM-ID (2007) was developed by the National Association for the Dually Diagnosed (NADD), in association with the American Psychiatric Association (APA). Both set out the guidelines for diagnosing anxiety disorders in those with an intellectual disability. Most recently, the International Classification of Diseases (ICD) 11 (World Health Organization, 2019) has further formalised the approach of using behavioural equivalents to diagnose mental illnesses in people with intellectual disabilities (Lemay et al. 2022; Reed et al. 2019).

Case Study 6.1 illustrates the presentation of anxiety in an individual with mild intellectual disability and autism.

> **Case Study 6.1**
>
> James, a 25-year-old with mild intellectual disability and autism, was referred to the psychiatrist through the community intellectual disability team with a history of agitation and behaviour that challenges. During the clinical interview, James reported feeling scared all the time and being worried about the wellbeing of his family members and carers. There was no history of persistently low mood, loss of interest in activities, or reduced energy levels, and no history suggestive of perceptual anomalies. James enjoys accessing the day centre, shopping, riding the bus, and collecting coins. Collateral history from his accompanying carer revealed several episodes of tremulousness, agitation, hyperactivity, vomiting, and diarrhoea, usually with no known trigger; these were persistent, although intensity could vary from time to time. Notably, these problems started a few weeks after his grandfather died following a massive stroke.
>
> Following a detailed assessment including a mental state examination, a diagnosis of generalised anxiety disorder was made. James and his carers were provided with easy-read information on anxiety disorder.

How Common Are Anxiety Disorders in People with Intellectual Disability?

In the general population, anxiety disorders constitute the most prevalent of mental disorders (Kessler et al. 2007), with lifetime prevalence figures reportedly as high as 31% (Katzman et al. 2014) and an incidence of 9.7 per 1,000 person-years in UK primary care (Martín-Merino et al. 2010). In people with intellectual disability, although anxiety disorders may be under-reported and under-diagnosed due to a variety of reasons, including communication difficulties and diagnostic overshadowing, prevalence rates are reported to be like the general population (Cooray et al. 2022). The figures show some variation, partly because of variations in the methodology. In a study involving Scottish adults with intellectual disability, Reid and colleagues (2011) reported a point prevalence of 3.8% (95% CI = 2.7–5.2%). Using the Mini PAS-ADD, Deb and colleagues reported a prevalence of 7.8% (Deb et al. 2001). In terms of anxiety symptoms, an estimated prevalence rate of 22% in comparison to 4–5% in the general population has been reported, indicating that people with intellectual disability are at higher risk compared with others (Edwards et al. 2022).

Treatments: The Evidence Base

General Population

In the general population the National Institute for Health and Care Excellence (NICE clinical guideline for generalised anxiety disorder and panic disorder (2011)) offers a comprehensive overview of the evidence base regarding therapeutic interventions. It proposes a stepped-care model with four steps.

- Step 1 is for all known and suspected cases of generalised anxiety and involves identification and assessment, education about the condition and its treatment options, and active monitoring.

- Step 2 is for those who have not improved after education and active monitoring in primary care and involves low-intensity psychological interventions, individual non-facilitated self-help, individual guided self-help, and psychoeducational groups.
- Step 3 is for those with an inadequate response to the step 2 interventions or who have marked functional impairment. This step involves a choice between cognitive behavioural therapy or applied relaxation or treatment with medication.
- Step 4 is for the complex treatment-refractory group with very marked functional impairment, such as self-neglect or a high risk of self-harm. This involves complex drug and/or psychological treatment regimens alongside input from multi-agency teams, crisis services, day hospitals, or inpatient care.

Regarding the use of medication for those who choose to have it, within this stepped-care model, NICE Clinical Guideline (CG)113 recommends:

- A selective serotonin reuptake inhibitor (SSRI), sertraline as the first choice.
- If sertraline is ineffective, an alternative SSRI or a serotonin–noradrenaline reuptake inhibitor (SNRI) as the next line.
- For those who could not tolerate SSRIs or SNRIs, pregabalin as the third line choice.
- The advice is not to use benzodiazepines in primary or secondary care, other than as a short-term measure.
- The advice is not to use antipsychotics in primary care.

> For a full account of the recommendations, associated caveats, and the relevant evidence base, please visit www.nice.org.uk/guidance/cg113/chapter/Recommendations.

People with Intellectual Disability

As described in Chapter 5, the clinical presentation of severe anxiety may be related to the experience of multiple traumas in people with intellectual disability and this possibility should be explored carefully. The specific evidence base for the treatment of anxiety in people with intellectual disabilities is limited to a relatively small number of empirical studies, along with case reports and theoretical reviews on the extension and modification of more well-studied treatments used for anxiety in the mainstream population (Davis et al. 2008). Like the general population, the range of effective interventions includes psychotherapy and pharmacotherapy, with psychological interventions being first line. The choice of treatment is determined by the intensity, duration, and severity of symptoms, associated distress and impairment, the presence of co-existing depressive symptoms, comorbid physical/ psychological disorders, patient characteristics and preferences, clinician experience, availability of proposed intervention, and other features such as a good response to, or poor tolerability of, previous treatments (Baldwin et al. 2014).

People with Intellectual Disability: Non-Medication Treatments

Psychological interventions such as reassurance, counselling, relaxation training, anger management, and self-help have been found to be useful in people with an intellectual disability (Stavrakaki& Mintsioulis, 1997). NICE Guideline NG54 (2016) recommends that in people with intellectual disabilities, clinicians should consider relaxation therapy to treat anxiety symptoms and graded exposure techniques to treat anxiety symptoms or phobias. In their systematic review, Dagnan and colleagues (2018) identified 19 studies (the majority of which were descriptive case studies); all but one reported a positive outcome. However, the currently available empirical evidence about the effectiveness of cognitive behavioural therapy (CBT) for treatment of anxiety disorders in people with an intellectual disability is weak due to methodological issues. Table 6.1 summarises the evidence base for psychotherapeutic treatment approaches for anxiety in people with intellectual disability.

People with Intellectual Disability: Medication Treatments

There are very few studies specifically looking at the pharmacological treatment of anxiety of people with intellectual disability. This is despite excess prescriptions of anxiolytics, antidepressants, and GABA agonists being reported in people with intellectual disabilities compared with the general population (Axmon et al. 2019). Table 6.2 summarises the studies which report the use of anxiolytics in people with intellectual disability.

Table 6.1 Non-medication treatments in intellectual disability

Psychotherapy	Evidence in intellectual disability
Relaxation therapy	In this pilot randomised controlled trial (RCT), relaxation reduced state anxiety and improved self-esteem and cognitive reappraisal, unlike in the control group (Bouvet and Coulet 2016)
Cognitive Behavioural Therapy	A 2018 systematic review identified 19 papers. The majority were descriptive case reports. Cognitive behavioural techniques (e.g., psychoeducation and interventions directly aimed at thoughts and beliefs) in most studies reported positive outcomes. In the better-controlled studies, the impact was less comprehensive (Dagnan et al. 2018)

Table 6.2 Medication treatments in intellectual disability

Medication	Evidence in intellectual disability
Antidepressants (SSRI citalopram & SNRI mirtazapine)	Retrospective study of 17 patients with pervasive developmental disorders aged 4–15 who were treated in an open-label trail of citalopram: 59% were judged to be much improved or very improved on anxiety and aggression, using the Clinical Global Impression (CGI) scale (Couturier & Nicolson, 2002).
	Retrospective chart review of 15 children and adolescent patients with pervasive developmental disorders, including Asperger's, autism, and PDD NOS treated with citalopram. Anxiety symptoms improved significantly in 66% of patients (Namerow et al. 2003).
	Patients with pervasive developmental disorders (n=26) treated in an open-label trial with the SNRI mirtazapine. Nine patients (34.6%) were judged much improved or very much improved on the CGI scale on anxiety and several other symptoms including aggression, self-injury, irritability, hyperactivity, depression, and insomnia (Posey et al. 2001).

Table 6.2 (cont.)

Medication	Evidence in intellectual disability
Risperidone	Double-blind, placebo-controlled trial of the atypical antipsychotic risperidone conducted in adults with pervasive developmental disorders and comorbid anxiety. Patients in the treatment group demonstrated significant reductions in anxiety and other psychiatric symptoms compared to the control group (McDougle et al. 1998).
	A case study of 14 children and adolescents with developmental disorders treated with risperidone: 10 of 14 patients demonstrated marked reductions in anxiety (Fisman & Steele 1996).
Buspirone	Twenty-two children aged 6–17 with pervasive developmental disorder were treated for anxiety in an open-label trial of buspirone. Nine showed a marked therapeutic response and 7 showed a moderate response on the CGI scale (Buitelaar et al. 1998).
	A study of 6 adults with intellectual disability demonstrated reductions in aggression and anxiety (Ratey et al. 1991).

These studies are mostly from those with autistic spectrum disorders and are quite dated now. The NICE clinical guideline for mental health problems in people with learning disabilities: prevention, assessment, and management (NICE 2016) recommended referring to the NICE guidelines on specific mental health problems for treatment guidance.

A large multi-centre, placebo-controlled, randomised controlled trial is currently under way in the United Kingdom and Australia to compare sertraline and placebo in the treatment of anxiety in autistic adults (Rai 2024). Until the results of that and similar studies are available, the advice from NICE to follow the guidelines for the general adult population, albeit with reasonable adjustments and caution in prescribing, will hold good.

Treatment Guideline and Algorithm in Intellectual Disability

Assessment

- A detailed diagnostic assessment (Alexander et al. 2010; Chester et al. 2023), as set out in Chapter 4, should be carried out. This will cover the degree of intellectual disability, cause of intellectual disability and any behaviour phenotypes, autism, other developmental disorders, mental illnesses including anxiety disorders, personality disorders, substance misuse, physical health conditions, the experience of trauma, and types of challenging behaviour.
- A psychological formulation using the 5-P model of the **p**resenting problem, **p**redisposing, **p**recipitating, **p**erpetuating, and **p**rotective factors (Macneil et al. 2012) or equivalent should be completed, along with using the HELP framework of **h**ealth,

environment, lived experience, and psychiatric problems (Green et al. 2018). Within the lived experience domain, particular attention must be paid to past experiences of multiple traumas as described in Chapter 5. If a clinical picture of complex-PTSD looks likely, the treatment approach should be as described in Chapter 5.

Non-Medication Treatments

- A stepped-care model of intervention, as set out earlier in this chapter (NICE CG113, 2011). In steps 1 and 2 of that model, focus on educational approaches for both patient and support staff.
- From step 3 onwards, use of relaxation training and/or cognitive behaviour therapy

Medication Treatments

- Assessment and treatment of anxiety disorders in intellectual disability must always be conducted within the context of a robust biopsychosocial understanding of illness and formulation.
- Careful medication history, including any use of over-the-counter remedies and self-medication with alcohol and/or drugs.
- Check for potential drug interactions and history of sensitivity to side effects.
- Detailed discussion with the patient and/or carers and family, as appropriate, about the target symptoms, the rationale for prescribing, and the monitoring and review arrangements.

Table 6.3 summarises the first, second, third, and fourth line of medication use.

Table 6.3 Medication choice for anxiety disorder in intellectual disability

Anxiety disorder	First line	Second line	Third line	Fourth line (no order of preference)
Generalised anxiety disorder	Cognitive behavioural therapy (CBT); other psychosocial and environmental interventions	Selective serotonin reuptake inhibitors (SSRIs)	Serotonin–noradrenaline reuptake inhibitor (SNRIs), then pregabalin	Tricyclic antidepressant (TCAs), buspirone, quetiapine, mirtazapine (consider propranolol if significant autonomic symptoms)
Panic disorder	CBT; other psychosocial and environmental interventions	SSRIs	SNRIs	TCAs, mirtazapine

Table 6.3 (cont.)

Anxiety disorder	First line	Second line	Third line	Fourth line (no order of preference)
Social phobia	CBT; other psychosocial and environmental interventions	SSRIs (atenolol helpful for autonomic symptoms in performance situations)	SNRIs	Olanzapine, benzodiazepines on an 'as required' (PRN) basis

- For individuals with acute, severe debilitating anxiety, consider the short-term use of benzodiazepines (for no longer than four weeks). Prescribers should be aware that the side effects of benzodiazepines may be under-recognised and under-reported in people with intellectual disability. The medication is used despite this disadvantage because, in the short term, this may improve their engagement with long-term psychosocial interventions.

Length of Treatment and Related Issues

- Since the launch of the NHS England 2016 programme Stopping Over-Medication of People with a Learning Disability (STOMP) (NHS England, 2016), clinicians have been reminded of the need to ensure medications are prescribed not only for appropriate indications but are also only continued for an appropriate time.
- As highlighted earlier, benzodiazepines should only be used for anxiety that is severe, disabling, or a cause of extreme distress to the patient; in these conditions, these drugs should be used at the lowest effective dose for no longer than four weeks.
- For selective serotonin reuptake inhibitors (SSRIs) and serotonin–noradrenaline reuptake inhibitor (SNRI), patients should begin to see some benefits within six weeks, and this continues to increase over time.
- Since the optimal duration for SSRI treatment of anxiety is still unclear, it is advised that treatment can continue for a year.
- Where effective, medical treatment should continue since abrupt discontinuation may precipitate relapse of symptoms or features suggestive of a discontinuation syndrome.
- For ongoing prescribing, conduct regular reviews at 3–6-month intervals (Royal College of Psychiatrists, 2016) or at least yearly (NICE 2016).

Case Study 6.2 continues with the individual discussed in Case Study 6.1 focusing on the treatment.

Case Study 6.2: Treatment

James was initially offered cognitive behaviour therapy, adapted for his communication needs. However, he was not able to engage with this due to his overwhelming anxiety. Considering the severity of the latter and the resulting functional impairments, James and his carers were provided with easy-read information on SSRI treatments to enable him to make an informed choice. He was subsequently commenced on sertraline, with intensive community nursing input to monitor symptoms and possible side effects of the medication, perform ongoing risk assessment, and implement supportive and positive behaviour strategies. The initial dose of sertraline was 25 mg per day, and this was gradually titrated up to 150 mg/day over a period of six weeks. James's anxiety improved and he was then able to engage in psychological therapy sessions.

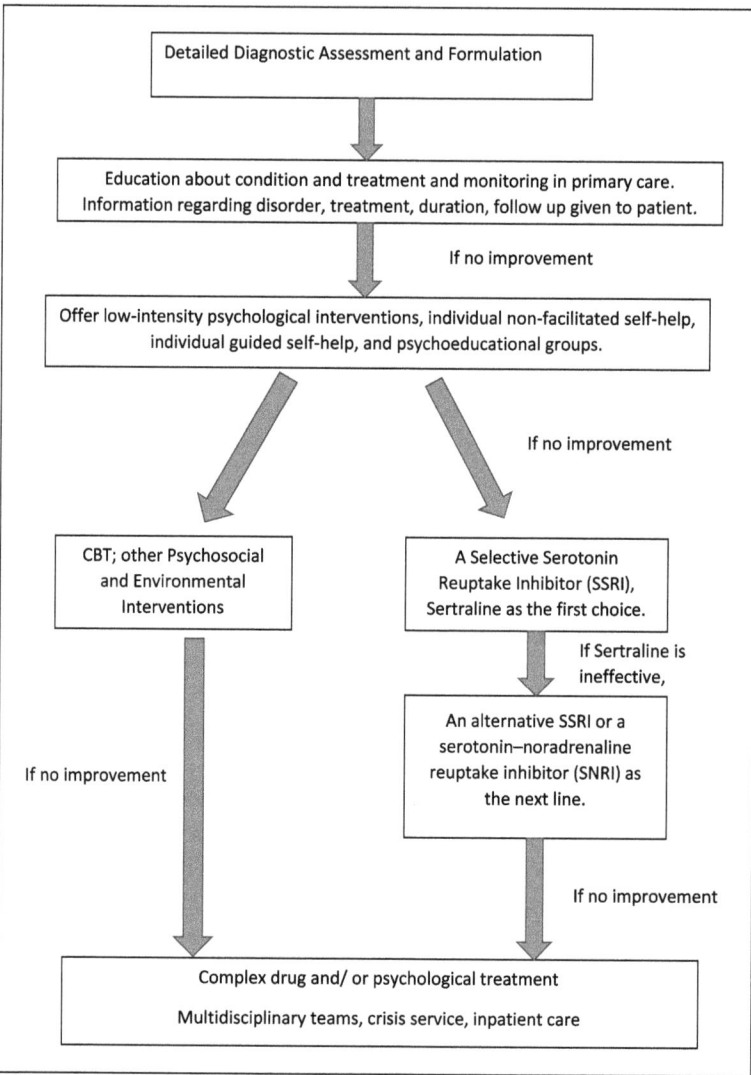

Figure 6.1 Algorithm for treatment of anxiety disorders in intellectual disability

The Frith Prescribing Guidelines Editors' Expert Group Consensus Statements

Statements of High Confidence
- The prevalence of anxiety *symptoms* in people with intellectual disability is higher although the prevalence of anxiety *disorders* may be similar.
- Careful diagnostic evaluation and a psychological formulation is a prerequisite for appropriate treatment.
- The treatment strategy can be a four-stage stepped approach, starting with education and progressing to psychological interventions followed by medication.
- The rationale for treatment, target symptoms, and arrangements for review should be discussed and agreed with the patient and or carers/family, as appropriate.

Statements of Medium Confidence
- Modified cognitive behavioural therapy may be a feasible and effective approach for the treatment of anxiety in intellectual disabilities.
- If medication is considered, then the SSRI sertraline is the first choice.

Statements of Low Confidence
- Relaxation therapy can be used to treat anxiety symptoms and graded exposure techniques used to treat anxiety symptoms or phobias in people with intellectual disabilities.
- Other SSRIs and SNRIs may be used as further options.

Resource Box

Rating Scales for Anxiety in Intellectual Disabilities

Glasgow Anxiety Scale for People with an Intellectual Disability (GAS-ID): https://onlinelibrary.wiley.com/doi/pdf/10.1046/j.1365-2788.2003.00457.x

Anxiety, Depression and Mood Scale (ADAMS): https://eprovide.mapi-trust.org/instruments/anxiety-depression-and-mood-scale

Easy-Read Documents

Royal College of Psychiatrists: Mental Health and Learning Disabilities:

www.rcpsych.ac.uk/docs/default-source/mental-health/problems-and-disorders/learning-disabilities-anxiety-disorder-leaflet.pdf?sfvrsn=10ac9d74_4

Foundation for People with Learning Disabilities: An Easy Read Guide to Anxiety:

www.learningdisabilities.org.uk/learning-disabilities/publications/easy-read-guide-anxiety

Easy-Read Documents for Medications

Choice & Medication: An information site (available through several NHS Trusts or individual subscriptions) which offers patient information about mental health conditions and the treatments available to help make informed decisions about choosing the right medicine. Options include Very Easy Read Leaflets (VERAs), designed for people with an intellectual disability. www.choiceandmedication.org/ SPECTROM Easy read medication leaflets: https://spectrom.wixsite.com/project/easy-read-medication-leaflets

Other Key Clinical Guidelines Referenced in This Chapter

National Institute for Clinical Excellence, 2011: *Generalised anxiety disorder and panic disorder in adults: management. Clinical guideline* [CG113] Published: 26 January 2011, updated 2019 & 2021 www.nice.org.uk/guidance/cg113/chapter/Recommendations

National Institute for Clinical Excellence, 2016: *Mental health problems in people with learning disabilities: prevention, assessment, and management* (NG54) Published: 14 September 2016 www.nice.org.uk/guidance/ng54/chapter/Recommendations

Taylor, D. M., Barnes, T. R., & Young, A. H., 2021. *The Maudsley prescribing guidelines in psychiatry*. John Wiley & Sons.

References

Alexander, R. T., Green, F. N., O'Mahony, B., et al. (2010). Personality disorders in offenders with intellectual disability: A comparison of clinical, forensic and outcome variables and implications for service provision. *Journal of Intellectual Disability Research*, **54**(7), 650–8.

American Psychiatric Association (2013). Neurodevelopmental Disorders. In *Diagnostic and statistical manual of mental disorders (DSM-5)*. 5th ed. American Psychiatric Association Publishing.

Axmon, A., El Mrayyan, N., Eberhard, J., & Ahlström, G. (2019). Pharmacotherapy for mood and anxiety disorders in older people with intellectual disability in comparison with the general population. *BMC Psychiatry*, **19**, 1–8.

Baldwin, D. S., Anderson, I. M., Nutt, D. J., et al. (2014). Evidence-based pharmacological treatment of anxiety disorders, post-traumatic stress disorder and obsessive-compulsive disorder: A revision of the 2005 guidelines from the British Association for Psychopharmacology. *Journal of Psychopharmacology*, **28**(5), 403–439.

Bhaumik, S. & Alexander, R. eds. (2020). *Oxford textbook of the psychiatry of intellectual disability*. Oxford University Press.

Bouvet, C. & Coulet, A. (2016). Relaxation therapy and anxiety, self-esteem, and emotional regulation among adults with intellectual disabilities: A randomized controlled trial. *Journal of Intellectual Disabilities*, **20**(3), 228–240.

Buitelaar, J. K., Van der Gaag, R. J., & Van der Hoeven, J. (1998). Buspirone in the management of anxiety and irritability in children with pervasive developmental disorders: Results of an open-label study. *Journal of Clinical Psychiatry*, **59**(2), 56–59.

Chester, V., Tharian, P., Slinger, M., Varughese, A., & Alexander, R. T. (2023). Overview of offenders with intellectual disability. In J. M. McCarthy, R. T. Alexander, & E. Chaplin. (Eds.), *Forensic aspects of neurodevelopmental disorders: A clinician's guide* (pp. 24–33). Cambridge University Press. https://doi.org/10.1017/9781108955522.003.

Cooray, S. E. & Bakala, A. (2005). Anxiety disorders in people with learning disabilities. *Advances in Psychiatric Treatment*, **11**(5), 355–61.

Cooray, S. E., Tassé, M. J., Barnhill, J., & Bhaumik, S. (2022). Anxiety and stress-related disorders in people with intellectual disability/disorders of intellectual development. In *Textbook of psychiatry for intellectual disability and autism spectrum disorder* (pp. 583–608). Springer.

Couturier, J. L. & Nicolson, R. (2002). A retrospective assessment of citalopram in children and adolescents with pervasive developmental disorders. *Journal of Child and Adolescent Psychopharmacology*, **12**(3), 243–8.

Dagnan, D., Jackson, I., & Eastlake, L. (2018). A systematic review of cognitive behavioural therapy for anxiety in adults with intellectual disabilities. *Journal of Intellectual Disability Research*, **62**(11), 974–91.

Davis, E., Saeed, S. A., & Antonacci, D. J. (2008). Anxiety disorders in persons with developmental disabilities: Empirically informed diagnosis and treatment. *Psychiatric Quarterly*, **79**(3), 249–63.

Deb, S., Thomas, M., & Bright, C. (2001). Mental disorder in adults with intellectual disability. 1: Prevalence of functional psychiatric illness among a community-based population aged between 16 and 64 years. *Journal of Intellectual Disability Research*, **45**(6), 495–505.

Duff, R., La Rocca, J., Lizzet, A. et al. (1981). A comparison of the fears of mildly retarded adults with children of their mental age and chronological age matched controls. *Journal of Behavior Therapy and Experimental Psychiatry*, **12**(2), 121–4.

Edwards, G., Jones, C., Pearson, E. et al. (2022). Prevalence of anxiety symptomatology and diagnosis in syndromic intellectual disability: A systematic review and meta-analysis. *Neuroscience & Biobehavioral Reviews*, 104719.

Fisman, S. & Steele, M. (1996). Use of risperidone in pervasive developmental disorders: a case series. *Journal of Child and Adolescent Psychopharmacology*, **6**(3), 177–90.

Fletcher, R., Loschen, E., Stavrakaki, C. & First, M. (2007). *DM-ID: diagnostic manual – intellectual disability: A textbook of diagnosis of mental disorders in persons with intellectual disability*. National Association for the Dually Diagnosed.

Green, L., McNeil, K., Korossy, M., et al. (2018). HELP for behaviours that challenge in adults with intellectual and developmental disabilities. *Canadian Family Physician*, **64** (Suppl 2), S23–S31.

Harrison, P., Cowen, P., Burns, T. & Fazel, M. (2017). *Shorter Oxford textbook of psychiatry*. Oxford University Press.

Katzman, M. A., Bleau, P., Blier, P., et al. (2014). Canadian clinical practice guidelines for the management of anxiety, posttraumatic stress and obsessive-compulsive disorders. *BMC Psychiatry*, **14**(1), 1–83.

Kessler, R. C., Angermeyer, M., Anthony, J. C., et al. (2007). Lifetime prevalence and age-of-onset distributions of mental disorders in the World Health Organization's World Mental Health Survey Initiative. *World Psychiatry*, **6**(3), 168.

Khreim, I. & Mikkelsen, E. (1997). Anxiety disorders in adults with mental retardation. *Psychiatric Annals*, **27**(3), 175–81.

Lemay, K. R., Kogan, C. S., Rebello, T. J., et al. (2022). An international field study of the International Classification of Diseases-11 behavioural indicators for disorders of intellectual development. *Journal of Intellectual Disability Research*, **66**(4), 376–91.

Lindsay, W.R., Neilson, C., & Lawrenson, H. (1997). Cognitive-behaviour therapy for anxiety in people with learning disabilities. In B. S. Kroese, D. Dagnan, & K. Loumidis (Eds.), *Cognitive behaviour therapy for people with learning disabilities*. Routledge, pp. 128–44.

Macneil, C. A., Hasty, M. K., Conus, P., & Berk, M. (2012). Is diagnosis enough to guide interventions in mental health? Using case formulation in clinical practice. *BMC Medicine*, **10**, 111. https://doi.org/10.1186/1741-7015-10-111.

Martín-Merino, E., Ruigómez, A., Wallander, M. A., Johansson, S., & García-Rodríguez, L. A. (2010). Prevalence, incidence, morbidity and treatment patterns in a cohort of patients diagnosed with anxiety in UK primary care. *Family Practice,* 27(1), 9–16.

McDougle, C. J., Holmes, J. P., Carlson, D. C., et al. (1998). A double-blind, placebo-controlled study of risperidone in adults with autistic disorder and other pervasive developmental disorders. *Archives of General Psychiatry,* **55**(7), 633–41.

Namerow, L. B., Thomas, P., Bostic, J. Q., Prince, J., & Monuteaux, M.C. (2003). Use of citalopram in pervasive developmental disorders. *Journal of Developmental & Behavioral Pediatrics,* **24**(2), 104–8.

National Institute for Health and Care Excellence (2011). Generalised anxiety disorder and panic disorder in adults: Management. Clinical Guideline [CG113]. www.nice.org.uk/guidance/CG113.

National Institute for Health and Care Excellence (2016). Mental Health problems in people with learning disabilities – prevention, assessment, and management [NG54]. www.nice.org.uk/guidance/ng54.

NHS England (2016). Stopping Over-Medication of People with a Learning Disability (STOMPLD) Pledge. www.england.nhs.uk/2016/06/over-medication-pledge/.

Posey, D. J., Guenin, K. D., Kohn, A. E., Swiezy, N. B., & McDougle, C. J. (2001). A naturalistic open-label study of mirtazapine in autistic and other pervasive developmental disorders. *Journal of Child and Adolescent Psychopharmacology,* **11**(3), 267–77.

Rai, D., Webb, D., Lewis, A., et al. (2024). Sertraline for anxiety in adults with a diagnosis of autism (STRATA): study protocol for a pragmatic, multicentre, double-blind, placebo-controlled randomised controlled trial. *Trials,* **25**(1), 37. https://doi.org/10.1186/s13063-023-07847-3.

Ratey, J., Sovner, R., Parks, A., & Rogentine, K. (1991). Buspirone treatment of aggression and anxiety in mentally retarded patients: a multiple-baseline, placebo lead-in study. *Journal of Clinical Psychiatry,* **52**(4), 159–162.

Reed, G. M., First, M. B., Kogan, C. S., et al. (2019). Innovations and changes in the International Classification of Diseases-11 classification of mental, behavioural and neurodevelopmental disorders. *World Psychiatry,* **18**(1), 3–19.

Reid, K. A., Smiley, E., & Cooper, S. A. (2011). Prevalence and associations of anxiety disorders in adults with intellectual disabilities. *Journal of Intellectual Disability Research,* **55**(2), 172–81.

Royal College of Psychiatrists (2001). *OP48 DC-LD: Diagnostic criteria for psychiatric disorders for use with adults with learning disabilities/mental retardation* (Vol. 48). Springer Science & Business.

Royal College of Psychiatrists (2016). Psychotropic drug prescribing for people with intellectual disability, mental health problems and/or behaviours that challenge: practice guidelines. Royal College of Psychiatrists.

Stavrakaki, C. & Mintsioulis, G. (1997). Anxiety disorders in persons with mental retardation: Diagnostic, clinical and treatment issues. *Psychiatric Annals,* **27**(3), 182–9.

Tambs, K., Czajkowsky, N., Neale, M. C., et al. (2009). Structure of genetic and environmental risk factors for dimensional representations of DSM-IV anxiety disorders. *The British Journal of Psychiatry,* **195**(4), 301–7.

World Health Organization (2019). International statistical classification of diseases and related health problems (11th ed.). https://icd.who.int/.

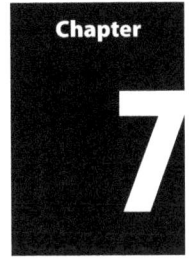

Chapter 7

Depression

Adelola Idowu and David M. L. Branford

Introduction

What Is Depression?

Depression is characterised by persistent low mood and/or loss of pleasure in most activities and a range of associated emotional, cognitive, physical, and behavioural symptoms. Depression can be categorised as mild, moderate, or severe, based on the presence of symptoms and how the individual is affected by these symptoms. For further details see fifth edition of the *American Psychiatric Association Diagnostic and Statistical Manual of Mental Disorders* (DSM-5) (2013).

How Common Is Depression in People with Intellectual Disability?

Depressive disorders are very common and are among the leading causes of disability worldwide. The worldwide prevalence of depression is estimated to be 4.4%; prevalence in the United Kingdom is 4.5%.

The point prevalence of affective disorder (a category of mental health conditions which includes depression) in a large population study with intellectual disability (n=1,023) was 6.6% based upon expert clinical assessment, compared with 5.7%, 4.8%, or 3.6% for diagnoses made according to various standard criteria respectively (Cooper et al. 2007).

Adults with epilepsy and intellectual disability had a more than seven-fold increased risk for developing psychiatric disorders, particularly depression, and unspecified disorders of presumed organic origin, including dementia (Turky et al. 2011).

Another study by Richard et al. (2001) found that intellectual disability was associated with a four-fold increase in risk of affective disorder, not accounted for by social and material disadvantage or by medical disorder.

Studies based on data generated by general practice (GP) prescribing systems give a much higher prevalence of depression (NHS Digital 2021) (see Table 7.1).

How Is Depression Different in People with Intellectual Disability?

Many conditions present differently in people with intellectual disability. Diagnosis is affected by communication problems, the influence of poor physical and social circumstances, and general lack of suitable diagnostic criteria. Psychiatric evaluation remains complex because of limitations in verbal abilities, atypical clinical presentation, and challenging behaviour (Richards et al. 2001). Clinical diagnosis is based upon history and

Table 7.1 Prevalence (%) of population diagnosed with depression: March 2016 and March 2021

	Percentage of population with depression diagnosis: 2016	Percentage of population with depression diagnosis: 2021	Percentage change
With intellectual disability	14.4	17.5	+22.0%
Without intellectual disability	14.9	17.2	+15.1%

Source: NHS Digital (2021).

Table 7.2 Clinical presentation of depression in intellectual disability

Core symptoms (similar to general population)	• tearfulness • social withdrawal • low mood • irritability • reduced energy • fatigue • increased/decreased appetite with increased/decreased weight • insomnia/hypersomnia
Behavioural symptoms (more common in intellectual disability)	• aggression • self-injurious behaviour • screaming • temper tantrums • incontinence
Other symptoms (more common in intellectual disability)	• hypochondriacal symptoms: headache, abdominal pain, vomiting • generalised deterioration in social relationships and self-care skills • pica (rare) (compulsive eating of non-edible things)

mental state examination. The symptoms of depression can be determined by talking with the person with intellectual disability and informants and careful clinical observation. People with intellectual disability can report or endorse symptoms of depression. The Diagnostic Criteria for Psychiatric Disorders for Use with Adults with Learning Disabilities (DC-LD) and Diagnostic Manual: Disorders of Intellectual Development (DM-ID) (Royal College of Psychiatrists 2001) have modified diagnostic criteria informed by the evidence base and expert consensus to account for differences in presentation due to cognitive, communication, and functional impairments. Symptoms that may suggest the presence of depression in people with intellectual disability are listed in Table 7.2.

When assessing a person with intellectual disability for depression, consideration of the following additional points would be helpful.
- The onset of depression and its symptoms tends to be more insidious in people with intellectual disability than in the general population
- The symptoms of depression may be mis-attributed to the intellectual disability itself – this is an example of diagnostic overshadowing
- Behavioural symptoms are more common in people with intellectual disability than in the general population as a manifestation of depression
- Clinicians may need to rely on observables signs rather than reported symptoms in people with intellectual disability because of limitations in verbal skills and emotional insight.

Many patients with depression and intellectual disability may not meet diagnostic criteria using DSM-5 or DM-ID because of limitations in verbal self-report of symptoms and inadequacy of caregiver report. We must therefore work with families and support staff to gather more accurate data and assure careful observation of all the areas important to assessment of psychiatric illness. In addition to the psychiatric diagnostic interview, clinicians must require further assessments using caregiver reported instrumentation, self-report instruments, and structured clinical interviews.

Rating Scales for Depression in Intellectual Disability
- Glasgow Depression Scale for People with a Learning Disability (GDS-LD): http://dx.doi.org/10.1192/bjp.182.4.347
- Carer supplement to GDS-LD: GDS-CS: http://dx.doi.org/10.1192/bjp.182.4.347

Case Study 7.1 contextualises the information provided so far about the presentation and diagnosis of depression in people with intellectual disability.

Case Study 7.1: Presentation

Amina, a 28-year-old woman with moderate intellectual disability and epilepsy, was referred by her GP to the local intellectual disability services with poor sleep, poor engagement in her usual activities, and hitting out at her carers.

She was reviewed by the psychiatrist at home, in the company of her support worker. History from her carers confirmed the aforenoted issues and revealed that she had recently moved into supported living accommodation. Over the preceding six weeks, she had gradually become more withdrawn and irritable, crying intermittently with no obvious triggers, sometimes refusing meals and support with personal care, and lashing out at staff. She was now refusing to go to the day centre, which had recently reported a sudden increase in her verbal outbursts and emotional distress.

Collateral history (information about the individual collected from other people) was obtained from her family regarding her pre-morbid functioning, and showed that she was very sociable and easy going, engaged well in her activities, and always looked forward to attending the day centre.

Following a comprehensive assessment, which included a mental state examination, a diagnosis of moderate depressive illness was made. The patient and her carers were provided with easy-read information on depression.

Antidepressant Prescribing in People with Intellectual Disability

Surveys of psychotropic medication prescribed for people with intellectual disability have been a common feature since the middle of the twentieth century. Aman (1988) reviewed 35 such USA based surveys and concluded that, typically, 30–50% received a psychotropic medication, of which antipsychotic prescribing was the main component. These older surveys showed relatively low use of antidepressants.

Since the turn of the twenty-first century, antidepressant use has increased greatly. In many parts of England antidepressants have now become the most widely prescribed psychotropic medication for people with intellectual disability. Details of the various studies on the prevalence of antidepressant use for people with intellectual disability are presented in Figure 7.1.

Other features of antidepressant prescribing in intellectual disability are:
- The percentage of people on antidepressants rises with age (Glover et al. 2015; Mehta & Glover, 2019; NHS Digital 2021)
- Antidepressants may be prescribed in combination with other psychotropic medications, such as antipsychotics and antiseizure medications.

The Evidence Base for Treatments

People with Intellectual Disability: Medication Treatments

There are very few studies of medication treatments of depression of people with intellectual disabilities. Most of the studies of antidepressant use in people with intellectual disability were undertaken in the 1990s and focused on the potential use for obsessive-compulsive disorder or behavioural management rather than depression. Most studies of antidepressants for depression involved very small numbers of patients. Table 7.3 details the available evidence.

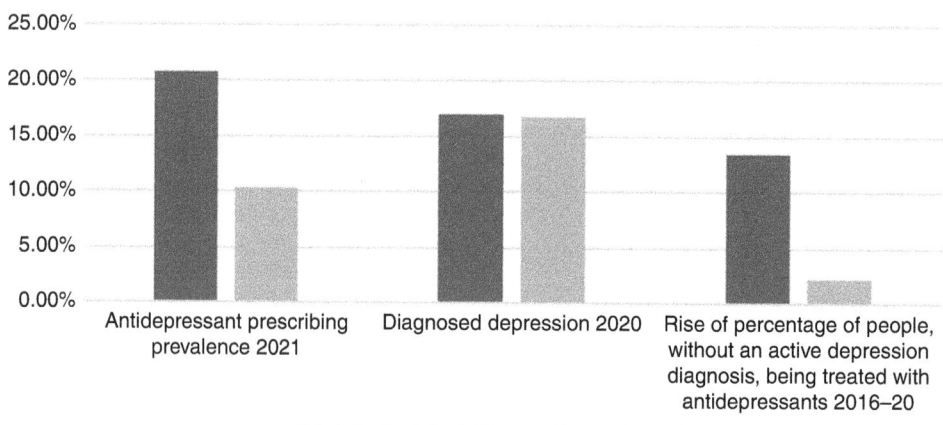

Figure 7.1 Prevalence (%) of prescribing of antidepressants and of diagnosis of active depression in adults with intellectual disability; general practice samples between 2016 and March 2021. Data from NHS Digital 2021

People with Intellectual Disability: Non-Medication Treatments

The evidence to support psychological treatments for depression in intellectual disability has developed significantly in the last ten years. However, access remains a problem, with few therapists trained to undertake the therapies for people with intellectual disability and depression. Historically, people with intellectual disability have been excluded from cognitive-based therapies such as cognitive behaviour therapy. However, recent research has shown that people with mild to moderate intellectual disability do have the capacity to engage in cognitive-based interventions (Bhaumik et al. 2011).

The American Psychiatric Association (APA) (2019) review of clinical practice guidelines for the treatment of depression across three age cohorts found that, in the general population, effectiveness studies demonstrated similar effects across five psychotherapies. Those that appear to have comparable effects include behavioural therapy; cognitive, cognitive behavioural, and mindfulness-based cognitive therapy; interpersonal psychotherapy; psychodynamic therapies; and supportive therapy. Table 7.4 provides an overview of the studies of psychological therapies in intellectual disability.

Table 7.3 Evidence for medication treatments in intellectual disability

- A 1992 open trial of fluoxetine, involving six individuals with intellectual disability who had depression, found a 'positive result' in all (Howland 1992)
- A 1992 review of the case notes of 149 adult in-patients with severe intellectual disability concluded that those with depressive, psychotic, and behavioural problems responded positively to tricyclics and tetracyclics (Langee and Conlon 1992)
- A 2001 open trial of citalopram in 20 patients with intellectual disability and depression found significant improvement in 12 of them (Verhoeven et al. 2001)
- A retrospective review of the case notes of 122 adults with intellectual disability found they responded to fluoxetine and paroxetine in depression (Bhaumik et al. 2000)
- A 2010 retrospective review of 241 treatment episodes showed a positive outcome in terms of clinical improvement at 6 weeks, 6 months, and 12 months, of 49.4%, 48.1%, and 49% respectively, and only 29 (12%) episodes of side effects were noted (Rai & Kerr 2010).

Table 7.4 Evidence for psychological therapies in intellectual disability

Psychotherapy	Evidence in intellectual disability
Cognitive, cognitive behavioural, and mindfulness-based cognitive therapy	A 2011 review suggested that people with intellectual disability have suitable skills to undergo cognitive behavioural therapy (CBT) (Bhaumik et al. 2011). Case studies have reported successful use of cognitive behavioural therapy techniques (with adaptations) in people with intellectual disability. A 2013 review and meta-analysis stated that CBT was efficacious for both anger and depression, while interventions aimed at improving interpersonal functioning were not effectual (Vereenooghe & Langdon 2013).

Table 7.4 (cont.)

Psychotherapy	Evidence in intellectual disability
	Small studies of CBT with computerised assisted cognitive behaviour therapy have found the combination helpful (Cooney et al. 2018)
Psychodynamic therapies	Small naturalistic studies (Beail et al. 2005)
Behavioural activation and guided self help	Behavioural activation was no better than a guided self-help intervention at improving depression at 12 months, although both groups improved during the trial (Jahoda et al. 2017)
Dialectical behaviour therapy (DBT)	An adapted DBT programme (aDBT-ID) was delivered to adults with mild-to-moderate intellectual disability (n = 20) and their caregivers (n = 20) Results suggest it was feasible and beneficial to deliver adapted dialectical behaviour therapy in the community (Jones et al. 2021) A 2017 systematic review and narrative analysis suggested that dialectical behaviour therapy could be successfully adapted for use by people with intellectual disability (Jones et al. 2021)

The Frith Treatment Guidelines for People with Intellectual Disability

General Guidance

There is a lack of specific depression guidelines for people with intellectual disability. Most key depression guidance documents make little (if any) reference to people with intellectual disability. However, general guidance on how to support people with intellectual disability is available from NICE (Guideline 54; 2016). This guideline provides general advice on how to assess and treat people with intellectual disability, including guidance on the type of psychological interventions useful in people with intellectual disability.

First-Line Medication Treatments

Tables 7.5–7.7 summarise information and guidance from a number of guidelines, including NICE (2022) Depression in adults: recognition and management (NG222), the British Association of Psychopharmacology (BAP) 2015 depression guideline, and the American Psychological Association (2019) clinical practice guideline for the treatment of depression across three age cohorts. NICE Guidance NG222 does not recommend a specific order of treatment, instead providing a range of options based on the degree of evidence for clinicians to choose from. The emphasis is on considering the personal circumstances, the choice of the person, and the nature of depression. Clinicians are encouraged to facilitate shared decision making. While shared decision making may seem difficult in people with intellectual disability, use of accessible information and involvement of carers will enable clinicians to keep in mind the view of the individual with intellectual disability in the treatment choice.

Table 7.5 First-line medication treatments

Presentation	Key statements on first-line medication treatment
Subthreshold depressive symptoms or mild depression	Do not use antidepressants routinely
Exceptions to above	History of previous episodes of moderate or severe depression or symptoms that persist subthreshold and have not benefitted from a low-intensity psychosocial intervention
Choice of medication	One of the selective serotonin reuptake inhibitors (SSRI) in a generic form
Factors that affect choice of selective SSRI	Risk of bleeding (if on other medications that interfere with clotting) Drug interactions (worse with fluoxetine and paroxetine) Higher incidence of discontinuation symptoms (paroxetine)
Length of treatment	Usually taken for at least 6 months (and for some time after symptoms remit)
Combined treatment	Combined treatment of choice – cognitive behavioural therapy plus an SSRI

Table 7.6 Key statements on second-line medication treatments

Presentation	Key statements on second-line treatment
Not responded at all after 4 weeks of antidepressant medication at a recognised therapeutic dose, or after 4–6 weeks for psychological therapy or combined medication and psychological therapy	Discuss whether: • Social factors • Physical or mental health conditions • Problems with medication or therapist
Continuing despite no response after 4 weeks	Only around 20% chance of remission at 12 weeks
Success of subsequent treatments	The chance of responding to a subsequent treatment declines with each failed treatment trial
Younger or older patient	No clinically significant difference between younger adults and elderly patients in the rate of improvement
Second-line choices	Wide variety of second-line antidepressants available when the individual does not respond to a selective serotonin reuptake inhibitor. These include venlafaxine, serotonin and norepinephrine reuptake inhibitors, or tricyclic antidepressants
Increasing dose	Lack of direct evidence for the efficacy of increasing the dose after initial treatment non-response

Table 7.6 (cont.)

Presentation	Key statements on second-line treatment
Switching antidepressants, including to the same class,	Associated with a wide range of response rates in different studies (12–70%)
Augmentation	Best evidence is for quetiapine, aripiprazole, risperidone, and lithium

Table 7.7 Key statements on medication treatments when there is medication resistance (non-response)

Presentation	Key statements on medication options when there is treatment resistance
Further augmentation strategies	Maudsley Guidelines (Taylor et al. 2021) provide the evidence for various augmentation strategies as first choice (lithium, olanzapine, quetiapine, bupropion, or mirtazapine) and second-line choices in refractory depression (ketamine, lamotrigine, buspirone, high dose venlafaxine, electro-convulsive-therapy (ECT), triiodothyronine, and risperidone)

Medication Treatments and Comorbid Illness

Many people with intellectual disability also have other medical illnesses (NICE, Clinical Guideline 91, 2009). Table 7.8 provides advice about prescribing for people with comorbid illness or chronic physical health problems.

Treatment Algorithms

In addition to the algorithm in the *Oxford Textbook for Intellectual Disability*, the Maudsley Guidelines provides algorithms, the National institute for Health and Care Excellence provides treatment algorithms, and the APA provides three algorithms:

- www.apa.org/depression-guideline/decision-aid-children-adolescents.pdf
- www.apa.org/depression-guideline/decision-aid-adults.pdf
- www.apa.org/depression-guideline/decision-aid-older-adults.pdf

Figure 7.2 provides a short algorithm drawn from the evidence base which can serve as a guide to the reader in their clinical decision making, in addition to the aforementioned texts.

Treatment of the individual with depression introduced in Case Study 7.1 is discussed in Case Study 7.2 to contextualise the information regarding treatment provided in the foregoing sections.

How Long Should Treatment Continue?

Since the launch of the Stopping Over-Medication of People with a Learning Disability (STOMP) programme (NHS England, 2016), there has been additional focus on providing clarity about how long treatments should continue.

Table 7.8 Key statements on antidepressant treatments with comorbid illness

Presentation	Key statements on antidepressant treatments with comorbid illness
Effectiveness	Antidepressants have small to moderate effects in people with comorbid medical illness
Choice of antidepressant	Should be guided by side-effect profile and potential for interaction with medication for other conditions
Different medical conditions	No evidence of a differential effect of antidepressants
Co-administered with aspirin/non-steroidal anti-inflammatory drugs	SSRIs modestly increase the risk of upper gastrointestinal bleeding
Myocardial infarction (MI)	Tricyclic antidepressants may be associated with an increased risk
Cardiovascular events following myocardial infarction	SSRIs, mirtazapine, and bupropion do not generally increase the risk
Epilepsy	SSRIs: fluoxetine is not the best choice due to its long half-life, a possibly greater incidence of seizures, and an increased risk of medication interactions
Hepatic impairment	Take into account the patient's reduced liver function and concomitant medications. For patients with chronic liver disease and hepatitis C, SSRIs appear to be the safest class of antidepressants
Renal impairment	Observational studies as well as small trials suggest that certain SSRIs may be safe to use in patients with advanced chronic kidney disease and end-stage renal disease. First choice sertraline requires no dose adjustment, but active metabolite is renally excreted. Alternative: fluoxetine
Diabetes	Sertraline, escitalopram, and fluoxetine; avoid tricyclic antidepressants and monoamine oxidase inhibitors

Most guidelines recommend that for people at low risk of relapse (e.g., first-episode patients without other risk factors) the duration of treatment should be at least 6–9 months after full remission.

For people who have remitted from depression when treated with antidepressant medication alone, but who have been assessed as being at higher risk of relapse, consider:

- continuing with their antidepressant medication for up to two years to prevent relapse
- maintaining the same dose unless there is good reason to reduce it (such as side effects)
- a course of CBT for people who do not wish to continue on antidepressant treatment
- or continuing with their antidepressant medication and a course of psychological therapy

Although there are no studies in intellectual disability of how long people remain on antidepressants, studies of the general population suggest that people are currently remaining on antidepressant treatment for longer. This is thought to be the main reason why antidepressant prescriptions have increased with treatment duration, roughly doubling every 10 years in the general population (Kendrick et al. 2021).

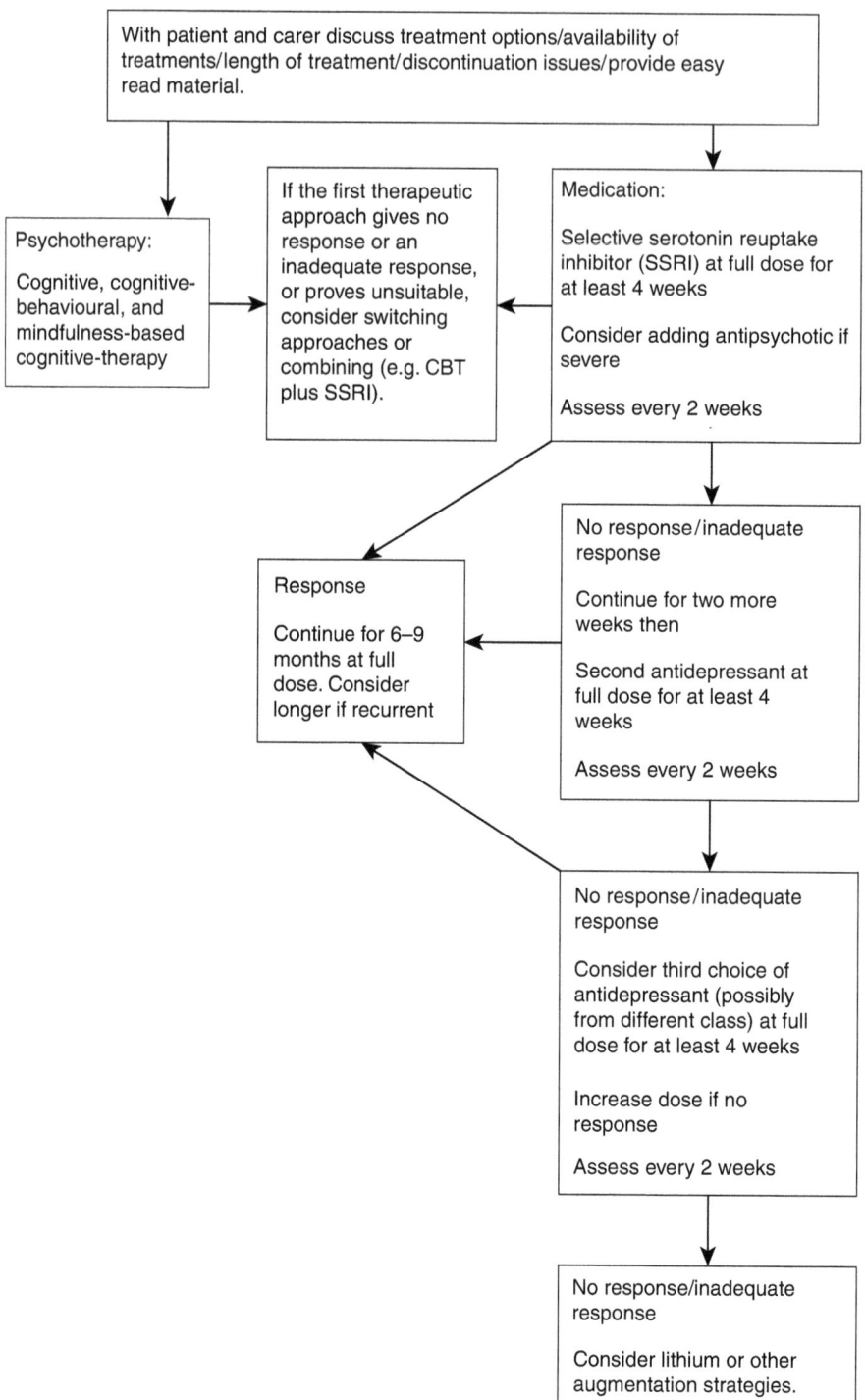

Figure 7.2 Depression treatment algorithm

Case Study 7.2: Treatment

For treatment of moderate depressive illness, the guidelines recommend a combination of antidepressant and psychological intervention. However, due to Amina's communication difficulties, it was not possible to offer psychological therapy. Amina, with the support of her parents and carers, was provided with information regarding antidepressant treatment, available in easy-read format, to enable her to make an informed choice. Due to her comorbid diagnosis of epilepsy, SSRI and monoamine oxidase inhibitors were the preferred choices. She was subsequently commenced on a low dose of sertraline. Community nurses were involved in her care to monitor her mood and any side effects of the medication, perform ongoing risk assessment, and implement supportive and positive behaviour strategies to help her, as well as educate her family and carers, about depressive disorders. Amina tolerated sertraline and there were no side effects; this was gradually increased to a therapeutic dose with positive therapeutic effect.

Stopping Antidepressant Medication

Prior to 2019, although problems with discontinuation of antidepressants was well documented, the withdrawal of antidepressants was not generally considered a major problem. Most guidelines recommended a relatively fast withdrawal and reassurance when problems emerged. However, increasing concern about problems associated with antidepressant discontinuation have led to changes to guidance.

If a person taking antidepressant medication stops taking it abruptly, miss doses, or does not take a full dose, they may have withdrawal symptoms (see Table 7.9).

Withdrawal symptoms can be mild, appear within a few days of reducing or stopping antidepressant medication, and go away within 1–2 weeks. However, they can last longer (in some cases, several weeks, and occasionally several months) and can sometimes be severe, particularly if the antidepressant medication is stopped suddenly.

People may need support to withdraw successfully, particularly if previous attempts have led to withdrawal symptoms or have not been successful.

If a person wants to stop taking antidepressant medication it is usually necessary to reduce the dose in stages over time, but most people do stop antidepressants successfully.

When stopping a person's antidepressant medication, ensure that the speed and duration of withdrawal is led by and agreed with the person taking the prescribed medication, and ensure that any withdrawal symptoms have resolved before making the next dose reduction.

If a person has more severe withdrawal symptoms, consider restarting the original antidepressant medication at the previous dose, and then attempt dose reduction at a slower rate with smaller decrements after symptoms have resolved.

The individual with intellectual disability and depression discussed in Case Studies 7.1 and 7.2 is followed up in Case Study 7.3, which focuses on stopping the antidepressant.

Table 7.9 Withdrawal symptoms associated with antidepressants

- restlessness or agitation
- problems sleeping
- altered feelings (e.g., suicidal thoughts, irritability, anxiety, low mood tearfulness, panic attacks, irrational fears, or confusion)
- unsteadiness, vertigo, or dizziness
- sweating
- abdominal symptoms (e.g., nausea)
- altered sensations (e.g., electric shock sensations)
- palpitations, tiredness, headaches, and aches in joints and muscles

Case Study 7.3: Stopping the Antidepressant

With support and encouragement from her carers, Amina was compliant with her medication and made gradual progress. After about 2–3 months, she was noted to appear a bit brighter in mood and was less withdrawn. She began to engage in activities within the home, though she still refused to attend the day centre. She mostly accepted her meals and ate more food from her dinner plate. Her emotional and verbal outbursts persisted. However, with continued support from the community nurses and her family and carers, Amina made a steady recovery over the subsequent year; she was reported to have settled well into the care home and was engaging well with all her activities, including attending the day centre.

Sertraline was continued for another year with no relapse. A multidisciplinary meeting that included Amina, her family, carers, and professionals was held to consider stopping the antidepressant.

The dose of sertraline was reduced very slowly and Amina was monitored for any signs of relapse or discontinuation symptoms. Following the initial reduction in the dose of sertraline, Amina developed mild withdrawal symptoms, which included sweating, some restlessness, and disturbed sleep; however, these were not distressing enough to necessitate reinstating the antidepressant dose. Time was given for these symptoms to subside before attempting a further slow reduction in dose, which Amina was fortunately able to tolerate. By the end of the following year, Amina had been completely weaned off sertraline with no evidence of relapse.

The Frith Prescribing Guidelines Editors' Expert Group Consensus Statements

Statements of High Confidence

Although the results from studies vary, it is likely that the prevalence of depression is at least as high in the intellectual disability population as in the general population.

The following principles of depression management from the general population apply to people with intellectual disability as well:

- Offering an initial choice between psychotherapy and pharmacotherapy, although access to psychotherapies may be limited for people with intellectual disability. Materials in easy-read formats are referenced in this chapter.

- For those that do not respond to the initial choice of therapy after 4–6 weeks, switch to an alternative psychotherapy or pharmacotherapy.
- SSRIs are the first antidepressants of choice.

In many parts of England, antidepressants have become the most widely prescribed psychotropic for people with intellectual disability.

Statements of Medium Confidence

Modified cognitive behavioural therapy may be a feasible and effective approach for the treatment of depression, anxiety, and other mood disorders in people with intellectual disability.

As in the general population, when withdrawing antidepressants it is usually necessary to reduce the dose in stages over time, but most people stop antidepressants successfully.

Statements of Low Confidence

For people with intellectual disability:

- Many patients with depression may not meet the diagnostic criteria detailed in DSM-5 or DM-ID
- Onset of depression tends to be more insidious and the changes less dramatic than in the general population, and symptoms are often attributed to the intellectual disability or onset of dementia
- Anxiety (a frequent comorbid symptom) may be expressed in the form of avoidance behaviour or autonomic features which are situation specific

Resource Box

Easy-Read Documents
What is Depression? https://leep1.co.uk/easy-read-resources/
  Choice and medication. www.choiceandmedication.org

Key Guidelines
National Institute for Health and Care Excellence (2009) Guidance for the treatment of depression in adults with chronic physical health problems (CG91). www.nice.org.uk/guidance/cg91.

British Association for Psychopharmacology (2015) Evidence-based guidelines for treating depressive disorders with antidepressants: A revision of the 2008 guidelines. www.bap.org.uk/pdfs/BAP_Guidelines-Antidepressants.pdf.

American Psychological Association (2019) Clinical practice guideline for the treatment of depression across three age cohorts: Recommendations for the general adult population from the APA Guideline Development Panel for the Treatment of Depression. www.apa.org/depression-guideline.

National Institute for Health and Care Excellence (2016) Guidance NG54: Mental health problems in people with learning disabilities: prevention, assessment, and management. www.nice.org.uk/guidance/ng54.

Taylor, D. M., Barnes, T. R. and Young, A. H. (2021). *The Maudsley prescribing guidelines in psychiatry*. John Wiley & Sons.

References

Aman, M., & Singh, N. (1988) Patterns of drug use, methodological consideration, measurement techniques, and future trends. In M. Aman and N. Singh (eds.), *Psychopharmacology of developmental disabilities* (pp. 1–29). Springer Verlag

American Psychiatric Association (2013). *Diagnostic and statistical manual of mental disorders (DSM-5 ®)*. 5th ed. American Psychiatric Association Publishing.

American Psychological Association (2019) Clinical practice guideline for the treatment of depression across three age cohorts: Recommendations for the general adult population from the APA Guideline Development Panel for the Treatment of Depression. www.apa.org/depression-guideline.

Beail, N., Warden, S., Morsley, K., & Newman, D. (2005). Naturalistic evaluation of the effectiveness of psychodynamic psychotherapy with adults with intellectual disabilities. *Journal of Applied Research in Intellectual Disabilities*, **18**(3), 245–51.

Bhaumik, S. & Alexander, R. eds. (2020). *Oxford textbook of the psychiatry of intellectual disability*. Oxford University Press.

Bhaumik, S., Branford, D., Naik, B. I. & Biswas, A. B. (2000) A retrospective audit of selective serotonin re-uptake inhibitors (fluoxetine and paroxetine) for the treatment of depressive episodes in adults with learning disability. *British Journal of Developmental Disabilities*, **46**, 131–9.

Bhaumik, S., Gangadharan, S., Hiremath, A., & Russell, P. (2011) Psychological treatments in disorders of intellectual development: The challenges of building a good evidence base. *British Journal of Psychiatry*, **198**(6), 428–30. https://doi.org/10.1192/bjp.bp.110.085084

Bhaumik, S., & Alexander, R. (2020) *Oxford textbook of the psychiatry of disorders of intellectual development*. Oxford University Press.

British Association for Psychopharmacology (2015) Evidence-based guidelines for treating depressive disorders with antidepressants: A revision of the 2008 guidelines. www.bap.org.uk/pdfs/BAP_Guidelines-Antidepressants.pdf.

Cooney, P., Jackman, C., Tunney, C., Coyle, D. & O'Reilly, G. (2018) Computer-assisted cognitive behavioural therapy: The experiences of adults who have an Disorders of intellectual development and anxiety or depression. *Journal of Applied Research in Intellectual Disabilities*, Nov; **31**(6), 1032–1045. https://doi.org/10.1111/jar.12459. Epub 2018 May 3. PMID: 29722919.

Cooper, S., Smiley, E., Morrison, J., Williamson, A., & Allan, L. (2007). An epidemiological investigation of affective disorders with a population-based cohort of 1023 adults with intellectual disabilities. *Psychological Medicine*, **37**(6), 873–82.

Digital NHS (2021). Health and Care of People with Learning Disabilities Experimental Statistics 2019 to 2020. www.gov.uk/government/statistics/health-and-care-of-people-with-learning-disabilities-experimental-statistics-2020-to-2021.

Glover, G., Williams, R., Branford, D., et al. (2015) *Prescribing of psychotropic drugs to people with learning disabilities and/or autism by general practitioners in England*. Public Health England

Howland, R. H. (1992) Fluoxetine treatment of depression in mentally retarded adults. *Journal of Nervous and Mental Disease*, **180**, 202–5.

Jahoda, A., Hastings, R., Hatton, C., et al. (2017) Comparison of behavioural activation with guided self-help for treatment of depression in adults with intellectual disabilities: a randomised controlled trial. *Lancet Psychiatry*, Dec; **4**(12), 909–19. https://doi.org/10.1016/S2215-0366(17)30426-1. Epub 2017 Nov 16. PMID: 29153873; PMCID: PMC5714593.

Jones, J., Blinkhorn, A., McQueen, M., et al. (2021) The adaptation and feasibility of dialectical behaviour therapy for adults with intellectual developmental disabilities and transdiagnoses: A pilot community-based randomized controlled trial. *Journal of Applied Research in Intellectual Disabilities*,

2021 May; 34(3), 805–17. https://doi.org/10.1111/jar.12860. Epub 2021 Feb 17. PMID: 33599087.

Kendrick, T. (2021) Strategies to reduce use of antidepressants. *British Journal of Clinical Pharmacology Themed Issue: Avoiding Harm from Over-Prescribing*, **87**(1), 23–33

Langee, H. R. & Conlon, M. (1992) Predictors of response to antidepressant medications. *American Journal of Mental Retardation*, **97**, 65–70.

McNair, L., Woodrow, C., & Hare, D. (2017) Dialectical behaviour therapy [DBT] with people with intellectual disabilities: A systematic review and narrative analysis. *Journal of Applied Research in Intellectual Disabilities*, Sep; **30**(5), 787–804. https://doi.org/10.1111/jar.12277. Epub 2016 Jul 26. PMID: 27456814.

Mehta, H., & Glover, G. (2019). *Psychotropic drugs and people with learning disabilities or autism*. Public Health England.

National Institute for Health and Care Excellence (2022), NICE Guideline 222: *Depression in adults: Treatment and management*. Published 29 June 2022. www.nice.org.uk/guidance/ng222/chapter/Recommendations#choice-of-treatments.

National Institute for Health and Care Excellence (2009) Guidance for the treatment of depression in adults with chronic physical health problems (CG91). www.nice.org.uk/guidance/cg91.

NHS Digital (2021) Health and Care of People with Learning Disabilities Experimental Statistics 2020 to 2021. https://digital.nhs.uk/data-and-information/publications/statistical/health-and-care-of-people-with-learning-disabilities/experimental-statistics-2020-to-2021/prescribing.

NHS England (2016) Stopping Over-Medication of People with a Learning Disability (STOMPLD) Pledge. www.england.nhs.uk/learning-disabilities/improving-health/stomp/.

Rai, P., & Kerr, M. (2010) Antidepressant use in adults with disorders of intellectual development. *The Psychiatrist*, **34**(4), 123–6. https://doi.org/10.1192/pb.bp.108.023325

Richards, M., Maughan, B., Hardy, R., et al. Long-term affective disorder in people with mild learning disability. *British Journal of Psychiatry* 2001 Dec; **179**, 523–7.

Royal College of Psychiatrists (2001). *DC LD: Diagnostic criteria for psychiatric disorders for use with adults with learning disabilities/mental retardation*, London, Royal College of Psychiatrists, Occasional Paper OP 48.

Fletcher, R., Loschen, E., Stavrakaki, C. & First, M. (2007). *DM-ID: diagnostic manual – intellectual disability: A textbook of diagnosis of mental disorders in persons with intellectual disability*. National Association for the Dually Diagnosed.

Rush, A. J., Fava, M., Wisniewski, S. R., et al. (2004) Sequenced treatment alternatives to relieve depression (STAR*D): rationale and design. *Controlled Clinical Trials*, Feb;**25**(1), 119–42. https://doi.org/10.1016/s0197-2456(03)00112-0. PMID: 15061154.

Turky, A., Felce, D. J., Jones, G. & Kerr, M. P. (2011). A prospective case control study of psychiatric disorders in adults with epilepsy and disorders of intellectual development. *Epilepsia*, **52**(7), 1223–30. https://doi.org/10.1111/j.1528-1167.2011.03044.x.

Vereenooghe, L. & Langdon, PE. (2013) Psychological therapies for people with intellectual disabilities: a systematic review and meta-analysis. *Research in Developmental Disabilities*, Nov; **34**(11), 4085–102. https://doi.org/10.1016/j.ridd.2013.08.030. Epub 2013 Sep 18. PMID: 24051363.

Verhoeven, W. M. A., Veendrik-Meekes, M. J., Jacobs, G. A. J., van den Berg, Y. W. M. M. & Tuinier, S. (2001) Citalopram in mentally retarded patients with depression: a long-term clinical investigation. *European Psychiatry*, **16**, 104–8.

Chapter 8

Bipolar Disorders

Prabhleen Jaggi, David M. L. Branford, and Regi T. Alexander

Introduction

What Are Bipolar Disorders?

Bipolar disorders are episodic mood disorders defined by the occurrence of manic, mixed, or hypomanic episodes/symptoms. Manic and hypomanic symptoms are characterised by a subjective experience of increased energy and activity, along with various other symptoms. Episodes typically alternate over the course of the disorder, with depressive episodes or periods of depressive symptoms, such as lowering of mood and decreased energy and activity (International classification of diseases (ICD-11), 2019; American Psychiatric Association's *Diagnostic and Statistical Manual of Mental Disorders* (DSM-5), 2013).

Both the DSM-5 and the ICD-11 broadly subclassify the condition as follows:

Bipolar I disorder:

- One or more manic episodes or mixed episodes.
- Individuals often have one or more major depressive episodes.

Bipolar II disorder:

- One or more major depressive episodes accompanied by at least one hypomanic episode.

How Common Are Bipolar Disorders?

In a *British Medical Journal* state-of-the-art review, Goes (2023) stated that bipolar disorders are recurrent and chronic disorders of mood that affect around 2% of the world's population.

In the context of intellectual disability, Cooper (2007) proposed that the prevalence rates for bipolar mania are between 3% and 4%, and bipolar disorder with depression are 0.1–0.5%, varying with diagnostic criteria and methods used, such as ICD-10, DSM-IV, DC-LD: Diagnostic Criteria for Psychiatric Disorders for Use with Adults with Learning Disabilities/Mental Retardation (2001), or clinical judgement. Cooper also proposed that depression has a higher prevalence in intellectual disability than in the general population, suggesting it is more enduring and undertreated.

In a 2018 paper, Cooper proposed that mania appears to occur at a considerably higher incidence in adults with intellectual disability than in the general population; this finding has not been previously reported as far as we are aware. Both these findings are further surprising, given the high proportion of the population who were taking mood stabilisers (mostly as anti-seizure medications for epilepsy).

How Is Bipolar Illness Different in People with Intellectual Disability?

Diagnosis of bipolar disorder in people with intellectual disability can be challenging due to limitations in communication skills, the influence of poor physical and social circumstances, and a general lack of suitable diagnostic criteria. In addition, differences in presenting symptoms (such as changes in behaviour) and the need to rely on observable symptoms (rather than the person being able to articulate their inner mental state) add to the diagnostic challenge. It may be difficult for carers/informants to distinguish mood symptoms from those which may arise as a consequence of developmental disability and/or from learned behaviours (Moss et al. 1998). Thus, the overall prevalence in this population may not be accurately estimated.

In a retrospective case study, Cain et al. (2003) stated that bipolar disorder can be recognised and distinguished from other behavioural and psychiatric diagnoses in individuals with intellectual disability and that DSM-IV criteria can be useful in the diagnosis of bipolar disorder. Matson et al. (2007) suggested that psychomotor agitation, decreased sleep, changes in mood, and aggression were significantly related to a diagnosis of mania. Observable behaviour, such as irritability, hyperactivity, and responses to environmental stimuli, can help in identification of a bipolar state (Valdovinos, 2019). Behaviours seen as challenging are the most commonly reported feature in patients with intellectual disability who are distressed, therefore such behaviour in itself has limited value as a specific indicator for bipolar disorder (Bertelli et al. 2022).

Other behavioural equivalents of mania in intellectual disability that have been suggested are excessive smiling, enthusiastic greeting of everyone, being easily provoked to scream or swear, and increased sexual behaviour, along with pacing and an increase in motor activity (Lowry 1998). Additionally, it has been noted that for adults with severe and profound intellectual disability, signs such as decreased need for sleep, restlessness, agitation, and irritability are associated with mania (Sturmey et al. 2010).

Mood is less likely to be euphoric or infectious and more likely to be irritable and accompanied at times by aggression. While pressure of speech may be present, more complex verbal symptoms such as flight of ideas or clang associations are rare. Grandiose ideas and delusions are usually in a simple form, and hallucinations are rare. Rapid cycling bipolar disorder (four or more episodes of affective illness in a year) is associated with severe behaviours seen as challenging in individuals with intellectual disability, particularly self-injurious behaviour (Bhaumik et al. 2015).

Screening Tools for the Psychopathology of Bipolar Disorder in People with Intellectual Disability

- Diagnostic Assessment for the Severity Handicapped-Revised (DASH-II) (Matson, 1997, 2007): an informant-based screening tool to assess psychopathology of individuals with severe and profound intellectual disability. The tool has 84 items, of which the following items are significant predictors of mania:

- Item 9. Restless or agitated
- Item 16. Decreased need for sleep
- Item 19. Wake frequently during night
- Item 26. Is cranky or irritable
- Item 39. Difficulty getting to sleep

- Parent version of the Young Mania Rating Scale (P-YMRS) (Matson, 2007, Youngstrom et al. 2003): based on the Young Mania Rating Scale, which is the most widely used tool for assessment in the general population, the Parent version of the Young Mania Rating Scale was originally developed to assess symptoms of bipolar disorder in youths based on ratings by their parents. A study of 45 patients with severe or profound intellectual disability with bipolar disorder and other psychiatric disorders found that 4 of the 11 items of the Parent version of the Young Mania Rating Scale directly assess symptoms easily identifiable by informants in people with more severe intellectual disability, and these items correspond with the DSM-IV criteria for mania (Matson, 2007). These items are elevated mood, motor activity, decreased need for sleep, and disruptive-aggressive behaviour.
- The Psychiatric Assessment Schedule for Adults with Developmental Disabilities Checklist (PAS-ADD Checklist) (Taylor, 2004): a screening instrument designed to help carers recognise likely mental health problems in people with intellectual disability. It helps assess symptoms across seven broad areas, including depression and hypomania. A study of 356 service users found high internal consistency in the sub-scales of affective/neurotic disorders (Matson 1998).

Case Study 8.1

Liam is a 21-year-old man with moderate intellectual disability. He lives with his parents and on weekdays attends college where he takes part in cooking classes and activities such as painting and horse-riding. While at home, Liam loves reading comics of his favourite super-heroes and helping in the kitchen.

Over a week, the staff at the day centre have noticed that Liam, who is usually reserved, has been disruptive and argumentative while participating in activities with other service users. On one occasion, Liam had to be removed from the painting class when he started to paint on the canvas of a fellow service user after having finished working on his own, causing the person much distress. At home, mum and dad have also observed Liam being more energetic than usual, waking up a couple of hours earlier, and always insisting on always wearing his favourite Spider-Man t-shirt. Although Liam's parents note these changes and the reports from the day centre, they think it is just a passing phase.

Over the next few days Liam appears increasingly agitated, shouting loudly and aggressively several times a day. He doesn't sleep for more than a couple of hours at night and has been trying to climb the walls and furniture at his home. Fearing for his safety, his parents reach out to his community mental health team. After psychiatric review, Liam is deemed to require admission for assessment to a mental health ward under section 2 of the Mental Health Act 1983. His father informs the treating clinical team that his sister was diagnosed with bipolar disorder in her twenties.

Following a comprehensive assessment, Liam is diagnosed with an episode of acute mania, and medication treatment is initiated in the mental health in-patient unit.

Evidence for Medication Treatment for Acute Mania in Intellectual Disability

At the time of writing, the authors were unable to source any studies on the pharmacological treatment of acute mania specifically for people with intellectual disability without other co-occurring neurodevelopmental disorders and aggression. However, various controlled trials and meta-analyses from the last four decades that have informed most treatment guidelines for the general population advocate the use of mood stabilisers, antipsychotics, or a combination of both.

General Recommendations for Treatment of Bipolar Disorder

Effective medication treatment for bipolar disorder, like any other mental health disorder, is dependent on the accuracy of its diagnosis; this is especially true in people with intellectual disability where there exist several challenges in diagnosis, such as limitations in communication and lack of suitable diagnostic criteria. Moreover, behaviours seen as challenging and neurodevelopmental conditions such as autism and attention deficit hyperactivity disorder (ADHD) are more common in people with intellectual disability, which may lead to misdiagnosis of mental health disorders (including bipolar disorder) due to diagnostic overshadowing arising from similarities in their presentation (Bertelli et al. 2022).

Effective treatment for bipolar disorder also relies on a therapeutic alliance between the clinician and the patient and carers. Apart from collaborating with the patient and the carers in medication-related treatment decisions which will include discussion of side effects, consideration of monitoring requirements, past adherence, and the experience and outcome of previous treatment(s), it is also necessary to discuss functional impairments and changes in sleep patterns. Where appropriate, the use of substances, for example cannabis and amphetamines, should also be discussed. The person with intellectual disability and their carers should also be educated about recognising emerging symptoms of manic or depressive episodes so that they know when to request early intervention (Goodwin et al. 2016).

Treatment of an Acute Manic Episode

Choice of medication for treatment of acute mania depends upon whether the person is currently taking medication for bipolar disorder or not. For a person not on medication, options include antipsychotics, mood stabilisers, or a combination of both. Most evidence recommends the use of second-generation antipsychotics such as risperidone or olanzapine as monotherapy or in combination, and valproate or lithium among mood stabilisers. When making this choice, prescribers should consider preferences for future prophylactic use and the side-effect profile. Prescribers should also consider:

- Prescribing an antipsychotic if there are severe manic symptoms or marked disturbances as part of the syndrome of mania.
- Prescribing valproate or lithium if symptoms have responded to these medications before and there has been good compliance with the medication and monitoring requirements.
- Avoiding valproate in people of childbearing potential. New MHRA regulations for sodium valproate came into force in the UK in 2024.
- Using lithium monotherapy in case of less-than-severe symptoms, as its onset of action is slower than valproate and antipsychotics.

- The person's likely compliance with medication monitoring, such as blood testing, which may not be easy in some people with intellectual disability.
- Short-term use of a benzodiazepine for initial management of acute behavioural disturbance or agitation in addition to the antimanic agent.

Monotherapy

- Second-generation (atypical) antipsychotics

Most atypical antipsychotics are effective in managing acute manic symptoms and preventing relapse; however, studies showing this are limited to prevention of manic episodes where the index episode was acute mania (Hayes 2016). They may be appropriate for the long-term management of bipolar patients, especially where non-mood-congruent psychotic features are prominent (Goodwin et al. 2016); however, their efficacy in prevention of depressive relapses is not well studied (Yatham et al. 2018).

Quetiapine as monotherapy or in combination with lithium or valproate has been found to be effective in prevention of relapse to either pole (Suppes et al. 2009); it has also been found to be particularly useful in managing mixed features (Vieta et al. 2012).

In some studies, olanzapine as monotherapy has shown a reduction in manic and depressive relapse (Vieta et al. 2012) and is an effective adjunct to lithium, but produces significant weight gain and adverse metabolic changes (Tohen 2006). Efficacy in prevention of depressive relapses is unknown.

- Lithium

Lithium has level 1 evidence for efficacy as well as tolerability and safety, and is considered the most effective long-term treatment for bipolar disorder (Yatham 2018; NICE 2020). Lithium is effective in preventing both manic and depressive episodes and has a degree of anti-suicidal effect. It should also be considered if there is an established family history of responsiveness to lithium in bipolar disorder. It has been reported useful for management of behaviours seen as challenging in people intellectual disability (Ali 2014).

Lithium therapy requires regular and frequent monitoring of serum-level concentrations as well as thyroid and kidney function, electrocardiography, and blood-electrolyte concentrations. Therefore, treatment with lithium must be carefully considered and discussed with the patients and/or carers, including whether its monitoring guidelines can be adhered to. Intermittent treatment with lithium can lead to worsening of the natural course of bipolar disorder, therefore lithium should not be initiated unless there is a clear intention to continue treatment for at least three years (Taylor 2021).

- Valproate

Meta-analyses and randomised controlled trials have found that there are no differences in efficacy between valproate (divalproex), quetiapine, and olanzapine in the maintenance treatment of bipolar disorder (Kessing et al. 2011). However, the BALANCE randomised open-label trial, which specifically compared valproate, lithium, and the combination, found lithium alone and in combination with valproate to be superior to valproate alone in reducing the rates of relapse in bipolar disorder (Geddes et al. 2009b).

Despite its established efficacy, valproate is recommended for use in the UK only when treatment with lithium alone does not produce desired results or is intolerable. The risk of foetal developmental malformations and adverse neurodevelopmental outcomes due to exposure during pregnancy with valproate are well known. In December 2022, the independent Commission on Human Medicines (CHM) advised that no person with childbearing potential should be prescribed valproate unless two specialists independently consider and document that there is no other effective or tolerated treatment and the Pregnancy Prevention Programme (PPP) is in place. In addition, the CHM has advised that no person under the age of 55 should be initiated on valproate unless no other treatment is deemed effective or tolerable by two independent specialists. The Medicines and Healthcare products Regulatory Agency (MHRA) updated its valproate prescription regulations to contraindicate valproate use in women/girls of childbearing age without restrictions (Watkins 2019).

Likewise, for people with intellectual disability, valproate should only be considered when they are on a PPP. Clinicians should be aware of the sexual lives and habits of people with intellectual disability and be mindful that people with intellectual disability are more prone to be subject to sexual violence and abuse. A recent United Kingdom investigation into use of valproate in women in the context of epilepsy that found that more than one-third of women using valproate had an intellectual disability and one-fifth could not consent to a sexual relationship. In one in three patients, valproate treatment did not comply with the MHRA regulations (Watkins 2019).

Valproate also requires regular monitoring of blood cell counts and liver function. Therefore, its use in people with intellectual disability may be limited to those patients who can adhere to frequent blood tests.

Combination Therapy with Antipsychotics

The risk of manic relapse is reduced when an antipsychotic is combined with lithium/valproate (Yatham et al. 2016). First-line adjunctive therapies include quetiapine with lithium or valproate (Suppes 2013, Vieta et al. 2012) and aripiprazole with lithium or valproate (Marcus 2011). Used in combination for the first six months following response offers clear benefit in preventing relapse, but benefits beyond this period of time remain uncertain. Therefore, clinicians should evaluate risks and benefits regularly to determine whether maintenance therapy in combination is justified.

Case Study 8.2

Julia is a 19-year-old woman with a mild intellectual disability who works in a charity shop. She has lived at her family home for most of her life. When she was 16, there were several short periods of less than two weeks when Julia was only sleeping for two hours a night, appeared excitable, was irritable with her family and talked loudly for long periods. She would leave home late in the evening with her friends and return in the early hours of the morning, and at times her parents could smell cigarette smoke and alcohol on her. Noting that this was out of character for their daughter, her parents contacted her general practitioner for help; however, by the time the GP's referral to the Child and Adolescent Mental Health Service (CAMHS) went through, Julia was back to her usual self and did not wish to seek treatment.

Three years later, when her younger brother left for college, Julia became withdrawn and appeared to lose interest in spending time with her family and friends. This continued for a number of weeks and her family persuaded her to seek help for her mental health. The treating team noted her previous referral to CAMHS. The team lead discussed the possibility of a bipolar illness and discussed various treatment options with Julia and her family. Julia chose lithium after understanding and agreeing to the frequent need for blood tests. She was also made aware of the risks associated with pregnancy and she agreed to take contraceptive injections. After lithium was started and optimised, Julia's mood stability improved. She regularly attended her GP appointments and underwent blood tests. Her lithium blood levels have remained steady between 0.5 and 0.7 mEq/l at a dose of 800 mg/day.

Medication Management of a Depressive Episode

Patients experiencing the first episode of bipolar depression are at risk of being misdiagnosed with major depressive disorder, especially if the episodes of hypomania or mania are particularly mild or do not require hospitalisation (Yatham 2018). This may be even more true in the case of people with intellectual disability where several diagnostic challenges exist, as explained in the previous sections. This distinction is important as the treatment would depend on whether the patient is receiving long-term treatment for bipolar disorder or not (Yatham 2018; Goodwin 2016). Most evidence recommends the use of quetiapine monotherapy and combinations of mood stabilisers, antipsychotics, and antidepressants.

Quetiapine

The effectiveness of quetiapine monotherapy in bipolar depression has been evidenced by a number of studies, including the Efficacy of Monotherapy Seroquel in BipOLar DEpressioN (EMBOLDEN) II study which compared it to paroxetine and placebo (McElroy 2010). Other studies have also found that quetiapine is effective in the attenuation of depressive symptoms in bipolar patients (Calabrese 2005; Thase 2006). Apart from its acute efficacy, quetiapine continuation is associated with fewer episodes of any polarity (Suppes 2013). Guidelines such as those by the Canadian Network for Mood and Anxiety Treatments and the British Association for Psychopharmacology recommend the first-line use of quetiapine in bipolar depression. However, metabolic adverse effects such as weight gain and significant increase in blood triglyceride levels necessitate regular monitoring which might not always be possible in people with intellectual disability. Sedation and somnolence are other adverse effects which may lead to treatment drop-out.

Lamotrigine

Lamotrigine has been found to have a modest benefit as monotherapy in bipolar depression (Geddes et al. 2009a); however, it has been found to be more effective in combination with quetiapine, lithium, or risperidone (Geddes et al. 2016). Additional benefits of lamotrigine include its efficacy in maintenance treatment, treatment of rapid cycling episodes (Bowden et al. 1999), and, in the context of intellectual disability, management of epilepsy.

Olanzapine and Fluoxetine

Olanzapine and fluoxetine (OFC) as a combination are approved by the FDA for the treatment of a depressive episode in bipolar I. Randomised controlled trials and meta-analyses show that combined olanzapine and fluoxetine has efficacy in treating bipolar depression (Detke et al. 2015; Bahji et al. 2020), and in the prevention of depressive relapse (Tohen et al. 2006). The National institute for Health and Care Excellence (NICE) guidelines recommend this combination as the first-line treatment for bipolar depression (NICE, 2020).

General Considerations for Maintenance Therapy

Bipolar disorder is understood to be a 'neuroprogressive' disease in which recurrences are associated with decrease in inter-episodic recovery, a higher rate and severity of relapse, and a reduced rate of treatment response. Therefore, maintenance treatment for bipolar disorder is required not only to prevent relapses and reduce residual symptoms, but also to minimise illness progression (Vieta et al. 2011; Malhi et al. 2013) which may be even more important in people with a developmental disability of the brain.

Apart from the need for concordance between the clinician's and the patient's/carers' views and a collaborative approach to treatment alliance, the prescriber needs to watch out for factors affecting non-adherence, comorbid substance use, and persistent subthreshold symptoms, all of which can increase the chances of a relapse (Yen 2016; Berk et al. 2010). Especially for long-term treatment, tolerability and safety become almost as important as efficacy (Grunze 2021).

Medications that have been found to be effective in the acute phase should be considered during the maintenance phase as most of them have prophylactic efficacy. Also, as the polarity of the index predicts the polarity of relapses, the acute phase medication is likely to be effective for prophylaxis (Popovic et al. 2012).

Treatment Recommendations for Long-Term Treatments

Tables 8.1 and 8.2 summarise long-term treatment options for bipolar I and II respectively.

Special Circumstances

- Carbamazepine has been found to be useful as monotherapy when patients do not respond to lithium or when the classical pattern of episodic euphoric mania is not observed (Goodwin et al. 2016).
- There is no specific treatment for rapid cycling. In such cases, underlying health conditions such as hypothyroidism or substance use may lead to the frequent episodes. These conditions should be identified and treated. Treatment with antidepressants can worsen the rapid cycling (Valentí et al. 2015).
- In patients with intellectual disability where non-compliance is an issue, long-acting injectable preparations of second-generation antipsychotics such as aripiprazole and olanzapine can be used as prophylactics (Yatham et al. 2018).

Treatment-Refractory Bipolar Disorder

Treatment refractoriness may be related to non-adherence to medication, failure to optimise medication, effects of comorbidities such as substance use, or true resistance to pharmacotherapy. A comprehensive assessment is needed to ascertain the factors leading to treatment refractoriness (Yatham et al. 2018).

Relative or marked treatment resistance may occur in bipolar depression; this would mean lack of response to an antidepressant along with first-line agents e.g. quetiapine,

Table 8.1 For the long-term treatment of bipolar I

Monotherapy	Lithium, quetiapine, olanzapine
Combination	Aripiprazole + valproate

Table 8.2 For the long-term treatment of bipolar II

Monotherapy	Lithium, quetiapine, lamotrigine
Combination	Olanzapine + fluoxetine

olanzapine, lamotrigine, either singly or in combination. Electroconvulsive therapy maybe an option in such cases, especially when there is high risk of suicide or other risks due to inanition (Goodwin et al. 2016; Bhaumik et al. 2015).

How Long Should Treatment Continue?

Bipolar disorder is understood to be a life-long condition, therefore the preferred management strategy in the general population is to prevent relapses with continuous treatment. Stopping medication presents risks of relapse towards either polarity. This may be especially true for some mood stabilisers, stopping which can lead to a relapse of mania (Goodwin et al. 2016). More recently, NICE has recommended the staged withdrawal of antidepressants and to make reductions in doses only when withdrawal symptoms from previous dose decreases are resolved (Iacobucci 2023). For people with intellectual disability, this treatment strategy presents the unique challenges explained in earlier sections; however, relapse prevention should be aimed for by continuing the fewest number of medications to minimise their long-term effects.

Stopping Medication for Bipolar Disorder

Since the launch of the Stopping Over-Medication of People with a Learning Disability (STOMP) programme (NHS England, 2016), there has been increased focus on providing clarity about how long treatments should continue. When considering the aforementioned recommendations on life-long treatment for bipolar disorder, an additional key consideration for people with intellectual disability is accuracy of diagnosis. In some cases, a past history of fluctuant mood in a person with intellectual disability that has been labelled as bipolar disorder may be open to re-examination if that presentation could be better explained by a previously undiagnosed neurodevelopmental disorder (autism or ADHD). Caution is needed, however, as dual diagnosis is of course more than possible in this patient group.

The issue of stopping individual medications is covered in Chapter 2.

People with Comorbid Medical Illness

Many people with intellectual disability also have other medical conditions (Cooper et al. 2015). Table 8.3 provides advice about prescribing for people with comorbid illness or chronic physical health problems.

Table 8.3 Key statements on mood stabiliser treatments with comorbid illness

Presentation	Key statements
Co-administered with aspirin/NSAIDs	Non-steroidal anti-inflammatory agents may increase lithium toxicity
	Aspirin may inhibit metabolism of valproate
Myocardial infarction (MI)	Risk of QT interval prolongation with some antipsychotics
Cardiovascular events following myocardial infarction	ACE inhibitors and thiazide diuretics may increase lithium toxicity.
	Risk of QT interval prolongation with some antipsychotics

Table 8.3 (cont.)

Presentation	Key statements
Epilepsy	Some antidepressants may impact on seizure frequency
Hepatic impairment	Caution with some antipsychotics in severe hepatic impairment
Renal impairment	Renal toxicity with lithium Valproate is regarded as drug of choice in renal failure as it is metabolised in the liver and only 1% is excreted through the kidney. However, a reduced dose of valproate is recommended
Diabetes	Increased risk of diabetes with some bipolar medications. Olanzapine and clozapine cause weight gain and thus contribute to or worsen diabetes. Lithium can cause diabetes insipidus, a disease unrelated to diabetes mellitus. Studies have shown a correlation between bipolar disorder and diabetes mellitus, but it is unclear if this correlation is a part of common pathophysiological pathways, or if medication for bipolar disorder has negative effects on blood sugar regulation (Charles et al 2016)

Case Study 8.3: Issues with Long-Term Treatment and the Need for Monitoring

Arthur is a 62-year-old man with moderate intellectual disability. During his childhood he was observed to have focal seizures and was started on carbamazepine titrated up gradually to 800 mg/day. Since his twenties, he has lived in different supported living homes across the county and his care has changed hands as many times. However, he has been regular with his medication.

Records show that in the early 1990s, following a move to a new care home, Arthur had a period of increased behaviour seen as challenging, including damage to property, verbal and physical aggression, and decrease in hours slept at night. After assessment by the psychiatrist a provisional diagnosis of mania was made and Arthur was started on olanzapine; a few weeks later, his symptoms had subsided.

A decade ago, Arthur lost his mother, and his carers noted a prolonged period where he appeared disinterested in going for walks and playing football, activities that he had previously loved. He was also observed to be tearful and aloof. He was then started with 10 mg of citalopram by his GP while the olanzapine and the carbamazepine were continued.

Around his 60th birthday, Arthur was moved to a new placement as the home he was staying at shut down. Despite the change, he adjusted and settled in well. A few months ago, when new service users moved in, Arthur's carers observed he had become irritable and 'difficult.' He is seen avoiding watching TV in the living room and prefers to have his meals in his bedroom. When this is brought to the attention of the psychiatrist, an increase in the dose of citalopram is trialled. While an improvement in the level of interaction is noted by his carers, they also note he is more forgetful and clumsier.

During his personal care routine one day, Arthur loses awareness and slumps to the bathroom floor. Paramedics are called and Arthur is rushed to the accident and emergency department, where his serum sodium levels are found to be 114 mmol/L. He receives treatment for hyponatraemia and is discharged a few days later. During the subsequent review by the psychiatrist, it is found that not only he is receiving three psychotropic medications, but that no seizure episode has been recorded for more than 25 years. The psychiatrist reduces the dose of the citalopram and also requests an urgent review by neurology. Arthur's carbamazepine is subsequently reduced, and he is also prescribed short-term sodium supplements. Regular reviews from both psychiatry and neurology are carried out, along with monthly blood tests to monitor his blood sodium levels which are now around 130 mmol/L.

Arthur's example shows the complexities in the management of mental health symptoms in intellectual disability and physical health disorders and how they can lead to over-medication and adverse effects. Arthur was started on mental health medication when he displayed behaviours associated with mania. However, it may be possible that these behaviours were a reaction to environmental changes or a manifestation of as-yet undiagnosed neurodevelopmental conditions. While the course of his history shows discrete episodes of mood fluctuations associated with bipolar disorder, there are indications that these mood changes could have resulted from life-events and changing environments. At these times, behavioural analyses and psychotherapeutic interventions could have complimented or been used instead of medication, especially following the bereavement. While medication may be necessary for mood changes, the NICE guidelines for medication optimisation in people with intellectual disability advocate their use only when psychological and other non-pharmacological interventions have not been effective.

In Arthur's case, the use of citalopram should have been preceded by such interventions and accompanied by blood tests as hyponatraemia is a recognised adverse effect when SSRIs are used with carbamazepine. Carbamazepine, which was started in childhood, was continued unreviewed for several years despite Arthur being seizure-free. This highlights the need for regular review of all medication by the prescriber regarding their indication and doses.

The Frith Prescribing Guidelines Editors' Expert Group Consensus Statements

Statements of High Confidence

The lack of studies of treatments for bipolar disorder in people with intellectual disability make it impossible to make specific recommendations; hence, the recommendations below are based on a strong evidence base in the non-intellectual disability population.

Atypical antipsychotic medications, and, where appropriate valproate, are the first-choice medications both in the acute phase and for long-term treatment in the general population and those with intellectual disability.

Most guidelines propose:

- Offering monotherapy for treatment of acute symptoms
- Those that do not respond to the initial choice of therapy after 4–6 weeks should switch to a different medication or combination therapy

For bipolar depression, quetiapine is effective in the attenuation of depressive symptoms. Lamotrigine is found to be effective in combination with quetiapine.

Statements of Medium Confidence
Mania appears to occur at a considerably higher incidence in adults with intellectual disability than in the general population.

Statements of Low Confidence
Behaviours seen as challenging are the most common presentation in people with intellectual disability who are distressed; therefore, this presentation in itself has limited value as a specific indicator for bipolar disorder.

Psychomotor agitation, decreased sleep, changes in mood, and aggression were significantly related to the diagnosis of mania in people with intellectual disability.

Resource Box

Key Guidelines

BAP_Guidelines: Bipolar: www.bap.org.uk/pdfs/BAP_Guidelines-Bipolar.pdf

Clinical Practice Guidelines for Management of Bipolar Disorder – PMC: www.ncbi.nlm.nih.gov/pmc/articles/PMC5310104/

2020 NICE Bipolar guidelines CG185 update: full text available here: www.nice.org.uk/guidance/CG185

Medscape: www.medscape.co.uk/viewarticle/bipolar-disorder-assessment-and-management-2022a10018nh

2023: April BMJ review article on Bipolar Disorder: www.bmj.com/content/381/bmj-2022-073591.abstract

2021: IDD-MH Prescriber guidelines for Bipolar Disorder in IDD. This guideline, from THE Centre for START services, Canada: https://centerforstartservices.org/IDD-MH-Prescribing-Guidelines/bipolar

Easy-Read Documents

Choice and Medication: www.choiceandmedication.org

From Norfolk County Council: https://brochure.norfolkslivingwell.org.uk/download/product/1345/downloads/Bipolar%20disorder%20-%20easy%20read%20201606.pdf

MindEd for families: https://mindedforfamilies.org.uk/Content/bipolar_disorder/course/assets/6fcc285eb8afe8a9714a676338d7b6939c62ccba.pdf

Leicestershire Partnership Trust: https://peterbates.org.uk/wp-content/uploads/2017/12/Bipolar-2.pdf

Health Awareness Group Devon: https://peterbates.org.uk/wp-content/uploads/2017/12/Bipolar-3.doc

2gether NHS Foundation Trust: https://peterbates.org.uk/wp-content/uploads/2017/12/Bipolar-1.pdf

References

Ali, A., Blickwedel, J., & Hassiotis, A. (2014) Interventions for challenging behaviour in intellectual disability, *Advances in Psychiatric Treatment: Cambridge University Press*, 20(3), 184–92. https://doi.org/10.1192/apt.bp.113.011577.

American Psychiatric Association (2013). *Diagnostic and statistical manual of mental disorders: DSM-5*. American Psychiatric Association.

Bahji, A., Ermacora, D., Stephenson, C., Hawken, E. R., & Vazquez, G. (2020) Comparative efficacy and tolerability of pharmacological treatments for the treatment of acute bipolar depression: A systematic review and network meta-analysis, *Journal of Affective Disorders*, 269, 154–84. https://doi.org/10.1016/j.jad.2020.03.030.

Berk, L., Hallam, K. T., Colom, F., et al. (2010). Enhancing medication adherence in patients with bipolar disorder. *Human Psychopharmacology: Clinical and Experimental*, 25(1), 1–16.

Bertelli, M. O., Deb, S., Munir, K., Hassiotis, A., & Salvador-Carulla, L. (2022) *Textbook of psychiatry for intellectual disability and autism spectrum disorder*. Springer.

Bhaumik, S., Gangadharan, S., Branford, D., & Barrett, M. (2015) *The Frith prescribing guidelines for people with intellectual disability*. John Wiley & Sons, Ltd.

Bowden, C. L. et al. (1999) 'The efficacy of lamotrigine in rapid cycling and non-rapid cycling patients with bipolar disorder', *Biological Psychiatry*, 45(8), 953–8. https://doi.org/10.1016/s0006-3223(99)00013-x.

Cain, N. N., Davidson, P. W., Burhan, A. M., et al. (2003) Identifying bipolar disorders in individuals with intellectual disability, *Journal of Intellectual Disability Research*, 47(1), 31–8. https://doi.org/10.1046/j.1365-2788.2003.00458.x.

Calabrese, J. R., Keck, P. E., Macfadden, W., et al. (2005) A randomized, double-blind, placebo-controlled trial of quetiapine in the treatment of bipolar I or II depression, *American Journal of Psychiatry*, 162(7), 1351–60. https://doi.org/10.1176/appi.ajp.162.7.1351.

Charles, E. F., Lambert, C. G., & Kerner, B. (2016) Bipolar disorder and diabetes mellitus: evidence for disease-modifying effects and treatment implications. *International Journal of Bipolar Disorder*, Dec; 4(1), 13. https://doi.org/10.1186/s40345-016-0054-4. Epub 2016 Jul 7. PMID: 27389787; PMCID: PMC4936996.

Cooper, S. A., McLean, G., Guthrie, B., et al. (2015). Multiple physical and mental health comorbidity in adults with intellectual disabilities: population-based cross-sectional analysis. *BMC Family Practice*, 16, 1–11.

Cooper, S.-A. et al. (2007) An epidemiological investigation of affective disorders with a population-based cohort of 1023 adults with intellectual disabilities, *Psychological Medicine*, 37(6), 873–82. https://doi.org/10.1017/s0033291707009968.

Cooper, S.-A., Smiley, E., Morrison, J., Williamson, A., & Allan, L. (2018) Incidence of unipolar and bipolar depression, and mania in adults with intellectual disabilities: Prospective cohort study, *British Journal of Psychiatry*, 212(5), 295–300. https://doi.org/10.1192/bjp.2018.12.

Detke, H. C., DelBello, M., Landry, J., & Usher, R. (2015) Olanzapine/fluoxetine combination in children and adolescents with bipolar I depression: A randomized, double-blind, placebo-controlled trial, *Journal of the American Academy of Child & Adolescent Psychiatry*, 54(3), 217–24. https://doi.org/10.1016/j.jaac.2014.12.012.

Geddes, J. R., Calabrese, J. R., & Goodwin, G. M. (2009a) Lamotrigine for treatment of Bipolar Depression: Independent meta-analysis and meta-regression of individual patient data from five randomised trials, *British Journal of Psychiatry*, 194(1), 4–9. https://doi.org/10.1192/bjp.bp.107.048504.

Geddes, J. R., Gardiner, A., & Rendell, J. et al. (2016) Comparative evaluation of Quetiapine plus lamotrigine combination versus quetiapine monotherapy (and folic acid versus placebo) in bipolar depression (CEQUEL): A 2 × 2 factorial randomised trial, *The Lancet*

Psychiatry, **3**(1), 31–9. https://doi.org/10.1016/s2215-0366(15)00450-2.

Geddes, J. R., Goodwin, G. M., & Rendell, J. (2009b). Lithium plus valproate combination therapy versus monotherapy for relapse prevention in bipolar I disorder (BALANCE): A randomised open-label trial. *The Lancet*, **375**(9712).

Goes, F. S. (2023). Diagnosis and management of bipolar disorders. *BMJ (Clinical research ed.)*, **381**, e073591. https://doi.org/10.1136/bmj-2022-073591.

Goodwin, G., Haddad, P. M. & Ferrier, I. N. (2016) Evidence-based guidelines for treating bipolar disorder: Revised third edition recommendations from the British Association for Psychopharmacology, *Journal of Psychopharmacology*, **30**(6), 495–553. https://doi.org/10.1177/0269881116636545.

Grunze, A., Amann, B. L. & Grunze, H. (2021) Efficacy of carbamazepine and its derivatives in the treatment of bipolar disorder, *Medicina*, **57**(5), 433. https://doi.org/10.3390/medicina57050433.

Hayes, J. F., Marston, L., Walters, K., et al. (2016) Lithium vs. valproate vs. olanzapine vs. quetiapine as maintenance monotherapy for bipolar disorder: A population-based UK cohort study using Electronic Health Records, *World Psychiatry*, **15**(1), 53–8. https://doi.org/10.1002/wps.20298.

Iacobucci, G. (2023) Clinicians should withdraw antidepressants gradually, says NICE, *BMJ (Clinical research ed.)*, **380**, 130. https://doi.org/10.1136/bmj.p130.

Kazdin, A. E. (1983) Assessment of depression in mentally retarded adults, *American Journal of Psychiatry*, **140**(8), 1040–3. https://doi.org/10.1176/ajp.140.8.1040.

Kessing, L. V., Hellmund, G., Geddes, J. R., Goodwin, G. M., & Andersen, P. K. (2011). Valproate v. lithium in the treatment of bipolar disorder in clinical practice: Observational nationwide register-based cohort study. *The British Journal of Psychiatry*, **199**, 47–63. https://doi.org/10.1192/bjp.bp.110.084822.

Lowry, M. A. (1998) Assessment and treatment of mood disorders in persons with developmental disabilities. *Journal of Developmental and Physical Disabilities*, **10**(4), 387–406. https://doi.org/10.1023/a:1021858622501.

Marcus, R., Khan, A. & Rollin, L. (2011) Efficacy of aripiprazole adjunctive to lithium or valproate in the long-term treatment of patients with bipolar I disorder with an inadequate response to lithium or valproate monotherapy: A multicenter, double-blind, randomized study, *Bipolar Disorders*, **13**(2), 133–44. https://doi.org/10.1111/j.1399-5618.2011.00898.x.

Matson, J. (1998) The convergent validity of the Matson Evaluation of social skills for individuals with severe retardation (messier), *Research in Developmental Disabilities*, **19**(6), 493–500. https://doi.org/10.1016/s0891-4222(98)00020-1.

Matson, J. L. & Smiroldo, B. B. (1997) Validity of the mania subscale of the Diagnostic Assessment for the severely handicapped-II (Dash-ii), *Research in Developmental Disabilities*, **18**(3), 221–5. https://doi.org/10.1016/s0891-4222(97)00005-x.

Matson, J. L., Gonzalez, M. L., Terlonge, C., Thorsn, R. B., & Laud, R. B. (2007) What symptoms predict the diagnosis of mania in persons with severe/profound intellectual disability in clinical practice?, *Journal of Intellectual Disability Research*, **51**(1), 25–31. https://doi.org/10.1111/j.1365-2788.2006.00897.x.

McElroy, S. L., Weisler, R. & Chang, W. (2010) A double-blind, placebo-controlled study of Quetiapine and paroxetine as monotherapy in adults with bipolar depression (embolden II), *The Journal of Clinical Psychiatry*, **71**(2), 163–74. https://doi.org/10.4088/jcp.08m04942gre.

Moss, S., Emerson, E., Kiernan, C., et al. (2000). Psychiatric symptoms in adults with learning disability and challenging behaviour. *British Journal of Psychiatry*, **177**, 452–6. https://doi.org/10.1192/bjp.177.5.452.

National Institute for Health and Care Excellence (2020). Bipolar disorder: Assessment and management. [NICE

Clinical Guideline CG185]. www.nice.org.uk/guidance/cg185.

Popovic, D., Reinares, M., Goikolea, J. M., et al. (2012) Polarity index of pharmacological agents used for maintenance treatment of bipolar disorder, *European Neuropsychopharmacology*, 22(5), 339–46. https://doi.org/10.1016/j.euroneuro.2011.09.008.

Popovic, D., Torrent, C., Goikolea, J. M., et al. (2013) Clinical implications of predominant polarity and the polarity index in bipolar disorder: A naturalistic study, *Acta Psychiatrica Scandinavica*, 129(5), 366–74. https://doi.org/10.1111/acps.12179.

Royal College of Psychiatrists (2001). *DC-LD: Diagnostic criteria for psychiatric disorders for use with adults with learning disabilities/mental retardation*, London, Royal College of Psychiatrists, Occasional Paper OP 48.

Sturmey, P., Laud, R. B., Cooper, C. L., Matson, J. L., & Fodstad, J. C. (2010) Mania and behavioral equivalents: A preliminary study, *Research in Developmental Disabilities*, 31(5), 1008–14. https://doi.org/10.1016/j.ridd.2010.04.017.

Suppes, T. & Vieta, E., Liu, S., Brecher, M., & Paulsson, B. (2009). Maintenance treatment for patients with bipolar I disorder: Results from a North American study of quetiapine in combination with lithium or divalproex (Trial 127). *American Journal of Psychiatry*, 166, 476–88. https://doi.org/10.1176/appi.ajp.2008.08020189.

Suppes, T., Vieta, E., Gustafsson, U., & Ekholm, B. (2013) Maintenance treatment with quetiapine when combined with either lithium or divalproex in bipolar I disorder: Analysis of two large randomized, placebo-controlled trials, *Depression and Anxiety*, 30(11), 1089–98. https://doi.org/10.1002/da.22136.

Taylor, D. M., Barnes, T. R., & Young, A. H. (2021) *The Maudsley prescribing guidelines in psychiatry*. Wiley Blackwell.

Taylor, J. L., Hatton, C., Dixon, L., & Douglas, C. (2004) Screening for psychiatric symptoms: PAS-add checklist norms for adults with intellectual disabilities, *Journal of Intellectual Disability Research*, 48(1), 37–41. https://doi.org/10.1111/j.1365-2788.2004.00585.x.

Thase, M. E., Macfadden, W., Weisler, R. H., et al. (2006) Efficacy of quetiapine monotherapy in bipolar I and II depression, *Journal of Clinical Psychopharmacology*, 26(6), 600–9. https://doi.org/10.1097/01.jcp.0000248603.76231.b7.

Tohen, M., Calabrese, J. R., Sachs, G. S., et al. (2006) Randomized, placebo-controlled trial of olanzapine as maintenance therapy in patients with bipolar I disorder responding to acute treatment with olanzapine, *American Journal of Psychiatry*, 163(2), 247–56. https://doi.org/10.1176/appi.ajp.163.2.247.

Valdovinos, M. G., Seibert, H. N., Piersma, D., et al. (2019) Characterizing mood states in individuals diagnosed with bipolar disorder and intellectual disability, *Journal of Mental Health Research in Intellectual Disabilities*, 12(1–2), 26–44. https://doi.org/10.1080/19315864.2018.1561770.

Valentí, M., Pacchiarotti, I., Undurraga, J., et al. (2015) Risk factors for rapid cycling in bipolar disorder, *Bipolar Disorders*, 17(5), 549–59. https://doi.org/10.1111/bdi.12288.

Vieta, E., Günther, O., Locklear, J. (2011). Effectiveness of psychotropic medications in the maintenance phase of bipolar disorder: a meta-analysis of randomized controlled trials. *International Journal of Neuropsychopharmacology*, 14(8), 1029–49. https://doi.org/10.1017/S1461145711000885.

Vieta, E., Montgomery, S., Sulaiman, A. H., et al. (2012) A randomized, double-blind, placebo-controlled trial to assess prevention of mood episodes with risperidone long-acting injectable in patients with bipolar I disorder, *European Neuropsychopharmacology*, 22(11), 825–35. https://doi.org/10.1016/j.euroneuro.2012.03.004.

Watkins, L., Cock, H., Angus-Leppan, H., et al. (2019) Valproate MHRA guidance: Limitations and opportunities, *Frontiers in Neurology*, 10. https://doi.org/10.3389/fneur.2019.00139.

World Health Organization (2019) *ICD-11: International Statistical Classification of Diseases and Related Health Problems.*

Yatham, L. N., Kennedy, S. H., Parikh, S. V., et al. (2018) Canadian network for mood and anxiety treatments (CANMAT) and International Society for Bipolar Disorders (ISBD) 2018 guidelines for the management of patients with bipolar disorder, *Bipolar Disorders*, **20**(2), 97–170. https://doi.org/10.1111/bdi.12609.

Yatham, L., Beaulieu, S., Schaffer, A. et al. (2016). Optimal duration of risperidone or olanzapine adjunctive therapy to mood stabilizer following remission of a manic episode: A CANMAT randomized double-blind trial. *Molecular Psychiatry*, **21**(1), 1050–6. https://doi.org/10.1038/mp.2015.158.

Yen, S., Stout, R., Hower, H., et al. (2016). The influence of comorbid disorders on the episodicity of bipolar disorder in youth. *Acta Psychiatrica Scandinavica*, **133**(4), 324–34.

Youngstrom, E. A., Gracious, B. L., Danielson, C. K., Findling, R. L., & Calabrese, J. (2003). Toward an integration of parent and clinician report on the Young Mania Rating Scale. *Journal of Affective Disorders*, **77**(2), 179–90. https://doi.org/10.1016/S0165-0327(02)00108-8.

Chapter 9
Schizophrenia

Dasari Michael, Amir Javaid, Muzammil Hayat, Ilyas Ali, Ayomipo J. Amiola, and Reena Tharian

Introduction

What Is Schizophrenia?

The conceptualisation of schizophrenia has evolved from its original descriptions in the nineteenth century through to the recent publication of the American Psychiatric Association's *Diagnostic and Statistical Manual of Mental Disorders* (DSM)-5 and the International Classification of Diseases (ICD)-11.

The ICD-11 describes a group of conditions called 'Schizophrenia spectrum and other primary psychiatric disorders' which includes schizophrenia, schizoaffective disorder, schizotypal disorder, acute and transient psychotic disorder, delusional disorder, and other specified schizophrenias or other primary psychotic disorders. All these conditions are characterised by impaired assessment of reality and behaviour, delusions, hallucinations, disorganised thinking and behaviour, experiences of passivity and control, negative symptoms, and psychomotor disturbances (Valle 2020, World Health Organization 2019). The ICD-11 specifies a symptom duration of at least one month and has removed the reliance on Schneiderian first rank symptoms, giving equal weight to any hallucinations or delusions. It has introduced a symptom specifier to replace the sub-types of schizophrenia and proposed a course specifier to map out the natural course of the illness (World Health Organization 2019).

The DSM-5 (American Psychiatric Association 2013) is like the ICD-11 in its description of symptom requirements to make a diagnosis. However, apart from the psychotic symptoms lasting for a month, it also requires prodromal or residual symptoms to be present for a total of six months and specifies the need for impaired functioning (Valle 2020).

What Causes Schizophrenia?

While the exact aetiology of schizophrenia is unknown, a combination of physical, genetic, psychological, and environmental factors have been proposed that make a person more likely to develop it (see www.nhs.uk/mental-health/conditions/schizophrenia/causes/). More recently, there have been studies suggesting a paradigm shift from schizophrenia being considered a neurodegenerative process occurring in early adult life towards one which sees it as a neurodevelopmental disorder starting well before birth (De Berardis et al., 2021).

How Is Schizophrenia Different in People with Intellectual Disability?

The potential difficulties of diagnosing complex psychopathology in people with intellectual disability is a theme throughout this book. Communication difficulties, diagnostic overshadowing, atypical presentations, and the presence of other comorbid conditions all contribute to this (Bhaumik & Alexander, 2020).

It has been suggested that the schizophrenic phenotype may be subtly different in the population with intellectual disability (Welch et al., 2011). While individuals with mild and, to a certain extent, moderate intellectual disability may be able to describe their psychopathology and therefore aid in the diagnosis, diagnosis of schizophrenia in individuals with severe or profound intellectual disability is unlikely to be made confidently (Einfeld et al., 2007; Dosen & Day, 2001).

Adults with moderate, severe, and profound intellectual disability, and schizophrenia may appear severely disturbed during episodes of schizophrenia. They can display disorientation, disorganised and bizarre behaviour, and agitation or aggression. In most cases, their language skills severely deteriorate. They are unavailable for social contact and display severely reduced global functioning. Thus, the patient has considerable problems with task performance, social interaction, and self-care. Due to their impaired ability to report their symptoms, they have an increased chance of their mental illness being overlooked (Mason & Scior, 2004). Disorganisation, both in speech and behaviour, may be identified both in patients with severe intellectual disability and among patients with autism. However, disorganised speech will be observable only in patients with at least minimal verbal skills (Cherry et al., 2000).

In people with mild to moderate degrees of intellectual disability, delusions of reference, persecution, and grandeur can be identified; however, it may be difficult to identify delusions of guilt. Based on verbal ability, patients can often report 'hearing voices' thus indicating auditory hallucinatory experiences. Clarifying the nature of this experience or whether they are in the second or third person is often difficult. Other hallucinatory experiences, such as in the visual, tactile, olfactory, and gustatory modalities, need to be specifically enquired about (Bhaumik et al., 2020). In people with severe to profound degrees of intellectual disability who do not report these unusual experiences, one may expect some sort of altered behaviour to be indicative of auditory hallucinations (Hurley, 1996).

Negative symptoms such as fatigue, apathy, lack of motivation, and social withdrawal may for the most part be observed as behavioural equivalents at all levels of intellectual disability. Clinical experience points to the phenomenon of aggravated social withdrawal being present when schizophrenia is suspected in patients with intellectual disability and autism. However, negative symptoms should not be assumed as indicative of schizophrenia unless apathy and loss of motivation represent a marked change in an individual's premorbid habitual functioning (Bakken, 2021).

The greater the degree of intellectual disability, the more the symptoms may appear as atypical (Ghazuiddin, 2005). Impaired language skills are closely related to occurrence of challenging behaviour and stereotyped activity. Repetitive behaviour and challenging behaviour (violence, damaging of objects, or self-mutilation) has been underpinned as atypical symptoms in individuals with autism (Tantam, 2000; Lainhart, 1999; Myers & Winters et al., 2002).

A recent review (Bakken, 2021) of behavioural equivalents of schizophrenia in people with intellectual disability and autism spectrum disorder echo these earlier findings. Disorganised speech and behaviour, negative symptoms, hallucinatory behaviour, and post-treatment reporting of delusions were described.

Presence of mood symptoms can confound the diagnosis of schizophrenia (Escamilla, 2001; Lindenmayer and Kay, 1989; Zisook et al., 1999), and side effects of medications, depression, or other chronic physical or mental illnesses can confound the picture of negative symptoms (Barabassy et al., 2018). In patients with epilepsy, pre- or post-ictal behavioural disorganisation or psychotic experiences should not be mistaken for schizophrenia (Ring et al., 2007; Hassiotis & Sinai, 2009).

As indicated elsewhere in this book, the Diagnostic Criteria for Psychiatric Disorders for use in Adults with Learning Disabilities (DC-LD 2001) was developed by the Royal College of Psychiatrists in the UK and the Diagnostic Manual – Intellectual Disability (DM-ID) (2007) was developed by the National Association for the Dually Diagnosed (NADD), in association with the American Psychiatric Association (APA). Both set out guidelines for diagnosing schizophrenia in those with an intellectual disability. Most recently, the ICD-11 (WHO, 2019) has further formalised the approach of using behavioural equivalents to diagnose mental illnesses in people with intellectual disability (Lemay et al., 2022).

The DASH-II (Diagnostic Assessment for the Severely Handicapped-II) is a questionnaire designed to identify psychopathology in adolescents and adults with severe or profound intellectual disability. The Moss Psychiatric Assessment Schedules (Moss-PAS; previously known as the Psychiatric Assessment Schedule for Adults with Developmental Disabilities (PAS-ADD)) offers a systematic approach to identifying psychopathology in adults with intellectual disability. It is designed to be used by staff who have received training in the measure. These can be accessed in both paper and digital formats (https://moss-pas.online/). Both of these tools may be useful in diagnosing schizophrenia in those at the severe end of the intellectual disability spectrum.

How Common Is Schizophrenia in People with Intellectual Disability?

In the general population, schizophrenia affects 1 in 300 people (0.32%) and 1 in 222 adults (0.45%) worldwide (Institute of health Metrics and Evaluation, 2021). In people with an intellectual disability the prevalence is significantly higher, with a recent systematic review and meta-analysis suggesting 3.45% (Aman et al., 2016). One of the biggest epidemiological studies in intellectual disability showed a 2-year incidence for psychosis of 2.4% and for first episode psychosis of 0.5%, amounting to a standardised incidence ratio of 10.0 (Cooper et al., 2007). The onset of the illness in those with intellectual disability appears to be earlier than is observed in those with normal intelligence (Humphries et al., 2020).

Treatments: The Evidence Base

General Population

In the general population, the NICE clinical guideline for psychosis and schizophrenia in adults: prevention and management CG:178 (NICE 2014) offers a comprehensive overview of the evidence base regarding therapeutic interventions. For a full account of the recommendations, associated caveats, and relevant evidence base, please visit www.nice.org.uk/guidance/cg178/chapter/Recommendations#first-episode-psychosis-2.

Assessment and management should be multi-disciplinary, with the full range of pharmacological, psychological, social, occupational, and educational interventions offered for people with psychosis. Oral antipsychotic medication should be offered in conjunction with psychological interventions such as family therapy and individual cognitive behavioural therapy (CBT). The choice of antipsychotic medication should be made collaboratively by the psychiatrist and the service user (including their carer) after discussing the likely benefits and possible side effects of each drug.

People with Intellectual Disability

Among people with intellectual disability, studies on schizophrenia are few. Most studies on schizophrenia actively exclude individuals with intellectual disability, for various reasons. Therefore, high-level evidence on the efficacy of antipsychotics for schizophrenia in people with intellectual disability is lacking (Duggan & Brylewski, 1999; Humphries et al., 2020; Korb and Hassiotis, 2022). Similarly, there is no high-level evidence for the efficacy of psychosocial options in the management of schizophrenia. Nevertheless, psychosocial interventions that work in the general population can be used in intellectual disability with reasonable adjustments, such as adapting therapy for the client's developmental stage, communication deficits, and individual needs. It is worth noting that antipsychotics are often prescribed to people without a recorded diagnosis of schizophrenia (and other psychotic disorders) but who have a record of challenging behaviour (Sheehan et al., 2015).

People with Intellectual Disability: Non-medication Treatments

Oathamshaw and Haddock (2006) suggested that people with intellectual disability and psychosis demonstrate the skills needed to undertake cognitive behaviour therapy similarly to those with intellectual disability without mental health problems. In keeping with this, individual and family CBT for psychosis has been modified for people with a mild intellectual disability who have a diagnosis of schizophrenia (Haddock et al., 2004). Other approaches found to be useful include acceptance and commitment therapy (Pankey & Hayes, 2003) and psychoeducational groups (Crowley et al., 2008). Table 9.1 details the evidence base for non-medication treatments for psychosis in people with intellectual disability.

Table 9.1 Non-medication treatments in intellectual disability

Psychotherapy	Evidence in intellectual disability
Cognitive behavioural therapy (CBT)	Modified individual and family cognitive behavioural therapy for psychosis for people with a mild intellectual disability and schizophrenia (Haddock et al., 2004)
	Case series of three men with intellectual disability engaging in CBT for psychosis (Kirkland, 2005)
	Case report outlining a method of adapting cognitive behavioural therapy for command hallucinations for people with a mild intellectual disability (Barrowcliff, 2008)
	Case report detailing the use of cognitive behavioural strategies for managing auditory hallucinations by a woman with mild intellectual disability (Leggett et al., 1997)

Table 9.1 (cont.)

Psychotherapy	Evidence in intellectual disability
Psychoeducational group	A preliminary study of psychoeducational groups for people with psychosis and mild intellectual disability (Crowley et al., 2008)
Acceptance and commitment therapy	A case report on acceptance and commitment therapy for a patient with intellectual disability and psychosis (Pankey and Hayes, 2003)

People with Intellectual Disability: Medication Treatments

A Cochrane Review (Duggan and Brylewski, 1999) identified only one relevant randomised trial (Foote 1958) which had four people with a dual diagnosis of schizophrenia and intellectual disability; in addition the group allocation of two was unclear. The review therefore found no trial evidence to guide the use of antipsychotic medication for those with both intellectual disability and schizophrenia. Clinical practice thus continues to be guided by evidence from trials involving people with schizophrenia who do not have intellectual disability (NICE 2016). Available evidence for the efficacy of antipsychotic medications in schizophrenia is from case reports, observational studies, retrospective chart reviews, and prospective clinical investigation.

Of the atypical (or second-generation) antipsychotics, risperidone is the one most often studied, and it is effective for both psychotic and non-psychotic disorders in people with intellectual disabilities (Malfa et al., 2006). In addition, consensus conferences appear to confirm the high efficacy and safety of atypical antipsychotics in both psychotic and behavioural disorders in people with intellectual disability. Hence, they are the drug of choice in the treatment of schizophrenia in people with intellectual disability, with risperidone and olanzapine as first-line and clozapine reserved for non-responders (Malfa et al., 2006). Table 9.2 details the evidence base for antipsychotic medication treatments for psychosis in people with intellectual disability.

Table 9.2 Medication treatments in intellectual disability

Medication	Study Type	Outcome
Olanzapine and risperidone	Prospective clinical investigation	Both drugs were well tolerated, risperidone more than olanzapine, but the difference was not statistically significant (Williams et al., 2000)
Risperidone and olanzapine	Retrospective study of prescription trends	Olanzapine tended to be prescribed mostly for psychotic disorders, and showed good rates of response, whereas risperidone was prescribed mostly for people with

Table 9.2 (cont.)

Medication	Study Type	Outcome
		behavioural disturbance associated with a psychiatric diagnosis. (Bokszanska et al., 2003)
Risperidone, olanzapine, clozapine and quetiapine	Retrospective chart review	Olanzapine is one of the most prescribed drugs, effective on psychotic and non-psychotic disorders, tolerated well, dystonia and dyskinesia especially in females are described (Friedlander et al., 2001)
Clozapine	Retrospective file review	Safe and effective in 24 people with schizophrenia spectrum disorders; three subjects had to stop it because of neutropenia (Thalayasingam et al., 2004)
Clozapine	Case series	In five patients with schizophrenia or schizoaffective disorder, no important side effects (Sajatovic et al., 1994)
Clozapine	Retrospective descriptive study	Effective on positive symptoms in 20 schizophrenic patients with violent behaviours. (Gelly et al., 1997)
Clozapine	Case report	Good response in an adolescent with a severe schizophrenic paranoid disorder (Sperner-Unterweger et al., 1998)
Clozapine	Case series	Good efficacy on two patients with VeloCardioFacial syndrome and schizophrenia (Gothelf et al., 1999)
Clozapine	Case report	Marked symptomatic improvement in a 32-year-old man with moderate intellectual disability, severe behavioural problems, and psychotic symptoms. (Kamal and Kelly, 1999)
Clozapine	Retrospective chart review	Significant improvement to the CGI scale in 26 resistant patients with schizophrenia spectrum disorders. (Antonacci and de Groot, 2000)

Treatment Guideline and Algorithm in Intellectual Disability

Assessment

- A detailed diagnostic assessment (Alexander et al., 2010; Chester et al., 2023), as set out in Chapter 4, should be carried out. This will cover the degree of intellectual disability, cause of intellectual disability, and any behaviour phenotypes, autism spectrum disorder, other developmental disorders, mental illnesses including anxiety disorders, personality disorders, substance misuse, physical health conditions, experience of trauma, and types of challenging behaviour.
- A psychological formulation using the 5-P model of the presenting problem, predisposing, precipitating, perpetuating, and protective factors (Macneil et al., 2012) or equivalent should be completed, along with using the HELP framework of Health, Environment, Lived experience and Psychiatric problems (Green et al., 2018)

Non-Medication Treatments

- Psychosocial interventions are more effective when delivered in conjunction with antipsychotic medication.
- Adaptations should be made in the delivery of psychological therapies, such as tailoring the intervention to the developmental level of the individual and ensuring appropriate adaptations to the treatment manual and the therapeutic environment.
- Provision of social support such as housing, daytime activities, and educational and occupational support.

Medication Treatments

- Assessment and treatment of schizophrenia in intellectual disability must always be conducted within the context of a robust biopsychosocial understanding of illness and formulation.
- Careful medication history, including any use of alcohol and/or illicit drugs.
- Pre-treatment investigations should include full anthropometric measurements (weight, height, body mass index, and waist circumference), including vital signs. Baseline blood tests such as full blood count, electrolytes, liver function tests, thyroid function tests, prolactin, blood glucose, and lipids should be conducted including an electrocardiograph to exclude congenital conduction abnormalities.
- Check for potential drug interactions and history of sensitivity to side effects.
- Detailed discussion with the patient and/or carers and family, as appropriate, about the target symptoms, the rationale for prescribing, and the monitoring and review arrangements.
- Typical (first-generation) antipsychotics are more likely to cause extrapyramidal side effects and worsen cognitive function. Atypical (second-generation) antipsychotics have a lower propensity to cause movement disorders; however, they can have metabolic side effects, such as obesity, insulin resistance, impaired glucose tolerance, and dyslipidaemia.

- Risperidone, olanzapine, and quetiapine (and other atypical antipsychotics) are first-line medications.
- Clozapine is licenced for treatment-refractory schizophrenia.
- Where there is hyperarousal, severe anxiety, insomnia, hostility, or a high risk of violence to self and others, benzodiazepines or antihistamines may be offered as adjunctive agents for a time-limited period.
- Use of doses beyond the BNF (British National Formulary) advisory maximum dose or combinations of antipsychotics is discouraged, due to increased adverse effect burden, including the risk of sudden cardiac death and lack of high-level evidence for effectiveness. It should only be considered in specialist settings if there is a documented lack of response to a single antipsychotic (including clozapine) prescribed at an optimum dose for an optimum length of time in conjunction with psychosocial interventions.

Length of Treatment and Related Issues
- Since the commencement in England of the Stopping Over-Medication of People with a Learning Disability (STOMP) programme (NHS England, 2016), clinicians have been reminded of the need to ensure medications are prescribed not only for appropriate indications but also continued only for an appropriate time, with regular reviews of the need for medications and their risk benefits.
- Response should ideally be monitored clinically with comprehensive symptom assessment scales. Trial of an initial dose may last up to two weeks, after which dose increases may be made.
- At the BNF advisory maximum dose, good response should be seen within six weeks. If not, a switch to another antipsychotic agent (not clozapine) is needed and the trial repeated.
- Where effective remission is achieved, maintenance treatment with antipsychotic medication at an optimum dose should be continued for at least two years as this reduces the risk of relapse.
- Long-acting injections or depot preparations should be offered if this will aid compliance.
- If a patient's illness does not remit despite adequate trials of two antipsychotic agents combined with appropriate psychosocial interventions, following a diagnostic reclarification as highlighted earlier, a trial of clozapine should be considered.
- For ongoing prescribing, regular reviews at 3-6-month intervals (Royal College of Psychiatrists, 2016) or at least yearly (NICE, 2016) should be held.
- If a patient's illness does not respond to an adequate trial of clozapine, other approaches such as clozapine augmentation, antipsychotic combination, and high-dose antipsychotic therapy may be considered. These should be initiated in specialist inpatient settings, as an individual patient trial with close and regular monitoring of symptoms and side effects.
- These treatments should only be continued after three months if there is clear clinical benefit that outweighs any risks.

Case Study 9.1

Navneet is a 21-year-old man with moderate intellectual disability. He has been living in a residential home for the last two years. He can communicate in a few words and can indicate his needs, and some staff support is needed for personal care. He attends a day centre four days a week and keeps himself busy at home with various activities. Navneet has been referred to the local intellectual disability service due to a change in behaviour over the last few weeks. He was noted to be screaming, shouting, and arguing, with hand gestures, when no one was around. He reported hearing voices talking about him and was getting agitated and confrontational with staff. Staff reported that Navneet has not been sleeping well, was refusing food, and was uncooperative with personal care.

Navneet was assessed by the intellectual disability psychiatrist, with support from community nursing and the speech and language therapy team. His mother and carers reported that the behaviour is completely out of character. A strong family history of schizophrenia was noted as his brother was recently diagnosed with schizophrenia. Navneet's physical examination, blood tests, and ECG were all normal. His behavioural observations were completed by the community nurse to identify any antecedents. Navneet was diagnosed with first-episode psychosis and a support package was put in place with the support of various members of the multi-disciplinary team.

Navneet was started on a low dose of risperidone which was gradually titrated up with close monitoring of side effects. He was provided information using an easy-read leaflet and the carers were provided with information on the therapeutic effects and side effects of risperidone. Navneet was visited by the community nurse regularly during the initial stages of the treatment and followed up at the outpatient clinic. He showed improvement in his behaviour and sleep, reduction in agitation and better engagement with staff at home and the day centre within 2–3 weeks of starting on risperidone. His behaviours settled completed after about three months.

Case Study 9.2

Shalewa is a 28-year-old woman with mild intellectual disability who lives with her mother in a bungalow. Her mother is her full-time carer. She is fairly independent but needs some support with her medication and personal hygiene. She was diagnosed with schizophrenia at the age of 22 and has been on first-generation antipsychotic medication since, supervised by her mother. She was discharged back to her GP a few years ago as her psychotic symptoms were in complete remission.

Shalewa was re-referred to the local intellectual disability psychiatrist as she was no longer going out of the house and had begun hiding under the bed covers in her room. She was irritable and angry with her mother, reported being watched by a camera in the house, and talked about being followed by people in the street. She also reported hearing the voices of several people who commented on everything she was doing and told her to harm the people who were following her.

Shalewa was assessed by the community psychiatrist, and it emerged that she had not taken her prescribed antipsychotic medication over the last three months due to extrapyramidal side effects, as well as due to her mother's ill health making it harder for her to supervise Shalewa. Shalewa's medication was reviewed and changed to olanzapine. She agreed to have carers coming in to support her with her antipsychotic medication and personal care. Regular reviews by the community nurse to improve compliance and to educate on the importance of compliance of medication with easy-read leaflets was agreed. Within two weeks of starting olanzapine, Shalewa showed marked improvement.

The Frith Prescribing Guidelines Editors' Expert Group Consensus Statements

Statements of High Confidence
- The prevalence of schizophrenia and psychosis in people with intellectual disability is higher than in the general population.
- The choice of antipsychotic medication should be made collaboratively by the psychiatrist and the service user (including their carer) after discussing the benefits and side effects of each medication.
- Adaptations should be made to psychological therapies, such as tailoring the intervention to the developmental level of the individual and ensuring appropriate adaptations to the treatment manual and the therapeutic environment.

Statements of Medium Confidence
- Oral antipsychotic medication should be offered in conjunction with psychological interventions such as family therapy and individual CBT.
- The first-line treatment can be monotherapy with a second-generation antipsychotic like risperidone and the second-line monotherapy with a different second-generation drug or a first-generation antipsychotic.
- Clozapine can be equally effective in treatment-resistant schizophrenia in those with intellectual disability as in the general population.

Statements of Low Confidence
- Clozapine augmentation can be done with second-generation antipsychotics like amisulpiride and aripiprazole or first-generation drugs like haloperidol.
- Combinations of antipsychotics or high-dose antipsychotic therapy may sometimes be useful in carefully monitored settings.

Resource Box

The Moss Psychiatric Assessment Schedules (MPAS): www.moss-pas.com/

Easy-Read Documents
Royal College of Psychiatrists: www.rcpsych.ac.uk/docs/default-source/mental-health/problems-and-disorders/learning-disability-psychosis-leaflet.pdf?sfvrsn=d0c5f825_4
Norfolk County Council: https://brochure.norfolkslivingwell.org.uk/product/schizophrenia-easy-read

Easy-Read Documents for Medications
Choice & Medication: An information site (available through several NHS trusts or individual subscriptions) which offers patient information about mental health conditions and the treatments available to help make informed decisions about choosing the right medicine. Options include Very Easy Read Leaflets (VERAs), designed for people with an intellectual disability. www.choiceandmedication.org/
SPECTROM Easy read medication: https://spectrom.wixsite.com/project/easy-read-medication-leaflets

Other Key Clinical Guidelines Referenced in This Chapter
National Institute for Health and Care Excellence (2014, Update 2021). Psychosis and schizophrenia in adults: Prevention and management (NICE Guideline CG178). National Institute for Health and Care Excellence. www.nice.org.uk/guidance/cg178.

National Institute for Clinical Excellence (2016) Mental health problems in people with learning disabilities: Prevention, assessment, and management (NG54). Published 14 September 2016. www.nice.org.uk/guidance/ng54/chapter/Recommendations.

Barnes, T. R., Drake, R., Paton, C., et al. (2020). Evidence-based guidelines for the pharmacological treatment of schizophrenia: updated recommendations from the British Association for Psychopharmacology. *Journal of Psychopharmacology*, **34**(1), 3–78.

Taylor, D. M., Barnes, T. R., & Young, A. H. (2021). *The Maudsley prescribing guidelines in psychiatry*. John Wiley & Sons.

References

Aman, H., Naeem, F., Farooq, S., & Ayub, M. (2016). Prevalence of nonaffective psychosis in intellectually disabled clients: Systematic review and meta-analysis. *Psychiatric Genetics*, **26**(4), 145–55. https://doi.org/10.1097/YPG.0000000000000137.

American Psychiatric Association (2013). *The Diagnostic and Statistical Manual of Mental Disorders* (5th ed). American Psychiatric Association.

Antonacci, D. J. & de Groot, C. M. (2000). Clozapine treatment in a population of adults with mental retardation. *Journal of Clinical Psychiatry*, **61**(1), 22–5.

Bakken T. L. (2021). Behavioural equivalents of schizophrenia in people with intellectual disability and autism spectrum disorder. A selective review. *International Journal of Developmental Disabilities*, **67**(5), 310–17. https://doi.org/10.1080/20473869.2021.1925402.

Barabassy, A., Szatmári, B., Laszlovszky, I., et al. (2018) Negative symptoms of schizophrenia: Constructs, burden, and management. Psychotic *disorders: An update*. InTech. https://Doi.org/10.5772/intechopen.73300.

Barrowcliff, A. L. (2008). Cognitive-behavioural therapy for command hallucinations and intellectual disability: A case study. *Journal of Applied Research in Intellectual Disabilities*, **21**(3), 236–45.

Bhaumik, S., Tromans, S., Gumber, R. and Gangavati, S., 2020. Clinical assessment including bedside diagnosis. In S Bhaumik, and R Alexander (eds.). Oxford *textbook of the psychiatry of intellectual disability*, Oxford University Press, 7–22.

Bokszanska, A., Martin, G., Vanstraelen, M., et al. (2003). Risperidone and olanzapine in adults with intellectual disability: a clinical naturalistic study. *International Clinical Psychopharmacology*, **18**(5), 285–91.

Cherry, K. E., Penn, D., Matson, J. L. & Bamburg, J. W. (2000). Characteristics of schizophrenia among persons with severe or profound mental retardation. *Psychiatric Services*, **51**(7), 922–4.

Cooper, S. A., Smiley, E., Morrison, J., et al. (2007). Psychosis and adults with intellectual disabilities. Prevalence, incidence, and related factors. *Social psychiatry and psychiatric epidemiology*, **42**(7), 530–6. https://doi.org/10.1007/s00127-007-0197-9.

Crowley, V., Rose, J., Smith, J., Hobster, K., & Ansell, E. (2008). Psycho-educational groups for people with a dual diagnosis of psychosis and mild intellectual disability: A preliminary study. *Journal of Intellectual Disabilities*, **12**(1), 25–39.

De Berardis, D., De Filippis, S., Masi, G., et al. (2021) Approach for a transitional model of early onset schizophrenia. *Brain Sciences*,

11(2), 275. https://doi.org/10.3390/brainsci11020275.

Dosen, A., & Day, K. (2001) Epidemiology, aetiology and presentation of mental illness and behaviour disorders in persons with intellectual disabilities. In A Dosen and K. Day (eds.), Treating *mental illness and behavior disorders in children and adults with intellectual disabilities*, pp. 3–24. American Association Books.

Duggan, L., & Brylewski, J. (1999). Effectiveness of antipsychotic medication in people with intellectual disability and schizophrenia: A systematic review. *Journal of Intellectual Disability Research*, 43(2), 94–104.

Einfeld, S., Tonge, B., Chapman, L., et al. (2007) Inter-rater reliability of the diagnoses of psychosis and depression in individuals with intellectual disabilities. *Journal of Applied Research in Intellectual Disabilities*, 20(5), 384–90.

Escamilla, M. A. (2001). Diagnosis and treatment of mood disorders that co-occur with schizophrenia. *Psychiatric Services*, 52(7), 911–19.

Fletcher, R., Loschen, E., Stavrakaki, C. & First, M. (2007). *DM-ID: diagnostic manual – intellectual disability: A textbook of diagnosis of mental disorders in persons with intellectual disability*. National Association for the Dually Diagnosed.

Foote, E. S. (1958) Combined chlorpromazine and reserpine in the treatment of chronic psychotics. *Journal of Mental Science*, 104(434), 201–5. https://doi.org/10.1192/bjp.104.434.201.

Friedlander, R., Lazar, S., & Klancnik, J. (2001). Atypical antipsychotic use in treating adolescents and young adults with developmental disabilities. *The Canadian Journal of Psychiatry*, 46(8), 741–5.

Gelly, F., Chambon, O. & Marie-Cardine, M. (1997). Long-term clinical experience with clozapine. *L'encephale*, 23(5), 385–96.

Ghaziuddin, M. (2005). *Mental health aspects of Autism and Asperger syndrome*. Jessica Kingsley Publishers.

Haddock, G., Lobban, F., Hatton, C., & Carson, R. (2004). Cognitive-behaviour therapy for people with psychosis and mild intellectual disabilities: A case series. *Clinical Psychology & Psychotherapy: An International Journal of Theory & Practice*, 11(4), 282–98.

Hassiotis, A., & Sinai, A. (2009) Psychotic illness. In A. Hassiotis, D A. Barron, & I. Hall (eds). *Intellectual disability psychiatry: A practical handbook*. Wiley, 67–83. https://doi.org/10.1002/9780470682968.

Humphries, L., Michael, D., & Hassiotisc, A. (2020) Schizophrenia and related psychoses in people with intellectual disability. In S. Bhaumik & R. Alexander (eds.), *Oxford textbook of the psychiatry of intellectual disability*. Oxford University Press, 91–103.

Hurley, A. D. (1996). The misdiagnosis of hallucinations and delusions in persons with mental retardation: A neurodevelopmental perspective. *Seminars in Clinical Neuropsychiatry*, 1, 122–33.

Institute of health Metrics and Evaluation (IHME) (2021). Global Health Data Exchange (GHDx). http://ghdx.healthdata.org/gbd-results-tool?params=gbd-api-2019-permalink/27a7644e8ad28e739382d31e77589dd7.

Kamal, M., & Kelly, M. (1999). The use of clozapine in an individual with moderate intellectual disability, aggressive behaviour and resistant psychosis. *Irish Journal of Psychological Medicine*, 16(1), 32–3.

Kirkland, J. (2005). Cognitive-behaviour formulation for three men with learning disabilities who experience psychosis: How do we make it make sense? *British Journal of Learning Disabilities*, 33(4), 160–5.

Korb, L., & Hassiotis, A. (2022). Psychotic disorders. In M. O. Bertelli S. Deb, K. Munir, A., Hassiotis, & L. Salvador-Carulla (Eds.), Textbook of *psychiatry for intellectual disability and autism spectrum disorder* (pp. 537–55). Springer International Publishing.

Lainhart, J. E. (1999). Psychiatric problems in individuals with autism, their parents and siblings, *International Review of Psychiatry*, 11(4), 278–8, DOI: 10.1080/09540269974177.

Laufer, N., Mozes, T., Hermesh, H., Weizman, A. & Frydman, M. (1999). Clinical characteristics of schizophrenia associated with velo-cardio-facial syndrome. *Schizophrenia Research*, 35(2), 105–12.

Lemay, K. R., Kogan, C. S., Rebello, T. J., et al. (2022). An international field study of the ICD-11 behavioural indicators for disorders of intellectual development. *Journal of Intellectual Disability Research*, 66(4), 376–91.

Lindenmayer, J. P., & Kay, S. R. (1989). Depression, affect and negative symptoms in schizophrenia. *The British Journal of Psychiatry*, 155(S7), 108–14.

Malfa, G. L., Lassi, S., Bertelli, M., & Castellani, A. (2006). Reviewing the use of antipsychotic drugs in people with intellectual disability. *Human Psychopharmacology: Clinical and Experimental*, 21(2), 73–89.

Mason, J. & Scior, K., 2004. 'Diagnostic overshadowing' amongst clinicians working with people with intellectual disabilities in the UK. *Journal of Applied Research in Intellectual Disabilities*, 17(2), 85–90.

National Institute for Health and Care Excellence (Great Britain). (2016). Mental health problems in people with learning disabilities: prevention, assessment and management (NG 54). National Institute for Health and Care Excellence.

NHS UK (2023). Causes – schizophrenia. 24 April. www.nhs.uk/mental-health/conditions/schizophrenia/causes/.

Oathamshaw, S. C., & Haddock, G. (2006). Do people with intellectual disabilities and psychosis have the cognitive skills required to undertake cognitive behavioural therapy? *Journal of Applied Research in Intellectual Disabilities*, 19(1), 35–46.

Pankey, J., & Hayes, S. C. (2003). Acceptance and commitment therapy for psychosis. *International Journal of Psychology and Psychological Therapy*, 3(2), 311–28.

Ring, H., Zia, A., Lindeman, S., & Himlok, K., 2007. Interactions between seizure frequency, psychopathology, and severity of intellectual disability in a population with epilepsy and a learning disability. *Epilepsy & Behavior*, 11(1), 92–7.

Royal College of Psychiatrists (2001). *DC-LD: Diagnostic criteria for psychiatric disorders for use with adults with learning disabilities/mental retardation*, London, Royal College of Psychiatrists, Occasional Paper OP 48.

Sajatovic, M., Ramirez, L. F., Kenny, J. T. & Meltzer, H. Y. (1994). The use of clozapine in borderline-intellectual-functioning and mentally retarded schizophrenic patients. *Comprehensive Psychiatry*, 35(1), 29–33.

Sheehan, R., Hassiotis, A., Walters, K., et al. (2015). Mental illness, challenging behaviour, and psychotropic drug prescribing in people with intellectual disability: UK population based cohort study. *British Medical Journal*, 351. www.bmj.com/content/351/bmj.h4326.

Sperner-Unterweger, B., Czeipek, I., Gaggl, S., Geissler, D., Spiel, G. & Fleischhacker, W. W. (1998). Treatment of severe clozapine-induced neutropenia with granulocyte colony-stimulating factor (G-CSF): remission despite continuous treatment with clozapine. *The British Journal of Psychiatry*, 172(1), 82–4.

Tantam, D. (2000). Adolescence and adulthood of individuals with Asperger syndrome. *Asperger syndrome*, 367–99.

Valle, R. (2020). La esquizofrenia en la CIE-11: comparación con la CIE-10 y el DSM-5/ Schizophrenia in ICD-11: Comparison of ICD-10 and DSM-5. *Revista de psiquiatría y salud mental*, 13(2), 95–104. https://doi.org/10.1016/j.rpsm.2020.01.001.

Welch, K. A., Lawrie, S. M., Muir, W., & Johnstone, E. C. (2011). Systematic review of the clinical presentation of schizophrenia in intellectual disability. *Journal of Psychopathology and Behavioral Assessment*, 33, 246–53.

Williams, H., Clarke, R., Bouras, N., Martin, J., & Holt, G. (2000). Use of the atypical antipsychotics olanzapine and risperidone in adults with intellectual disability. *Journal of Intellectual Disability Research*, 44(2), 164–9.

World Health Organization (2019). *International statistical classification of diseases and related health problems (11th ed.)*. https://icd.who.int/.

Zisook, S., McAdams, L. A., Kuck, J., et al. (1999). Depressive symptoms in schizophrenia. *American Journal of Psychiatry*, 156(11), 1736–43.

Chapter 10

Aggression and Self-Injurious Behaviour

Peter E. Langdon, Kris Roberts, Danielle Adams, Farshad Shaddel, and Mary Barrett

Introduction

This chapter focuses upon the management of two behaviours: aggression and self-injury. At points we have also used the term 'behaviours seen as challenging' to encompass both these and a wider set of behaviours. We recognise that terminology in this area has long been controversial, with concerns about labelling, stereotyping, and diagnostic overshadowing, with suggestions to move to alternatives such as 'behaviours of concern' (Chan et al., 2012). Our choice of 'behaviours seen as challenging' aims to acknowledge the current classificatory approach (ICD-11: 'Problem or challenging behaviours') alongside considering differing perspectives on behaviour, rather than solely viewing behaviour as innate to the person.

What Is Aggression?

Aggression is often defined with reference to the intended consequences of an act exhibited by a person. Anderson and Bushman (2002) defined aggression as any behaviour exhibited by a person where they intentionally acted to cause harm to another. Behaviours which cause harm but without associated intent tend not to be defined as aggression. Some people with intellectual disability may engage in behaviours with intent to cause harm to another, while for others, especially those with severe to profound intellectual disability, an absence of intent may exist. Nevertheless, the topography and consequences of behaviour may be similar regardless of the capacity to form intent. Aggressive behaviour exhibited by people with intellectual disability can take the form of verbal threats; physical aggression directed towards others, including punching, kicking, slapping, and biting, among other behaviours; and/or property damage and destruction. Aggressive behaviour can cause serious harm to others which may be life-threatening and result in social exclusion and a reduced quality of life.

How Common Is Aggression in Intellectual Disability?

Prevalence studies regarding aggressive behaviour exhibited by people with intellectual disability have adopted a variety of definitions, often without reference to intent, and inclusive of behaviours that are more broadly defined as behaviour that is seen to be challenging. Crocker et al. (2006) completed a survey of aggressive behaviour among Quebec citizens with intellectual disability receiving services. They cited L'Abbé and Morin's definition of aggressive behaviour: 'verbal and/or motor behaviour directed towards oneself, one's environment or others. It can be manifested directly or indirectly and can be more or less planned' (L'Abbé and Morin, 2001, p. 16). Crocker et al. reported that 53.9% of adults with intellectual disability engaged in aggressive behaviour, inclusive of sexually aggressive behaviour. The behaviour most seen was verbal aggression, and the behaviour least frequently seen was sexual aggression. Intellectual disability of increasing severity was associated with lower rates of aggressive behaviours.

Others have made use of diagnostic criteria to define aggressive behaviour exhibited by people with intellectual disability; for example, the Diagnostic Criteria for Psychiatric Disorders for Use with Adults with Learning Disabilities (DC-LD, Royal College of Psychiatrists, 2001) includes definitions for physically aggressive behaviour, destructive behaviour, and verbally aggressive behaviour. Using these definitions, along with the diagnostic criteria for problem behaviour, Cooper et al. (2009b) reported a prevalence of 9.8% for aggressive behaviour among Scottish adults with intellectual disability, which is substantially lower than that reported by Crocker et al. (2006). Davies and Oliver (2013) synthesised prevalence data for aggression across 11 studies involving children and adults with intellectual disability, reporting that the prevalence ranged from 0% to 33% across different age groups. They concluded that there may be a curvilinear relationship between age and aggression, with the increase in prevalence occurring during childhood and into adulthood, followed by a decrease among those who are older.

There are a variety of reasons for the differing estimates of the prevalence of aggressive behaviour among people with intellectual disability. These include differences in: (1) the definition of aggression, (2) the methods used to capture data (e.g., survey methods vs. clinical interview vs. observations), (3) the nature of the participant sample (e.g., children, adults, total population surveys vs. participants known to clinical services, co-morbidity including genetic disorders).

Several factors have been shown to increase the risk of engaging in aggressive behaviour, which include: increasing or decreasing severity of intellectual disability, highlighting an inconsistency across studies (e.g., Cooper et al., 2009b; Crocker et al., 2006, Tyrer et al., 2006; Crocker et al., 2007), being female (Cooper et al., 2009b), being male (Schroeder et al., 2014; Tyrer et al., 2006), not living in the family home with a carer (Cooper et al., 2009b), or living in the family home (Crocker et al., 2007), not living independently (Crocker et al., 2007), parental income (Schroeder et al., 2014), urinary incontinence and other physical health problems (Cooper et al., 2009b; Crocker et al., 2007), sensory and communication problems (Schroeder et al., 2014), not having specific genetic syndromes (e.g., Down syndrome, Cooper et al., 2009b; Tyrer et al., 2006), having hyperkinesis (persistent hyperactivity, impulsivity, or mental illness (Cooper et al., 2009b, Crocker et al., 2007), impulsivity and restricted and repetitive behaviours (Davies and Oliver, 2016), use of psychotropic medication (Deb et al., 2001), and age (Tyrer et al., 2006; Davies and Oliver, 2013). It is also the case that aggressive behaviours may present as atypical symptoms of mental illness among people with intellectual disability.

What Is Self-Injurious Behaviour?

Self-injurious behaviour exhibited by people with intellectual disability can take the form of deliberate minor scratches upon the skin, headbanging, skin-picking, pica (compulsive eating of non-edible items), insertion of foreign objects, deep cuts or other types of physical injury including broken bones, disfigurement, and impaired vision related to the intensity and severity of self-injurious behaviour. Self-injurious behaviour is sometimes referred to as auto-aggression when the form involves slapping, punching, or using objects to cause harm to oneself. Auto-aggression and other types of self-injurious behaviour may also have a repetitive and sensory related quality (e.g., repetitive motion). There is a risk of infection, scarring, sensory impairments, disfigurement, poorer quality of life, and death associated with self-injurious behaviour.

Self-injurious behaviour needs to be differentiated from self-harm. NHS Scotland describes self-harm as 'an expression of personal distress' which can be linked to mental health conditions such as depression and anxiety. Self-harming behaviours involve a person intentionally damaging or injuring their body 'as a way of expressing deep emotional feelings such as low self-esteem, or a way of coping with traumatic events' (www.nhsinform.scot/illnesses-and-conditions/mental-health/self-harm/). Common presentations include self-cutting and taking intentional overdoses of medication. People undertaking self-harming behaviour may describe a temporary relief from internal tension and distress when they engage in the behaviour.

How Common Is Self-Injurious Behaviour in Intellectual Disability?

Estimates of prevalence of self-injurious behaviour have varied widely. The aforementioned reasons for the variation in the estimated prevalence of aggression are also relevant for self-injurious behaviour. Cooper et al. (2009a) reported a prevalence of self-injurious behaviour of 4.9% among adults with intellectual disability and went on to report that greater severity of intellectual disability, not living with family, having hyperkinesis, visual impairment, and not having Down syndrome were associated with the presence of self-injurious behaviour. There is evidence of a relationship between specific disorders and an increased prevalence of self-injurious behaviour, including autism (Oliver et al., 2017), Fragile X (Oliver et al., 2017), and Lesch–Nyhan syndrome (Juneja et al., 2019), as well as others including Cornelia de Lange syndrome, Prader–Willi syndrome, Rett syndrome, and Smith–Magenis syndrome.

Dimian and Symons (2022) completed a systematic review of risk factors associated with the development of self-injurious behaviour among people with intellectual disability. They found that the incidence of self-injurious behaviour across studies varied from 1.3% to 22% for children up to 17 years of age, and 0–22% for adolescents and adults, while prevalence estimates ranged from 4.9–100%. Risks for engaging in self-injurious behaviour included: being young, having poorer self-care, having self-injurious behaviour directed at the head, frequency and severity of self-injurious behaviour, autism, social and communication difficulties, more severe intellectual disability, hyperkinesis, and parental criticism.

What Causes Self-Injurious Behaviour?

The causes of self-injurious behaviour among people with intellectual disability are related to a combination of genetic, social, and psychological factors, including operant conditioning. However, for those with mild intellectual disability, factors related to self-harming behaviours commonly seen among those without intellectual disability are also relevant: for example, childhood abuse, problem-solving ability, impulsivity, and distress tolerance (Rees & Langdon, 2016).

Clinical Subtypes of Self-Injurious Behaviour

More than 20 years ago, but remaining relevant today, Mace and Mauk (1995) developed a model to classify self-injurious behaviour and outline the associated treatment based upon

Table 10.1 Clinical subtypes of self-injurious behaviour (Mace & Mauk, 1995)

Subtype	Central Feature	Neurotransmitter System
Extreme self-inflicted tissue damage	Insensitivity to pain	Opiate
Repetitive & stereotypic	Features of autism	Dopamine
Agitation when self-injurious behaviour is interrupted	Obsessive-compulsive behaviour	Serotonin
Heightened anxiety	High arousal (agitation & self-injurious behaviour co-occur)	Noradrenaline
Mixed	Two or more of above subtype	Multiple

clinical presentation. Table 10.1 illustrates key elements of their model; how this model informs treatment is further considered in Table 10.5. Finally, and as is the case with aggressive behaviour, self-injurious behaviour may present as atypical symptoms of mental illness.

When choosing a medication, it is vital to be clear what behaviour(s) you are targeting. Table 10.1 summarises the key subtypes of self-injurious behaviour that need targeting for optimum treatment.

Case Study 10.1 describes the example of an individual with intellectual disability and behaviours seen as challenging to contextualise the information discussed so far in this chapter.

Case Study 10.1

Michael is a 43-year-old man diagnosed with mild intellectual disability and bipolar affective disorder. He is prescribed risperidone for management of mood and anxiety. He lives in a shared home with another man with mild intellectual disability and they receive carer support for six hours per day. He has been settled in mood and behaviour for the last three years.

Michael has a history of behaviour seen as challenging, including shouting, swearing, throwing objects at others, and banging his arms on surfaces (resulting in bruising). A number of triggers have been identified, including carers arriving late, having new carers, his housemate taking Michael's snacks, becoming physically unwell, and missing doses of medication.

His neighbours contact social services as they are concerned that they hear shouting and banging coming from Michael's home in the evening. A social worker visits and ascertains that Michael is worried about the change in carers. Michael is noted to have a few bruises on his arms which have come from him hitting the table. There are also some broken cups and plates which Michael says he threw at the wall. Michael also admits he has not taken his evening medication for three days as he was not sure if the new carers were 'doing it right'. There are no immediate safety concerns for Michael and his housemate; however, the social worker calls an urgent multidisciplinary meeting to discuss Michael's support.

The following plan is agreed:

- The new carers will shadow the existing staff to allow a smooth transition and gradual introduction of new carers.
- The existing staff agree to provide short-term evening calls to support Michael with his medication until he is familiar with the new carers.

- The intellectual disability nursing team review and update the existing Positive Behaviour Support guidelines and provide training for the new carers on communicating and supporting Michael when he becomes agitated.
- Michael is seen by a general practitioner for an annual health check and monitoring completed for risperidone and lithium.
- The intellectual disability psychiatrist reviews Michael's mental health and answers questions about his medication. The psychiatrist provides accessible information about the medication to Michael and his care team and this is used to reassure Michael when he is offered his evening tablets.

With this combined approach, Michael gradually settles and develops a good relationship with his new carers.

The Evidence Base for Treatments

Psychological Therapies for Self-Injurious Behaviour and Aggression

When attempting to treat self-injurious behaviours or aggression, a behavioural programme should be tried first as medication may be associated with serious side effects. If psychotropic medicine is subsequently initiated, the behavioural programme should remain in place. This should include systematic direct observations and the use of rating scales – for example, the Behaviour Problems Inventory (Mascitelli et al., 2015; Rojahn et al., 2012).

Morano et al. (2017) completed a meta-analysis of single case studies, reporting that behavioural interventions for self-injurious behaviour were associated with a large reduction in self-injurious behaviour, while medication was associated with a smaller reduction, and suggested that medication may not be effective, although there are questions about the validity of these data. Denis et al. (2011), in an earlier meta-analysis of single case designs, also reported that behaviour interventions focused upon the use of reinforcement were effective in reducing self-injurious behaviour among people with intellectual disability, and medication did not moderate this effect. Similar meta-analytic work using single-case experimental designs has been completed for behaviour seen as challenging more broadly. For example, Heyvaert et al. (2010) reported a moderate effect size for 'biological, psychotherapeutic or contextual interventions' for behaviour seen as challenging. This group went on to complete a multilevel meta-analysis and reported there was evidence to support the conclusion that interventions for behaviour seen as challenging are associated with a large effect size, but this many not be consistent for all patients, and there was evidence of publication bias. They also reported that interventions were not as effective for patients presenting with aggression, but were more effective when they incorporated antecedent control strategies (Heyvaert et al., 2012).

Medication should only be used after behavioural methods and other approaches have been tried, as recommended by the National Institute for Health and Care Excellence (NICE, 2015).

The evidence to support the treatment of behaviours that are seen as challenging, including aggression is problematic. Many of the studies have focused upon problem behaviours or behaviours seen as challenging, which include a wide topography. Many studies have made use of the Aberrant Behaviour Checklist (ABC) irritability subscale as the primary outcome measure. There is a paucity of recent controlled studies.

Medication for Aggression

In adults, the National Institute for Health Research–funded NACHBID trial is the most quoted study. Within the NACHBID study, Tyrer and colleagues (2008) conducted a three-arm, parallel-group, randomised trial comparing haloperidol, risperidone, and placebo in patients with intellectual disability who were showing disruptive behaviour. Despite major methodological problems, including under-recruitment, all three arms in the study achieved a parallel drop in the severity of the behaviours within days of the intervention. They concluded that antipsychotics should no longer be considered an acceptable routine therapy for patients with an intellectual disability exhibiting aggressive behaviour, which is inconsistent with other studies. There remains a desperate need for further trials to clarify whether this conclusion is valid.

The available data involving controlled trials is summarised in Table 10.2.

Table 10.2 Evidence base for medication treatment of aggressive behaviours in intellectual disability

Part 1: Trials in children

Medication	Overview of evidence from specific medication trials of benefits in aggressive behaviours	Grade
Antipsychotic medications		
Risperidone Usual doses in trials 1–2mg daily.	Some evidence of benefit for aberrant behaviour checklist (ABC) subscales of irritability, hyperactivity, and social withdrawal. These must, however, be considered against adverse effects, most prominently weight gain. Five placebo-controlled trials between 2002 and 2013. High rate of discontinuation in trials.	High
Aripiprazole Usual doses in trials 5–10mg	Some evidence of benefit for ABC subscales of irritability. This must, however, be considered against adverse effects, most prominently weight gain. Two placebo-controlled trials in 2009. ABC irritability subscale used and diagnosis predominantly autism. Side effects did not seem to cause discontinuation from trials.	High
Risperidone vs aripiprazole head-to-head	Cohen et al. (2013) completed a meta-analysis of studies (8 studies, N = 782) and demonstrated no significant effect between the two drugs and concluded they are equally effective for behavioural disturbances in children with autism or intellectual disability. Adverse effects are common, and include extra-pyramidal side effects, weight gain and sedation.	High

Part 2a: Trials in adults

Medicine	Overview of evidence from specific medication trials of benefits in aggressive behaviours	Grade
Risperidone	Some evidence of benefits. Three placebo-controlled trials since 1998. Only Tyrer et al. (2008) specifically targeted aggression and failed to show any benefits for risperidone over placebo. McDougle et al. (1998) showed greatest benefits, but the sample was predominantly those with autism.	High
Haloperidol Usual doses 1–2mg daily	Licenced for short-term adjunctive management of psychomotor agitation, excitement, and violent and dangerous impulsive behaviour. Haloperidol has been found effective for reducing behavioural symptoms such as hyperactivity, aggression, stereotypies, affective lability, and tantrums. Haloperidol is associated with a high incidence of tardive and withdrawal dyskinesias, and clinical use is significantly limited due to these side effects.	High
Risperidone and haloperidol head-to-head	No significant difference between groups in terms of improvement, quality of life, or adverse events.	High
Quetiapine	A number of very small open trials using low doses have shown limited short-term effects on symptoms such as aggression.	Moderate
Olanzapine	Very limited evidence base. Small trials have shown benefit in alleviating some behavioural symptoms (irritability, hyperactivity/ noncompliance and lethargy/withdrawal) associated with autism. Concerns about weight gain and metabolic side effects.	Moderate
Olanzapine and risperidone head-to-head	Amore et al. (2011) undertook a clinical trial where patients had been previously prescribed first-generation antipsychotics and were switched to either olanzapine and risperidone. Participants were randomly allocated to one of two groups. Both olanzapine and risperidone were effective in reducing aggression in people with intellectual disability. Those who were	Moderate

(cont.)

Medicine	Overview of evidence from specific medication trials of benefits in aggressive behaviours	Grade
	randomly allocated to olanzapine had very few incidents of verbal aggression relative to those who were allocated to risperidone.	

Part 2b: Withdrawal studies in adults

Medication	Overview of evidence from specific medication trials of benefits in aggressive behaviours	Grade
Zuclopenthixol	Three withdrawal studies. Withdrawal of zuclopenthixol associated with significant increase in aggression and behaviour disorders and reduced adaptive social functioning.	Moderate
Patient's regular psychotropic medication	One discontinuation vs continuation study (Ahmed et al., 2000) showed that 48% of discontinuation group had medication reinstated.	Low

Part 3: Other medication

Medication	Overview of evidence from specific medication trials of benefits in aggressive behaviours	Grade
Lithium	One old study (Craft et al., 1987) showed significant reduction in aggressive behaviours.	High
SSRIs	Most studies show sustained reductions in aggressive behaviours. Sohanpal et al. (2007) completed a systematic review to examine the evidence for the treatment of behaviour problems with antidepressant medication. They reported improvement of aggression and self-injurious behaviour on average in less than 50% of cases; the remaining cases showed no improvement or showed deterioration in behaviours.	Moderate
Valproate	One open-label study (Ruedrich et al., 1999) and two in children, with inconclusive results.	Low

Medication for Self-Injurious Behaviour

The evidence for the treatment of self-injurious behaviour using medication is limited; the available data are summarised in Table 10.3. Prescription of various agents appears to follow certain trends, with an increased propensity for prescribing antidepressant medication and second-generation antipsychotic medications in recent years (Costello et al., 2022).

Rana et al. (2013) completed a systematic review of the treatment of self-injurious behaviour using medication and synthesised the findings from 5 double-blind randomised

Table 10.3 Evidence base for medication as a treatment for self-injurious behaviour in people with intellectual disability

Medication	Overview of evidence from specific medication trials of benefits in self-injurious behaviour	Grade
Antipsychotics		
Risperidone *Usual doses 1–2mg daily*	In a small double-blind crossover trial of 20 people with intellectual disabilities, risperidone was compared to placebo, resulting in a reduction in aggression and self-injury (McAdam et al., 2002; Zarcone et al., 2001; Zarcone et al., 2004). Risperidone appeared effective for the short-term treatment of aggression, temper outbursts, and self-injurious behaviour. Significant improvements in conduct, prosocial behaviour, and self-injury was reported by Aman et al. (2002) using doses that ranged from 0.006 to 0.092mg/kg vs placebo in 115 children. Two participants who received risperidone experienced extra-pyramidal symptoms, while average weight gain with risperidone was 2.2 kg. There was also an initial increase in heart rate associated with the first two weeks of risperidone treatment.	High
Aripiprazole	Limited evidence. No randomised controlled trials. Two open-label studies (small numbers) 92–100% response rate.	Moderate
Olanzapine	Limited evidence base. Hollander et al. (2006) reported global improvement of function using doses of 10mg/day vs placebo in a pilot study with 11 children with pervasive developmental disorder (PDD). Concerns over sedation, weight gain, and metabolic side effects.	Low
Ziprasidone	Limited evidence. No randomised controlled trials. Two open-label studies with small numbers. A 50–70% response rate was noted.	Low
Quetiapine	Limited evidence. No randomised controlled trials. Four open-label studies with small numbers. A response rate between 22% and 60% was reported.	Low
Antidepressants		
SSRIs	Some evidence of benefit. Sohanpal et al. (2007), within their systematic review, reported	High

Table 10.3 (cont.)

Medication	Overview of evidence from specific medication trials of benefits in self-injurious behaviour	Grade
	an improvement in aggression or self-injurious behaviour, on average, in less than half of cases. The remaining cases showed either no improvement or deterioration. Enhanced effect was noted with a comorbid diagnosis of anxiety or obsessive-compulsive disorder. However, the evidence is biased. An open trial of sertraline using a single-case experimental design demonstrated a decrease in self-injurious behaviour when the medication was used in combination with a behavioural intervention.	
Clomipramine	Rana et al. (2013) completed a systematic review and reported no statistically significant benefit for clomipramine versus placebo, which included self-injurious behaviour rate and intensity, stereotypy, and adverse events. However, there was evidence to indicate a clinically significant improvement in the rate and intensity of self-injurious behaviour and stereotypy.	Low
Opiate antagonists		
Naltrexone	Rana et al. (2013) reported inconsistent evidence for the efficacy of naltrexone in the management of self-injurious behaviour in patients with intellectual disability. One of the naltrexone versus placebo trials reported that naltrexone had clinically significant effects ($\geq 33\%$ reduction) on the daily rates of the most severe self-injurious behaviour among three of four participants, and modest to substantial reductions in self-injurious behaviour for all participants; however, this study did not report statistical significance. Another trial reported that naltrexone attenuated self-injurious behaviour in all four participants, with 25mg and 50mg doses producing a statistically significant decrease. Another trial, with eight participants, indicated that naltrexone administration was associated with significantly fewer days of high-frequency self-injury and significantly more days with low-	Medium

Table 10.3 (cont.)

Medication	Overview of evidence from specific medication trials of benefits in self-injurious behaviour	Grade
	frequency self-injury. Naltrexone had different effects depending on the form and location of self-injury. Another trial with 26 participants found that neither single-dose (100mg) nor long-term (50 and 150mg) naltrexone treatment had any therapeutic effect on SIB.	

controlled trials involving a total of 50 participants. They found weak evidence that naltrexone leads to a reduction in self-injurious behaviour and no evidence that clomipramine is effective. However, the majority of included trials were judged to be at high risk for bias, meaning that the conclusions may lack validity.

The Frith Treatment Guidelines for People with Intellectual Disability

NICE has published guidance about the treatment and support for all people with intellectual disability who have behaviour that is seen as challenging: Challenging behaviour and learning disabilities: prevention and interventions for people with learning disabilities whose behaviour challenges (NICE, 2015).

The guidance emphasises the importance of partnership working between services and with people with intellectual disability of all ages and their carers. Readers should refer to this guidance in full alongside this chapter for further detail; however, the key recommendations are included here.

Assessment and Formulation

Thorough assessment of the intensity and frequency of the behaviour and associated risks using a biopsychosocial approach is required to develop a formulation which then directly informs the choice of intervention. An individual with high-risk behaviour, or an individual who has the physical ability and tendency to cause physical injuries, would need a more active approach, including consideration of the use of medications to minimise the risk.

NICE Guidance Key Assessment Recommendations

- Those involved in providing care should understand factors that increase the risk of behaviour that is seen as challenging. These include:
  - Personal risk factors (e.g., severity of intellectual disability, autism, dementia, communication and sensory difficulties, physical health problems)
  - Environmental risk factors (e.g., restrictive environments, sensory stimulation, changes in the environment, the culture of staff teams)

- Behaviour that is seen to be challenging should be appropriately assessed and include a focus upon a person's abilities and needs, physical and mental illness, medication and side effects, previous interventions and response, quality of life, independent living skills, social history, culture, life events, sensory needs, and the physical and care environment.
- The behaviour should be well described and include information about the severity, frequency, duration, and impact upon the person and others.
- The factors that are identified as leading to the development and maintenance of the behaviour should be well described as part of the completion of a functional assessment inclusive of direct measurement of the behaviour.
- A risk assessment should be completed.

Treatment

Development of a behavioural support plan is the mainstay of treatment for behaviours that are seen as challenging. Support strategies include proactive, secondary prevention and reactive strategies; examples of these are detailed in Table 10.4.

Table 10.4 Examples of behavioural support strategies

Strategy type	Purpose	Can be defined as treatment	Examples
Proactive	These are interventions that are meant to be rehabilitative. This is the treatment you are providing which has been informed by your formulation.	Y	Broad-based ecological strategies where you make changes to the environment to reduce the probability of a behaviour being triggered; antecedent control strategies where you modify or remove triggers; teaching functional equivalent skills where we teach new skills that serve the same function as the behaviour we are trying to change; teaching new skills which could be specialist therapies, including communication or coping strategies; focused support strategies that involve using changing and using reinforcement; medication to treat e.g., anxiety.

Table 10.4 (cont.)

Strategy type	Purpose	Can be defined as treatment	Examples
Secondary prevention	Used to further reduce the probability of behaviour that we wish to change occurring when the risk has increased.	Y	Strategies that you would use when someone is displaying early warning signs indicating that behaviour is likely to occur. They are used to reduce risk. Secondary prevention can be some of the strategies that are also defined as proactive. For example, you might modify a trigger to reduce risk. Distraction and prompting are also examples of secondary prevention. For example, you might prompt someone to use a previously taught coping strategy.
Reactive	Used when the behaviour has occurred. Used to help keep the person and others safe.	N	Strategies used to enable a safe response when the behaviour that you are trying to change has already occurred. They should be graded from least to most restrictive and can involve seeking help from others, continuing to prompt, changing triggers further, or the use of pro-re-nata (PRN) medication.

The use of medication for aggression and self-injurious behaviour should only be considered when accompanied by a defined set of psychological and other interventions as outlined by NICE. When choosing a medication, it is vital to be clear what behaviour(s) you are targeting: for example, Table 10.5 summarises the key subtypes of self-injurious behaviour that need targeting for optimum treatment.

The treatment plan should be closely monitored and updated as required, and the formulation should be revised in tandem.

Table 10.5 Clinical features of self-injurious behaviour and associated suggested treatment (derived from Mace and Mauk (1995))

Subtype	Clinical features	Psychotropic medications (aim for monotherapy if possible)
Extreme self-inflicted tissue damage (opiate)	*History of severe self-injurious behaviour* Fractures, extensive scarring, lacerations > 3x3 cm^2, cauliflower ear, auto-amputation, loss of consciousness. Signs of little distress when inflicting self-injury – crying, screaming. Targeting the head/face/hands/fingers.	Opioid antagonists Naltrexone
Repetitive & stereotypic (dopamine)	*History of repetitive & stereotypic self-injurious behaviour* Topography of actions are similar, not variable (e.g., hand mouthing, repeated rubbing). Short duration between repetitive action (1–10 seconds). Tissue damage occurs due to repetitive injury Other non-self-injurious behaviour stereotypic behaviours are also present.	Antipsychotics (small doses) *Atypical antipsychotics*: Risperidone Amisulpride Quetiapine Olanzapine *Older medications*: Haloperidol Levomepromazine Chlorpromazine
Agitation when self-injurious behaviour is interrupted (serotonin)	Obsessive-compulsive behaviour. Agitation or distress when self-injurious behaviour is interrupted (e.g., crying, hyperventilation, aggression, pacing). Mean rate of SIB is usually > 100 incidents per hour. Self-injurious behaviour stops during another activity but resumes within 30 seconds of its completion.	SSRIs TCAs (tricyclics) Clomipramine
Heightened anxiety (noradrenaline)	High arousal: tachycardia, raised BP, pacing, agitation, screaming. Self-injurious behaviour rates vary considerably (>50%) between sessions and settings.	*Anxiolytics* Propranolol Pregabalin *TCAs* Amitriptyline (low dose)

Table 10.5 (cont.)

Subtype	Clinical features	Psychotropic medications (aim for monotherapy if possible)
	Topographies consist of hitting self, head banging. Sleep and/or appetite disturbance. Slowing of processing of information presented. Anxious affect. Preoccupied in deep thoughts.	*Mood stabilisers* Lithium carbonate Carbamazepine Sodium Valproate
Mixed (multiple)	A combination of features in two or more of the subtypes described earlier Commonest presentation	One or more medication classes depending on predominant subtype

NICE Guidance Key Treatment Recommendations

- Interventions should be least restrictive and focused upon reducing behaviour that is seen as challenging, improving quality of life, and increasing skills.
- Clinicians should have training in the development and delivery of proactive interventions.
- Clinicians should also be able to develop and deliver reactive strategies.
- A behavioural support plan should be developed and implemented informed by your formulation and include proactive, secondary prevention, and reactive strategies.
- Anger management based upon cognitive behavioural therapy should be considered where appropriate.
- Antipsychotic medication should be considered only when psychological and other interventions have not produced the desired results within an agreed timescale, treatment of any comorbid mental or physical illness has not led to a reduction in behaviour, and the behaviour is associated with a severe risk to the person and/or others. Antipsychotic medication should only be offered in combination with psychological or other interventions.
- Prescribe a single medication and start at a low dose, while monitoring side effects. Document your rationale for prescribing the medication, how long you anticipate them taking the medication, and a strategy for regularly reviewing the medication. You must record the response to the medication.
- You should review the benefits and side effects every three to four weeks initially, and stop if there is no response at six weeks. If you continue, you should review within a multidisciplinary team at three months and then every six months going forward.
- You should only continue to prescribe the medication when there is a clear benefit supported by evidence.
- People with intellectual disability should have their physical and mental health regularly monitored. Treatments for any coexisting physical or mental health problem should be accordance with additional NICE guidance.

Algorithm: Assessment and Treatment of Aggression and Self-Injurious Behaviour

The algorithm presented in Figure 10.1 may be helpful in navigating the pathway from assessment to treatment.

Assessment

- Assess for co-morbid conditions

Physical illness	Including any conditions that can cause pain/discomfort, dental issues, headache/migraine, menstrual pain, constipation, gastro-oesophageal reflux, hay fever, UTI, ENT and eye conditions, epilepsy.
Mental illness	Including mood disorders, anxiety, psychosis, dementia, post-traumatic stress disorder.
Neurodevelopmental disorders	Including autism and ADHD.
Genetic syndromes	Including but not limited to Lesch-Nyhan, Prader-Willi, Cornelia de Lange, Rett syndrome, Smith-Magenis syndrome, tuberous sclerosis.
Medication side effects	Consider all medications, not just psychotropics.

- Assess behaviour
    - Adopt a multidisciplinary holistic approach.
    - Include risk assessment including risk of abuse and/or neglect.
    - Complete functional assessment of behaviour to understand the reasons why the behaviour is occurring including an assessment of psychosocial and environmental factors, life events, and communication. Determine the factors that trigger the occurrence of behaviour.
    - Assess capacity and undertake best interest assessment if required.

Formulation

- Develop a bio-psycho-social formulation that directly informs and justifies treatment incorporating an understanding of the function of the behaviour.

Treatment

- Develop a behavioural support plan drawing together proactive, secondary prevention and reactive strategies (Table 13.3).
- Medication for aggression and self-injurious behaviour should only be used when accompanied by a defined set of psychological and other interventions as outlined by NICE. This would ideally be a behavioural support plan.
- Treatment should be closely monitored and updated as required resulting in revisions to the formulation.

Figure 10.1 Algorithm: Assessment and treatment of aggression and self-injurious behaviour

Case Study 10.2 provides an example of how an individual with intellectual disability and behaviours seen as challenging is assessed and supported, illustrating some of the principles discussed earlier.

Case Study 10.2: Treatment

Fatima is a 46-year-old woman with moderate intellectual disability and cerebral palsy. She lives in a residential home for adults with intellectual disability and her family visit regularly. Prior to the COVID-19 pandemic, Fatima had a regular routine of accessing the community on a daily basis to enjoy a wide range of activities. When COVID-19 restrictions came into force, Fatima became very distressed, struggling to understand why she couldn't go out and why her usual activities had stopped. She also found the increased noise and busyness of the home environment, due to all the other residents staying in as well, overwhelming. Video calls with her family also proved difficult, as Fatima couldn't understand why they did not visit in person.

Fatima began to hit out at staff, scream and cry for prolonged periods, throw objects, and bite her wrists. She began awakening at night and shouting, which disturbed other residents. She became incontinent of urine at times but declined support to have her clothing changed.

A GP assessed Fatima and prescribed treatment for a urinary tract infection; staff also supported Fatima to use the toilet on a regular basis and this produced an improvement in urinary incontinence, but the other issues continued. The GP then referred Fatima to the intellectual disability team, and she was initially seen by a community nurse who worked with the staff team to create a Positive Behaviour Support plan and implement this consistently. A Positive Behaviour Support plan using a person-centred approach builds on the strength of the individual and uses positive approaches to reduce a behaviour of concern. The emphasis is on a positive approach reducing the need for restrictive interventions. More information on Positive Behaviour Support can be found via the Challenging Behaviour Foundation: www.challengingbehaviour.org.uk/information-and-guidance/positive-behaviour-support/.

Fatima was then seen by a psychiatrist who noted high anxiety levels and low mood. Due to her level of intellectual disability, Fatima was unable to engage with psychological treatment for mood and anxiety, so the psychiatrist recommended treatment with a selective serotonin reuptake inhibitor (SSRI); this was optimised and produced an improvement in mood, anxiety, and sleep. A consistent positive behavioural support approach, coupled with improvements in mental state, were noted to have contributed to a gradual reduction in aggression and self-injury.

As COVID restrictions lifted, Fatima began to access the community again. She found returning to busy environments overwhelming and began to have 'meltdowns', which included aggression and self-injury again. Observations were carried out that highlighted Fatima to be shaky, sweaty, and pale at these times. The GP assessed and found no evidence of a physical cause. A psychiatry review highlighted the new presentation as being consistent with panic attacks. No further benefit could be obtained by adjusting the dose of SSRI, so the psychiatrist recommended cautious introduction of propranolol, which produced a notable reduction in the 'meltdowns', including aggression and self-injury. Fatima was then gradually able to resume a full community programme, with carer support.

Medication Withdrawal

Psychotropic deprescribing should be carried out in a safe and effective way, taking the risk of discontinuation symptoms into account. Despite NICE recommending that only one antipsychotic medicine should be prescribed for a limited time for the management of behaviour that is seen as challenging, with regular review, and plans for stopping this medication, there is evidence of the overprescribing of several classes of psychotropic medicines together with polypharmacy. Although antipsychotics appear to be the most common class of psychotropic medicines overprescribed, there is now evidence that there is also considerable overprescribing of antidepressants and mood stabilisers for people with intellectual disability.

For individuals with intellectual disability who are prescribed psychotropic medicines for behaviour that is seen as challenging, the lowest effective dose should be prescribed for the minimum length of time, together with regular review and monitoring. Opportunities for starting conversations about psychotropic deprescribing include routine medication reviews and primary care health checks. Prescribing and deprescribing interventions should be based on shared decisions between clinicians and the individual with intellectual disability. For good practice in psychotropic deprescribing, see Table 10.6.

Table 10.6 Good practice psychotropic deprescribing guidelines

Review outcomes of previous psychotropic deprescribing attempts.

Discuss potential risks and benefits of psychotropic deprescribing with patient and carers.

A behavioural support plan should be in place as a framework for the delivery of treatment, driven by a robust formulation.

Ensure access and optimisation of non-pharmacological interventions (e.g., environmental, behavioural, and psychological interventions).

Consider the best time to begin dosage reductions to avoid concurrent changes in circumstances or routines (e.g., accommodation, care team).

Develop and document a deprescribing plan together with the patient and their carers to include responsibilities for monitoring, frequency of monitoring, addressing discontinuation effects, and delivery of staff (carer) training. Communicate this plan with all stakeholders.

Ideally, only one psychotropic medicine should be reduced at a time in order that the effect of the deprescribing intervention, the emergence of new behaviours, relapse of behaviour that is seen as challenging, or the emergence of discontinuation (withdrawal) symptoms can be fully monitored and evaluated.

To minimise the effects of discontinuation symptoms, the psychotropic medicine should be tapered slowly over several weeks or months, with regular review. For antipsychotics, these symptoms may include relapse of challenging behaviour, dyskinesias and sleep problems, the reduction of high prolactin levels to normal levels, and possible reversal of amenorrhea.

The speed at which the psychotropic medicine can be deprescribed may change over time and should be determined through shared decision making with the patient and the carer together with input from the multidisciplinary team and routine medication monitoring and review.

Sometimes physical health medicines are prescribed to address the side effects of psychotropic medicines (e.g., laxatives for constipation). These medicines will need to be reviewed as the psychotropic medicine dose is reduced.

Table 10.6 (cont.)

Deprescribing decisions should be documented and communicated clearly to all stakeholders (including the GP and the community pharmacy) to avoid prescription and dispensing errors during the deprescribing process when there may be several dose changes.

There should be access to appropriate, easy-read material.

After the psychotropic medicine has been stopped or the maximum dose reduction has been achieved, the monitoring of physical health parameters and behaviours should continue regularly.

Case Study 10.3 illustrates the process of the withdrawal of medications used for the management of behaviours.

Case Study 10.3: Deprescribing in a Community Patient

Rohan is a 20-year-old man with diagnoses of moderate intellectual disability, autism, and attention deficit hyperactivity disorder (ADHD). He attends a residential college in the week and lives with his family during weekends and holidays. College staff report that Rohan gets very anxious if things change; when anxious, he lashes out, punches walls and doors, and hits his head. Rohan has a Positive Behaviour Support plan and risk assessment in place; however, there are usually several incidents reported each month when behavioural measures have not been sufficiently effective. Rohan's family state they don't have these problems when he is at home, as he 'just does his own thing'.

Rohan is prescribed a combination of guanfacine 3mg daily, risperidone 4mg daily, promethazine 25mg at night, and as required (PRN) lorazepam. He struggles to settle to sleep and has been noted to be tired in the mornings. His family are keen for his medication to be reduced; however, staff at the college are anxious in case he then becomes more unsettled.

Rohan is referred to the intellectual disability behaviour support team. The team complete a full reassessment, including functional analysis of Rohan's behaviour. The assessment highlights that Rohan's presentation fits with the pathological demand avoidance (PDA) profile of autism. His Positive Behaviour Support plan is rewritten in line with PDA management strategies. There was a significant reduction in aggression and self-injury and a drop in the use of lorazepam (PRN: used on as and when basis), when staff started using the aforementioned strategies. A risperidone reduction plan is then commenced, and the dosage has been successfully reduced by 50% so far.

Staff are also able to start taking Rohan out in the community and support him to increase his exercise levels. He starts to settle more easily at night so promethazine is switched to PRN and then stopped.

Rohan is noticeably more alert and able to engage with activities, including activities of daily living. At a recent multidisciplinary review both college staff and family reported positive progress in his level of independence, and it was agreed that a longer-term supported living placement should be worked towards.

Case Study 10.4: Deprescribing in a Complex Inpatient

John is a 36-year-old man with established diagnoses of mild intellectual disability and autism associated with significant behaviour that is seen as challenging, including unpredictable episodes of physical aggression, targeted violence toward vulnerable peers, and occasional head banging and threating to tie ligatures since age nine. As a result, John has mostly resided in supported accommodation and secure specialist psychiatric services since a young age, moving around multiple times throughout adolescence and adulthood. He is currently managed in a low secure unit.

John is prescribed zuclopenthixol decanoate depot injection 500mg every two weeks (for his aggression), melatonin modified release 2mg at night, and clonazepam 1mg three times daily. On this regime he is sleeping about 16 hours per day and is drowsy when awake. Despite this combination, he still needed IM lorazepam and haloperidol about 3 times a week because of behaviours seen as challenging. He had limited access to adapted psychological and occupational therapy due to being over-sedated. John was generally fit and well, but his body mass index was at obese range.

Observations indicated a clear link between John's behaviours and his favourite activities. He was usually settled and safe on the day before his weekly shopping and more aggressive after returning to the unit.

Further to capacity and best-interest discussions, John was moved to an individual care suite, where his care plan and medication could be reviewed and optimised safely without putting other patients at risk. John himself had reported a worsening of his anxiety previously when he was cared for on an open ward. This relocation to a suitable placement immediately reduced the frequency of incidents to about once every fortnight. John reported feeling over-sedated and his psychiatrist agreed to gradually reduce his medication.

First, his melatonin was stopped with no adverse impact on his behaviours and an improvement to his alertness and ability to engage with different activities he likes, especially going to parks and outdoor gyms. This in turn helped John to lose some weight and have a better therapeutic relationship with staff. The frequency of incidents reduced to almost once every other month.

At this stage, his clonazepam was reduced to twice a day. John continued to do well and therefore after four weeks the dose was reduced again, to once a day. Staff reported a noticeable increase in John's restlessness and anxiety in the following weeks with no clear physical or psychological reason. The frequency of incidents increased again to once every 3–4 weeks. The incidents did not respond to non-pharmacological interventions such as adding more activities and they did not subside in the following four weeks. Therefore, his clonazepam was put back to 1mg twice daily with a positive effect on John's presentation.

Functional analysis of incidents by a clinical psychologist further suggested a possible link between headaches and John's unprovoked aggression. As a result, his care plan and behavioural support plan were updated, and staff would regularly and proactively ask him about headaches and offer him pain killers if he was suffering from one. As a result, the frequency and intensity of incidents reduced to one low-risk incident every six months which would respond to verbal de-escalation/staff withdrawal without needing reactive strategies, including 'as and when required' (PRN) medication. These medications, including intramuscular haloperidol and lorazepam, were stopped and he remained well. John was then deemed ready for discharge to a bespoke community placement.

The Frith Prescribing Guidelines Editors' Expert Group Consensus Statements

Statements of High Confidence
- A well-developed strategy for measuring and monitoring behaviour should remain in place during treatment with psychotropic medication.

- Psychotropic medication for aggression and self-injurious behaviour should only be considered when psychological and other interventions have not produced the desired results within an agreed timescale, treatment of any comorbid mental or physical illness has not led to a reduction in behaviour, and the behaviour is associated with a severe risk to the person and/or others.
- There is a paucity of recent randomised controlled trials examining psychological interventions for challenging behaviour, including aggression and self-injurious behaviour.
- The evidence base for medication treatment for aggressive and self-harming behaviours in isolation remains scarce. There is a desperate need for further trials to guide our practice in this area.

Statements of Medium Confidence

- In general, behavioural interventions have been found effective in reducing self-injurious behaviour, and to a lesser extent for reducing aggression, although effect sizes vary.
- Risperidone is the most-studied antipsychotic for aggression and self-injurious behaviour in both children and adults with intellectual disability and/or autism; many of the studies reported evidence of benefit for behavioural symptoms, however adverse effects were also common, even at low doses.
- For treatment of aggression, aripiprazole may be an alternative choice of antipsychotic in children and low-dose haloperidol in adults; however, side effects again limit their use.
- SSRI treatment may be helpful for aggression and/or self-injurious behaviour.

Statements of Low Confidence

- The clinical subtypes introduced by Mace and Mauk (1995) may inform the choice of medication group for treatment of self-injurious behaviour.
- There is limited evidence on the impact of deprescribing of psychotropic medication for behaviours seen as challenging; good practice guidelines are provided to support clinicians around this.

Resource Box

Resources for Professionals

National Institute for Health and Care Excellence (2015): Challenging behaviour and learning disabilities: Prevention and interventions for people with learning disabilities whose behaviour challenges. www.nice.org.uk/guidance/ng11

Faculty of Intellectual Disability & British Psychological Society (2016): Challenging behaviour: A unified approach – update. FR/ID/08. www.nottingham.ac.uk/healthsciences/documents/challenging-behaviour-a-unified-approach.pdf

British Institute for Learning Disabilities (2022): What does good PBS look like now? www.bild.org.uk/wp-content/uploads/2022/08/Bild-What-Does-Good-PBS-Look-Like-Print.pdf

Resources for Carers

- The Challenging Behaviour Foundation: Quick Read: Challenging Behaviour Guide www.challengingbehaviour.org.uk/wp-content/uploads/2021/03/quickreadchallengingbehaviourguidev6.pdf

- The Challenging Behaviour Foundation: Understanding Challenging Behaviour: Part 1. www.challengingbehaviour.org.uk/wp-content/uploads/2022/12/001-Understanding-Challenging-Behavour-Part-1.pdf
- The Challenging Behaviour Foundation: Finding the Reasons for Challenging Behaviour: Part 2. www.challengingbehaviour.org.uk/wp-content/uploads/2022/12/002-Finding-the-Reasons-for-Challenging-Behaviour-Part-2.pdf
- The Challenging Behaviour Foundation: Positive Behaviour Support Planning: Part 3. www.challengingbehaviour.org.uk/wp-content/uploads/2022/12/003-Positive-Behaviour-Support-Planning-Part-3.pdf

References

Ahmed, Z., Fraser, W., Kerr, M. P., et al. (2000). Reducing antipsychotic medication in people with a learning disability. *The British Journal of Psychiatry*, **176**, 42–6.

Aman, M. G., De Smedt, G., Derivan, A., et al. (2002). Double-blind, placebo-controlled study of risperidone for the treatment of disruptive behaviors in children with subaverage intelligence. *American Journal of Psychiatry*, **159**, 1337–46.

Amore, M., Bertelli, M., Villani, D., Tamborini, S., & Rossi, M. (2011). Olanzapine vs. risperidone in treating aggressive behaviours in adults with intellectual disability: A single blind study. *Journal of Intellectual Disability Research*, **55**, 210–18.

Anderson, C. A., & Bushman, B. J. (2002). Human aggression. *Annual Review of Psychology*, **53**, 27–51.

Chan, J., Arnold, S., Webber, L., Riches, V., & Parmenter, T. (2012). Is it time to drop the term 'Challenging Behaviour'? *Learning Disability Practice*, **15**, 36–8.

Cohen, D., Raffin, M., Canitano, R., et al. (2013). Risperidone or aripiprazole in children and adolescents with autism and/or intellectual disability: A Bayesian meta-analysis of efficacy and secondary effects. *Research in Autism Spectrum Disorders*, **7**, 167–75.

Cooper, S. A., Smiley, E., Allan, L. M., et al. (2009a). Adults with intellectual disabilities: prevalence, incidence and remission of self-injurious behaviour, and related factors. *Journal of Intellectual Disability Research*, **53**, 200–16.

Cooper, S. A., Smiley, E., Jackson, A., et al. (2009b). Adults with intellectual disabilities: prevalence, incidence and remission of aggressive behaviour and related factors. *Journal of Intellectual Disability Research*, **53**, 217–32.

Cooper, S. J., Reynolds, G. P., Barnes, T., et al. (2016). BAP guidelines on the management of weight gain, metabolic disturbances and cardiovascular risk associated with psychosis and antipsychotic drug treatment. *Journal of Psychopharmacology*, **30**, 717–48.

Costello, A., Hudson, E., Morrissey, S., et al. (2022). Management of psychotropic medications in adults with intellectual disability: A scoping review. *Annals of Medicine*, **54**, 2486–99.

Craft, M., Ismail, I., Krishnamurti, D., et al. (1987). Lithium in the treatment of aggression in mentally handicapped patients: A double-blind trial. *The British Journal of Psychiatry*, **150**, 685–9.

Crocker, A. G., Mercier, C., Allaire, J. F., & Roy, M. E. (2007). Profiles and correlates of aggressive behaviour among adults with intellectual disabilities. *Journal of Intellectual Disability Research*, **51**, 786–801.

Crocker, A. G., Mercier, C., Lachapelle, Y., et al. (2006). Prevalence and types of aggressive behaviour among adults with intellectual disabilities. *Journal of Intellectual Disability Research*, **50**, 652–61.

Davies, L. E., & Oliver, C. (2016). Self-injury, aggression and destruction in children with severe intellectual disability: Incidence, persistence and novel, predictive behavioural risk markers. *Research in Developmental Disabilities*, **49–50**, 291–301.

Davies, L., & Oliver, C. (2013). The age related prevalence of aggression and self-injury in persons with an intellectual disability: A review. *Research in Developmental Disabilities*, **34**, 764–75.

Deb, S., Thomas, M., & Bright, C. (2001). Mental disorder in adults with intellectual disability. 2: The rate of behaviour disorders among a community-based population aged between 16 and 64 years. *Journal of Intellectual Disability Research*, **45**, 506–14.

Denis, J., Van Den Noortgate, W., & Maes, B. (2011). Self-injurious behavior in people with profound intellectual disabilities: A meta-analysis of single-case studies. *Research in Developmental Disabilities*, **32**, 911–23.

Dimian, A. F., & Symons, F. J. (2022). A systematic review of risk for the development and persistence of self-injurious behavior in intellectual and developmental disabilities. *Clinical Psychology Review*, **94**, 102158.

Heyvaert, M., Maes, B., & Onghena, P. (2010). A meta-analysis of intervention effects on challenging behaviour among persons with intellectual disabilities. *Journal of Intellectual Disability Research*, **54**, 634–49.

Heyvaert, M., Maes, B., Van Den Noortgate, W., Kuppens, S., & Onghena, P. (2012). A multilevel meta-analysis of single-case and small-n research on interventions for reducing challenging behavior in persons with intellectual disabilities. *Research in Developmental Disabilities*, **33**, 766–80.

Hollander, E., Wasserman, S., Swanson, E. N., et al. (2006). A double-blind placebo-controlled pilot study of olanzapine in childhood/adolescent pervasive developmental disorder. *Journal of Child, & Adolescent Psychopharmacology*, **16**, 541–8.

Juneja, D. K., Sultan, A., Juneja, A., & Siddiqui, M. (2019). Lesch–Nyhan syndrome: A rare occurrence. *Journal of Behavioral Health*, **8**, 122–5.

L'Abbé, Y., & Morin, D. (2001). *Comportements Agressifs et Retard Mental: Compréhension et Intervention*, 2nd ed. QC, Éditions behaviora.

Mace, F. C., & Mauk, J. E. (1995). Bio-behavioral diagnosis and treatment of self-injury. *Mental Retardation and Developmental Disabilities Research Reviews*, **1**, 104–10.

Mascitelli, A. N., Rojahn, J., Nicolaides, V. C., et al. (2015). The Behaviour Problems Inventory-Short Form: Reliability and factorial validity in adults with intellectual disabilities. *Journal of Applied Research in Intellectual Disabilities*, **28**, 561–71.

McAdam, D. B., Zarcone, J. R., Hellings, J., Napolitano, D. A., & Schroeder, S. R. (2002). Effects of risperidone on aberrant behavior in persons with developmental disabilities: II. Social validity measures. *American Journal on Mental Retardation*, **107**, 261–9.

McDougle, C. J., Holmes, J. P., Carlson, D. C., et al. (1998). A double-blind, placebo-controlled study of risperidone in adults with autistic disorder and other pervasive developmental disorders. *Archives of General Psychiatry*, **55**, 633–41.

Morano, S., Ruiz, S., Hwang, J., et al. (2017). Meta-analysis of single-case treatment effects on self-injurious behavior for individuals with autism and intellectual disabilities. *Autism, & Developmental Language Impairments*, **2**, 2396941516688399.

National Institute for Health and Care Excellence (2015). *Challenging behaviour and learning disabilities: prevention and interventions for people with learning disabilities whose behaviour challenges*, National Institute for Health and Care Excellence.

Oliver, C., Licence, L., & Richards, C. (2017). Self-injurious behaviour in people with intellectual disability and autism spectrum disorder. *Current Opinion in Psychiatry*, **30**, 97–101.

Rana, F., Gormez, A., & Varghese, S. (2013). Pharmacological interventions for self-injurious behaviour in adults with intellectual disabilities. *Cochrane Database of Systematic Reviews*, **4**, CD009084.

Rees, J., & Langdon, P. E. (2016). The relationship between problem-solving ability and self-harm amongst people with mild intellectual disabilities. *Journal of Applied*

Research in Intellectual Disabilities, 29, 387–93.

Rojahn, J., Rowe, E., Sharber, A., et al. (2012). The Behavior Problems Inventory-Short Form for individuals with intellectual disabilities: Part I: development and provisional clinical reference data. *Journal of Intellectual Disability Research*, **56**, 527–45.

Royal College of Psychiatrists (2001). *DC-LD: Diagnostic criteria for psychiatric disorders for use with adults with learning disabilities/mental retardation*, London, Royal College of Psychiatrists, Occasional Paper OP 48.

Ruedrich, S., Swales, T., Fossaceca, C., Toliver, J., & Rutkowski, A. (1999). Effect of divalproex sodium on aggression and self-injurious behaviour in adults with intellectual disability: A retrospective review. *Journal of Intellectual Disability Research*, **43**, 105–11.

Schroeder, S. R., Marquis, J. G., Reese, R. M., et al. (2014). Risk factors for self-injury, aggression, and stereotyped behavior among young children at risk for intellectual and developmental disabilities. *American Journal on Intellectual and Developmental Disabilities*, **119**, 351–70.

Sohanpal, S., Deb, S., Thomas, C., et al. (2007). The effectiveness of antidepressant medication in the management of behaviour problems in adults with intellectual disabilities: A systematic review. *Journal of Intellectual Disability Research*, **51**, 750–65.

Tyrer, F., McGrother, C. W., Thorp, C. F., et al. (2006). Physical aggression towards others in adults with learning disabilities: Prevalence and associated factors. *Journal of Intellectual Disability Research*, **50**, 295–304.

Tyrer, P., Oliver-Africano, P. C., Ahmed, Z., et al. (2008). Risperidone, haloperidol, and placebo in the treatment of aggressive challenging behaviour in patients with intellectual disability: A randomised controlled trial. *The Lancet*, **371**(9606), 57–63.

Zarcone, J. R., Hellings, J. A., Crandall, K., et al. (2001). Effects of risperidone on aberrant behavior of persons with developmental disabilities: I. A double-blind crossover study using multiple measures. *American Journal on Mental Retardation*, **106**, 525–38.

Zarcone, J. R., Lindauer, S. E., Morse, P. S., et al. (2004). Effects of risperidone on destructive behavior of persons with developmental disabilities: III. Functional analysis. *American Journal on Mental Retardation*, **109**, 310–21.

Chapter 11

Personality Disorders

Ayomipo J. Amiola, Sreeja Sahadevan, Reena Tharian, Sadie Clarke, and Regi T. Alexander

Introduction

What are Personality Disorders?

Personality refers to the innate and enduring characteristics that influence an individual's attitudes, their behaviours, and their experience of themselves, others, and the world. Historically, personality disorders were conceptualised as enduring and pervasive disturbance in an individual's patterns of thinking, feelings, and behaviours. This disturbance results in significant disturbance in their psychosocial functioning and interpersonal relationships (Cooray et al., 2022).

Traditionally, a categorical system was used to identify personality disorders. For example, the American Psychiatric Association's *Diagnostic and Statistical Manual of Mental Disorders* DSM-IV (1994) identified 10 personality disorders across 3 clusters. Paranoid, schizoid, and schizotypal personality disorders were part of cluster A; antisocial, borderline, histrionic, and narcissistic personality disorders were part of cluster B; and obsessive-compulsive, avoidant, and dependent personality disorders part of cluster C.

The International Classification of Diseases (ICD 10) categorisation (1993) was similar, albeit with small differences. Schizotypal disorder was classified as a schizophrenia spectrum condition and not a personality disorder. Antisocial personality disorder was called 'dissocial'. Instead of the category of borderline personality disorder, there were two sub-types of emotionally unstable personality disorder: borderline and impulsive. Narcissistic personality disorder was not recognised.

The American Psychiatric Association's *Diagnostic and Statistical Manual of Mental Disorders* DSM-5 (2013) retained the categorical approach, albeit limiting it to 6 categories (antisocial, borderline, narcissistic, schizotypal, avoidant, and obsessive-compulsive) from the 10 named in the DSM-IV. It also introduced an alternate model which could be used. This model incorporated a dimensional approach and was organised as a four-stage process: identification of the deficits in self; assessment of their severity; comparison of the personality traits of the patient with those of the six personality disorder types named earlier; and, finally, identification of maladaptive personality traits.

In a radical departure from ICD-10, ICD-11 (2019) abolished all categories except for a general description of personality disorder. Clinicians could classify three levels of severity (Mild Personality Disorder, Moderate Personality Disorder, and Severe Personality Disorder). Five personality trait domains (negative affectivity, dissociality, anankastia, detachment, and disinhibition) could be specified in addition to a borderline pattern qualifier. The ICD-11 shows considerable alignment with the DSM-5's alternative model for personality disorders (Bach et al., 2022; Mulder, 2021, Bach and First, 2018). Its dimensional model is still relatively new and there is limited evidence for its clinical utility. Prescribing decisions still tend to rely mostly on categorical diagnostic models.

What Causes Personality Disorders?

While the exact aetiology of personality disorders is unknown; a complex combination of genetic and environmental factors, including gene–environment interactions, have been proposed as making a person more likely to develop one (Cooray et al., 2022). Risk factors such as physical and sexual abuse, growing up in an antisocial family, violent parenting, lack of consistent rules in the family, and early conduct problems have been identified as significant risk factors (Harrison et al., 2017).

How Are Personality Disorders Different in People with Intellectual Disability?

The diagnosis of personality disorders in people with intellectual disability is complicated for many reasons (Alexander & Cooray, 2003). Firstly, there is a delay in the development of lasting personality traits in people with intellectual disability. Secondly, there is a significant overlap between the features of autism spectrum conditions and some cluster A personality disorders, and in the consequences of trauma and negative life experiences often present in people with intellectual disability and the criteria for some cluster B personality disorders. Similarly, the criteria for cluster C dependent or anxious-avoidant personality disorders are very similar to the realistic dependency needs of people with intellectual disability. A third complicating factor is that in people with intellectual disability there is a significant difficulty in eliciting information about subjective thoughts and emotions, especially in those with severe to profound forms of intellectual disability (Cooray et al., 2022). Therefore, it was recommended that, clinically, a diagnosis of personality disorders in people with intellectual disability should not be made until at least 21 years of age, it should be limited to cluster B (emotionally unstable and dissocial) and should be made only in those with mild to moderate intellectual disability (Naik et al., 2002).

Symptoms such as anger outbursts and violence to self and others can be present in many people with intellectual disability. However, when these are associated with features such as persistent and potentially fatal behaviours, inadequate reactions to the suffering of others; a pervasive tendency to irritability; a limited range of emotional responses; a persistent drive for self-gratification; interactions aimed primarily at deriving a secondary advantage; alternating between idealisation of staff and subsequent devaluation; manipulative behaviour; impulsive behaviour; overestimation of the intimacy of relationships; a pattern of stormy, emotionally charged and short-lived relationships, etc., it should warrant an assessment for the presence of a personality disorder (Bertelli et al., 2012).

Case Study 11.1: Presentation

Shobna is a 32-year-old female who was a frequent attender at her local accident and emergency unit for overdose attempts, self-harming behaviours, and police involvement for challenging behaviours. Shobna is diagnosed with a mild learning disability, challenging behaviour, episodes of low mood, and poor sleep. Her mother died when Shobna was six years old. Her father was imprisoned when Shobna was eight and she became a looked-after child. Shobna was subjected to multiple placement breakdowns due to difficulties with managing her challenging behaviours and there is history of childhood physical and emotional abuse by the foster family. Shobna was diagnosed with depression at the age of 25 years by her general practitioner and was prescribed sertraline, which improved her episodes of low mood. However, Shobna continued to present with impulsive behaviours, including self-harm, substance misuse, and violent outbursts. When stressed, she hears voices telling her to kill herself and hurt others. When settled, she will often report feeling lonely and desperate, and will get involved in quite turbulent and short-lived intimate relationships.

How Common are Personality Disorders in People with Intellectual Disability?

The worldwide pooled prevalence for all personality disorders is 7.8% (95% CI 6.1–9.5), the prevalence of clusters A, B, and C being 3.8% (95% CI 3.2, 4.4%), 2.8% (1.6, 3.7%), and 5.0% (4.2, 5.9%) respectively (Winsper et al., 2020). However, a significant level of heterogeneity was noted based on the study design, the income of the country, and the interview administration (clinician vs trained graduate).

The literature regarding the prevalence of personality disorders in intellectual disability shows an uncertainty in prevalence, both in community (1–91%) and inpatient settings (22–92%). This wide range was partly attributable to the setting, the complexity in diagnosis, and symptom overlaps, and was too large to reflect true variability (Cooray et al., 2022; Alexander and Cooray, 2003).

A study done in the forensic inpatient setting using American Psychiatric Association's *Diagnostic and Statistical Manual of Mental Disorders* DSM-IV-TR criteria for people with intellectual disability showed that antisocial personality disorder was the most common personality disorder (62.8%), followed by personality disorder not otherwise specified (30.6%), schizotypal personality disorder (8.6%), paranoid personality disorder (7.6%), schizoid personality disorder (7.6%), borderline personality disorder (7.6%), narcissistic personality disorder (7.6%), histrionic personality disorder (3.8%), and anxious-avoidant personality disorder (3.3%) (Cooray et al., 2022).

Among people with mild intellectual disability, Wieland et al. found cluster B personality disorders to be the most common (9.2%) (antisocial 0%, borderline 7.9%, histrionic 0.7%, narcissistic 0.7%), followed by cluster C at 2.6% (avoidant 2.0%, dependent 0.7%, obsessive-compulsive 0%), personality disorder not otherwise specified (PD NOS) at 21.7%, and cluster A at 0%. In the same study among people with borderline intellectual functioning, PD NOS was the most frequent diagnosis (28.1%), followed by cluster B (17.4%) (antisocial PD 1.7%, borderline PD 15.3%, histrionic PD 0%, narcissistic PD 1.3%) and cluster C (8.1%) (avoidant 2.6%, dependent 4.7%, obsessive-compulsive 1.3%), with an absence of cluster A (Cooray et al., 2022; Wieland et al., 2015).

Among people with intellectual disability with severe challenging behaviours, the prevalence noted for paranoid personality disorder was 64%, schizoid 50%, dissocial 53%, emotionally unstable 50%, histrionic 33%, anankastic 22%, avoidant 50%, and dependent 28% (Flynn et al., 2002; Cooray et al., 2022).

Treatments: The Evidence Base

General Population

In the general population, the National Institute for Health, and Care Excellence (NICE) has published two clinical guidelines. The first was borderline personality disorder: recognition and management (2009) and the second, Antisocial personality disorder: prevention and management (2013). In addition, the guidance for Personality disorders: borderline and antisocial QS88 (NICE, 2015) sets out the standards in assessing and managing personality disorders.

For all patients, diagnosis should be made using a structured clinical assessment, psychological interventions should be provided in a collaborative manner, and pharmacological agents should only be for short-term crisis management or treatment of comorbid conditions. In the long term, care providers and patients should agree on a structured and phased plan prior to any form of change or end of services. In addition, care plans should incorporate long-term goals for education and employment. Lastly, length and frequency of supervision should be agreed collaboratively.

In terms of treatments, psychotherapy may be effective in reducing borderline symptom severity, self-harm, suicide-related outcomes, and depression, while also improving psychosocial functioning. Dialectical behavioural therapy (DBT) appears to be better at reducing borderline severity and self-harm and improving psychosocial functioning compared to usual treatment. Mentalisation-based treatments (MBT) appear to be more effective than usual treatment at reducing self-harm and suicidality (Völlm et al., 2020).

In the UK, the NICE treatment guidelines for emotionally unstable and dissocial personality disorders (2009, 2013) recommend that apart from short-term sedating medication during crises in emotionally unstable personality disorder, drug treatment should not be used.

The American Psychiatric Association guidelines, however, recommend the use of psychotropic medication based on the prominent symptom domains, and name antidepressant medication for affective instability, mood stabilisers for impulsive-aggression, and antipsychotics for cognitive-perceptual disturbances (American Psychiatric Association 2001).

In 2010, a Cochrane collaboration systematic review and meta-analysis suggested that drug treatment, especially with mood stabilisers and second-generation antipsychotics, may be effective for treating several core symptoms and associated psychopathology of personality disorder. It found some evidence that mood stabilisers reduce affective dysregulation and impulsive-aggression while antipsychotics reduce cognitive-perceptual symptoms and affective dysregulation (Leib et al., 2010).

In 2022, a review with updated trials found that no pharmacological therapy seems effective in specifically treating borderline pathology (Stoffers-Winterling et al., 2022).

A nationwide retrospective cohort study examining the prescribing of antipsychotics among people with recorded personality disorder in primary care in the UK involved 46,210 people and found that antipsychotics are frequently and increasingly prescribed for extended periods to people with a personality disorder who had no serious mental illnesses. It called for an urgent review of clinical practice, and an examination of the effectiveness of such prescribing and the need to monitor for adverse effects (Hardoon et al., 2022).

People with Intellectual Disability

Among people with intellectual disability, the evidence base for the management of personality disorders, although growing, is relatively limited (Williams & Rose, 2020). Like the general population, the gold standard of treatment remains psychotherapy. Several factors impact the success of therapy in people with intellectual disability. These range from cognitive abilities, presence of comorbid diagnoses, level of insight, and individual motivation to change (Gentile et al., 2022).

When there are coexisting major mental illnesses or symptoms that can potentially benefit from medications, these should be judiciously prescribed together with psychotherapeutic and behavioural strategies (Lew et al., 2006). In addition, five predominant symptom domains (cognitive-perceptual, affective dysregulation, behavioural dyscontrol, anxiety, and self-injurious behaviour) with potential for pharmacological management have been proposed for people with intellectual disability and comorbid personality disorder (Alexander et al., 2007).

People with Intellectual Disability: Non-Medication Treatments

Methodological flaws limit the evidence base for these treatments. DBT, schema therapy, nidotherapy, therapeutic community treatment models, and rehabilitation approaches have been found to be beneficial, although these are mostly based on small case reports and case series. Table 11.1 provides a summary of the non-medication treatments used for people with intellectual disability and personality disorder.

Table 11.1 Non-medication treatments in intellectual disability

Psychotherapy	Evidence in intellectual disability
Standard dialectical behavioural therapy (DBT)	Full dialectical behavioural therapy programme aimed at individuals with intellectual disability presenting with 'problem behaviours' and underserved by community services. It incorporated weekly individual therapy, 69 group sessions, a consultation team, a telephone coaching service, and involvement of allied services and family members to develop environments which could support the therapy (Lew et al., 2006). An adapted DBT programme for male offenders with intellectual disabilities at a high-secure intellectual disability service. The programme included 60 group sessions, weekly individual therapy, and coaching via 'dialectical behavioural therapy-aware' inpatient staff (Morrissey & Ingamells, 2011). Full DBT programme incorporating a group skills component (adapted versions of all four modules offered in standard DBT), individual therapy, a consulting team, and a carers' component substituting 24-hour coaching (Hall et al., 2013)
Stand-alone adapted DBT skills groups	Forensic client group with intellectual disability, therapy based on DBT principles, and a coping skills programme. It included 13 90-minute sessions focusing on the quality of life and addressing risk

Table 11.1 (cont.)

Psychotherapy	Evidence in intellectual disability
	factors for challenging and/or offending behaviour. Other components included environment structuring, residential staff training to assist with homework, and strategies to encourage joint learning and generalisation (Sakdalan et al., 2010).
	Ten adult women with intellectual disability and PD recruited from two inpatient units. Details of adaptations to DBT not available (Roscoe et al., 2016)
Integrated biopsychosocial interventions	A four-stage model of behavioural management, pharmacotherapy, staff training, and development of dialectical behavioural therapy-informed coping strategies (Wilson, 2001).
	A case study illustrating combined behavioural, psychological, and pharmacological treatment of comorbid personality disorder in intellectual disability (Esbenson & Benson, 2003).
	Integrated and personalised intervention including maintaining consistent therapeutic environments, staff training regarding personality disorder, behavioural interventions, psychotherapy, relaxation, skills to reduce self-harm, and pharmacotherapy (Wink et al., 2010)
Psychoeducational groups	A 'living with personality disorder group' for women in a secure forensic service aimed at increasing knowledge of personality, personality disorders, and their treatment, including 'non-disordered' parts of self. Twelve group sessions plus two individual sessions based on DBT principles. Additional 'drop-in' sessions were available to support with homework (Morris & Gray, 2015).
	A therapeutic community intervention for men with a primary diagnosis of personality disorder, living in a high-secure intellectual disability service (Morrissey et al., 2012)
Occupational therapy	A work-based learning programme designed for patients within a forensic hospital for people with intellectual disability. The partnership between the hospital, a workplace, and a further education college became a crucial part of the patient's treatment programme (Smith et al., 2010).
	A personally meaningful programme of activities was utilised as a basis for developing positive, trusting relationships between participants and staff in a medium-secure unit (Withers et al., 2012)

People with Intellectual Disability: Medication Treatments

There are no randomised controlled trials conducted to assess the usefulness of medications in the management of personality disorders in people with intellectual disability. Hence, the evidence for medication treatment of personality disorders in intellectual disability is limited to case reports and small case series as highlighted in Table 11.2.

Table 11.2 Medication treatments in Intellectual disability

• A case series of 20 people with intellectual disability and personality disorder with history of offending behaviour which showed that 70% were prescribed psychotropic medications (hypnotics, anxiolytics, antidepressants, and antipsychotics)	Day, 1988
• In a case report of two people with intellectual disability and personality disorder, medication treatment included a low-dose antipsychotic and an selective serotonin reuptake inhibitor antidepressant	Goldberg et al., 1995
• Significant clinical improvement was reported with olanzapine + fluoxetine + semisodium valproate combination in patients with intellectual disability and personality disorder	Mavromatis, 2000
• In a sample of adults with intellectual disability and personality disorder, although only 30% had comorbid mental illnesses, 90% were receiving psychotropic medication	Naik et al., 2002
• A case series of 24 patients with intellectual disability and mental health difficulties who were treated with clozapine, of which 3 had a personality disorder and a favourable response to treatment	Thalayasingam et al., 2004
• Significant and sustained improvement in both mood and impulsivity over a period of four years in a person with intellectual disability and personality disorder receiving treatment with clozapine	Biswas et al., 2006
• Case series on the long-term outcome of treatment for 5 patients with intellectual disability and personality disorder at the end of 36 months of treatment with clozapine	Kiani et al., 2015

Treatment Guidelines in Intellectual Disability

Assessment

- A detailed diagnostic assessment (Alexander et al., 2010; Chester et al., 2023) as set out in Chapter 4 should be carried out. This will cover the degree of intellectual disability, cause of intellectual disability, and any behaviour phenotypes, autism spectrum disorder, other developmental disorders, mental illnesses, personality disorders, substance misuse, physical health conditions, experience of trauma, and types of challenging behaviour.
- A psychological formulation using the 5-P model of the presenting problem, predisposing, precipitating, perpetuating and protective factors (Macneil et al., 2012) or equivalent should be completed along with using the HELP framework of Health, Environment, Lived experience and Psychiatric problems (Green et al., 2018).
- Particular attention should be paid to the experience of past trauma. The therapeutic approach to that is examined in detail in Chapter 5 of this book.

Non-Medication Treatments

- Psychological interventions are the mainstay of treatment.
- While there is no clear superiority for any school of therapy, DBT or dialectical behavioural therapy-based approaches are widely used.

- Adaptations should be made to adapt existing psychological, behavioural, and social treatments available in the general population.
- Provision of coping skills, including practical social support such as housing, educational and occupational assistance.
- Staff support and training is also important in designing treatment programmes.

Medication Treatments

- Where present, comorbid acquired mental illnesses should be managed appropriately based on the guidelines specific for that illness.
- In the absence of a mental illness, psychotropic medication is not recommended for people with intellectual disability and a personality disorder. The conditions for using any psychotropic medication, particularly antipsychotics, in this situation would be like those listed in Chapter 4 of this book in relation to challenging behaviour (NICE, 2015; Royal College of Psychiatrists, 2016); for example, when:
    - psychological or other interventions alone have not produced the desired outcome within an agreed reasonable time; or
    - treatment for any coexisting mental or physical health problem has not led to a reduction in the behaviour; or
    - the risk to the person or others is severe.
- Five symptom domains have been described (Alexander et al., 2007; Alexander & Tharian, 2021; Cooray et al., 2022). They are:
    - Cognitive, perceptual (e.g., chronic, low-level features like ideas of reference, pseudo-hallucinations, persecutory or self-referential ideas, fleeting hallucinations, etc.)
    - Affective dysregulation (e.g., affective instability, mood swings, chronic dysthymia-like features, emotional detachment, etc.)
    - Behaviour dyscontrol (e.g., types of aggression including affective, predatory, and ictal)
    - Anxiety (e.g., cognitive and somatic)
    - Self-injurious behaviour (e.g., including repetitive stereotyped behaviour, extreme tissue damage, co-occurring self-injury and aggression, self-injury with agitation when interrupted, mixed type)
- A narrative account of which of these domains are present and those that are the targets of treatment should be recorded.
- The goal for medication treatment should be discussed, agreed, and recorded collaboratively before commencing treatment.
- Both the anticipated effects and potential side effects of the proposed treatment should be discussed with the patient and, where appropriate, their family members and carers.
- The medications of choice for each symptom domain are as follows:
    - Cognitive-perceptual domain:
        - For low-level, chronic symptoms, consider low-dose antipsychotics.
        - For acute psychotic relapses, follow treatment guidelines for psychosis.

- Affective dysregulation domain:
  - For chronic dysthymia-like symptoms, consider antidepressant medication/SSRIs as first line followed by mood stabilisers.
  - For mood swings not amenable to non-pharmacological treatments, consider mood stabilisers as first line followed by low-dose antipsychotic medication.
- Behaviour dyscontrol domain:
  - Affective aggression (characterised by impulsivity, angry outbursts, rapid mood changes, and often a normal ECG): consider antidepressant medication, SSRIs, or mood stabilisers as first line.
  - Predatory aggression (relatively rare in people with intellectual disability and characterised by hostile and cruel behaviour associated with low emotional or physiological arousal): consider antipsychotic medication. Although there is randomised controlled trial evidence supporting the use of oral Zuclopenthixol for aggression, clinicians and patients may prefer atypical antipsychotics due to a better side-effect profile.
  - Ictal aggression domain (characterised by episodic, stereotyped aggression and often associated with epilepsy or abnormal electroencephalographs: consider mood stabilising antiepileptics as first line).
- Anxiety domain:
  - For cognitive anxiety symptoms, selective serotonin reuptake inhibitors can be the first line. For very severe symptoms, short-term benzodiazepine use may be needed.
  - For somatic anxiety symptoms, a beta blocker such as propranolol can be considered.
- Self-injurious behaviour domain:
  - Follow guidelines for self-injurious behaviour as set out in Chapter 10 of this book.

Length of Treatment and Related Issues

- Since the instigation of the Stopping Over-Medication of People with a Learning Disability (STOMP) programme (NHS England, 2016), clinicians have been reminded of the need to ensure medications are prescribed only for appropriate indications and only continued for an appropriate time.
- Prescribing of psychotropic medication in those with personality disorders is off label, and hence prescribers should follow recommendations set out by the regulatory bodies for such prescribing (Good practice in prescribing and managing medicines and devices 2021;www.gmc-uk.org/professional-standards/professional-standards-for-doctors/good-practice-in-prescribing-and-managing-medicines-and-devices).
- Any such prescribing should be for the shortest possible time. It should be considered an individual treatment trial and must be reviewed regularly, with a set length of time collaboratively agreed.
- There should be regular follow-ups to monitor progress, screen for side effects, and check for worsening of symptoms (minimum recommended frequency of 3–6 months).

- The response to treatment should be recorded with objective instruments such as the Clinical Global Impression Scale (Guy, 1976), the Liverpool University Neuroleptic Side Effect Rating Scale (LUNSERS) (Day et al., 1995), or equivalents.
- Treatments should only be continued if there is clear clinical benefit that outweighs any risks; otherwise, medications should be discontinued.

Case Study 11.2: Treatment

Following multiple relationship breakdowns, Shobna took a significant overdose and was admitted to a specialist hospital for people with intellectual disability and mental health difficulties. Following full diagnostic assessment, Shobna was diagnosed with a personality disorder. She had a psychological formulation and positive behaviour support plans. She had both group and individual psychotherapy sessions incorporating dialectic behavioural therapy principles, mindfulness, coping strategies, and practical problem-solving skills. Due to the prominence of affective and transient psychotic symptoms when stressed, she was commenced on quetiapine for both its mood stabilising and its antipsychotic effect. Shobna participated in ward and day unit activities, excelling at sewing, dance, and art. She also began to volunteer at a local charity shop, and, following a period of mutual familiarisation with community support team, she was discharged back home. Quetiapine was tapered off and stopped within six months of discharge.

The Frith Prescribing Guidelines Editors' Expert Group Consensus Statements

Statements of High Confidence

In the absence of a mental illness, psychotropic medication is not recommended for people with intellectual disability and a personality disorder.

Prescribing of psychotropic medication in those with personality disorders would be off label, and hence prescribers should follow recommendations set out by the regulatory bodies for such prescribing.

There should be regular follow-ups to monitor progress and side effects (minimum recommended frequency of 3–6 months).

Treatments should only be continued if there is clear clinical benefit that outweighs any risks, otherwise medications should be discontinued.

Statements of Medium Confidence

Five symptom domains have been described in personality disorders in intellectual disability: cognitive-perceptual, affective dysregulation, behaviour dyscontrol, anxiety, and self-injurious behaviour.

Statements of Low Confidence

The first- and second-line medications for each of the aforementioned symptom domains that have been proposed may be effective for short-term management.

Resource Box

Antisocial personality disorder: prevention and management. National Institute for Health and Care Excellence Clinical guideline [CG77]. Published: 28 January 2009; last updated: 27 March 2013. https://www.nice.org.uk/guidance/cg77

Borderline personality disorder: recognition and management. National Institute for Health and Care Excellence Clinical guideline [CG78]. Published: 28 January 2009. www.nice.org.uk/guidance/cg78

Lieb, K., Völlm, B., Rücker, G., Timmer, A., & Stoffers, J. M. (2010). Pharmacotherapy for borderline personality disorder: Cochrane systematic review of randomised trials. *British Journal of Psychiatry*, Jan;196(1), 4–12. https://doi.org/10.1192/bjp.bp.108.062984. PMID: 20044651.

Medication Treatments chapter (pp. 84–91) in Working in community settings with people with learning disabilities and autistic people who are at risk of coming into contact with the criminal justice settings. A resource for health and social care staff (2021). Health Education England. http://wrap.warwick.ac.uk/156472/7/WRAP-Working-community-learning-disabilities-autistic-risk-criminal-justice-system-2021.pdf

National Institute for Health and Care Excellence (2015). Personality disorders: borderline and antisocial. Quality standard [QS88]. www.nice.org.uk/guidance/qs88

Taylor, D. M., Barnes, T. R. and Young, A. H. (2021). *The Maudsley prescribing guidelines in psychiatry*. 14th ed. John Wiley & Sons.

Easy-Read Documents

Borderline personality disorder (BPD): https://www.rethink.org/advice-and-information/about-mental-illness/learn-more-about-conditions/borderline-personality-disorder-bpd/

Helping You understand Personality Disorder: https://view.officeapps.live.com/op/view.aspx?src=https%3A%2F%2Fpeterbates.org.uk%2Fwp-content%2Fuploads%2F2017%2F12%2FPersonallity-disorder.doc&wdOrigin=BROWSELINK

Personality Disorders: https://www.mind.org.uk/media/7568/personality-disorders-2020-downloadable-pdf-version.pdf

References

Alexander, R. & Cooray, S. (2003). Diagnosis of personality disorders in learning disability. *The British Journal of Psychiatry*, 182(S44), s28–s31

Alexander, R. T., Green, F. N., O'Mahoney, B., et al. (2010). Personality disorders in offenders with intellectual disability: A comparison of clinical, forensic and outcome variables and implications for service provision. *Journal of Intellectual Disability Research*, 54(7), 650–8.

Alexander, R. T., Tajuddin, M., & Gangadharan, S. K. (2007). Personality disorders in intellectual disability: Approaches to pharmacotherapy. *Mental Health Aspects of Developmental Disabilities*, 10(4), 129–37.

Alexander, R., & Tharian, R. (2021). Medication Treatments, in P. E. Langdon & G. H. Murphy (ed.) *Working in community settings with people with learning disabilities and autistic people who are at risk of coming into contact with the criminal justice settings. A resource for health and social care staff.* Health Education England. http://wrap.warwick.ac.uk/156472/7/WRAP-Working-com

munity-learning-disabilities-autistic-risk-criminal-justice-system-2021.pdf, pp. 84–91.

American Psychiatric Association (1994). *Diagnostic and statistical manual of mental disorders* (4th ed.) American Psychiatric Association.

American Psychiatric Association (2001). Practice guideline for the treatment of patients with borderline personality disorder. *The American Journal of Psychiatry*, **158** (Suppl10), 1–52. https://doi.org/10.1176/appi.ajp.158.1.1.

American Psychiatric Association (2013). *Diagnostic and statistical manual of mental disorders* (5th ed.) American Psychiatric Association.

Bach, B. & First, M. B. (2018). Application of the ICD-11 classification of personality disorders. *BMC Psychiatry*, **18**(1), 351. https://doi.org/10.1186/s12888-018-1908-3. PMID: 30373564; PMCID: PMC6206910.

Bach, B., Kramer, U., Doering, S., et al. (2022). The ICD-11 classification of personality disorders: A European perspective on challenges and opportunities. *Borderline Personality Disorder and Emotion Dysregulation*, **9**(1), 1–11.

Bertelli, M., Scuticchio, D., Ferrandi, A., et al. (2012). Reliability and validity of the SPAID-G checklist for detecting psychiatric disorders in adults with intellectual disability. *Research in Developmental Disabilities*, **33**(2), 382–90.

Biswas, A., Gibbon, S. & Gangadharan, S. (2006), Clozapine in borderline personality disorder and intellectual disability: A case report of four-year outcome. *Mental Health: Aspects of Developmental Disabilities*, **9**(1), 13.

Chester, V., Tharian, P., Slinger, M., Varughese, A. & Alexander, R. T. (2023). Overview of offenders with intellectual disability. In J. M. McCarthy, R. T. Alexander, & E. Chaplin. (Eds.), Forensic *aspects of neurodevelopmental disorders: A clinician's guide* (pp. 24–33). Cambridge University Press.

Cooray, S. E., Alexander, R., Purandare, K., Chester, V., & Tyrer, P. (2022). Personality disorder in people with intellectual disability or those with intellectual disability and autism spectrum disorder. In M.O. Bertelli, S. Deb, K. Munir, A. Hassiotis, & L. Salvador-Carulla (eds.) Textbook of *psychiatry for intellectual disability and autism spectrum disorder*. Springer.

Day, J. C., Wood, G., Dewey, M., & Bentall, R. P. (1995). A self-rating scale for measuring neuroleptic side-effects: Validation in a group of schizophrenic patients. *The British Journal of Psychiatry*, **166**(5), 650–3.

Day, K. (1988). A hospital-based treatment programme for male mentally handicapped offenders. *The British Journal of Psychiatry*, **153**(5), 635–44.

Esbensen, A. J., & Benson, B. A. (2003). Integrating behavioral, psychological and pharmacological treatment: A case study of an individual with borderline personality disorder and mental retardation. *Mental Health Aspects of Developmental Disabilities*, **6**, 107–13.

Flynn, A., Matthews, H. & Hollins, S. (2002). Validity of the diagnosis of personality disorder in adults with learning disability and severe behavioural problems: Preliminary study. *The British Journal of Psychiatry*, **180**(6), 543–6.

Gentile, J. P., Bhatt, N. V., Cannella, J. P., Harper, K., & Johnson, J. (2022). Personality disorders in patients with intellectual disability. *Innovations in Clinical Neuroscience*, **19**(7–9), 17–21.

Goldberg, B., Gitta, M. Z., & Puddephatt, A. (1995). Personality and trait disturbances in an adult mental retardation population: Significance for psychiatric management. *Journal of Intellectual Disability Research*, **39**(4), 284–94.

Green, L., McNeil, K., Korossy, M., et al. 2018. HELP for behaviours that challenge in adults with intellectual and developmental disabilities. *Canadian Family Physician*, **64** (Suppl 2), S23–S31.

Guy, W. (1976). ECDEU assessment manual for psychopharmacology. US Department of Health, Education, and Welfare, Public Health Service, Alcohol, Drug Abuse, and Mental Health Administration, National Institute of Mental Health,

Psychopharmacology Research Branch, Division of Extramural Research Programs.

Hall, L., Bork, N., Craven, S., & Woodrow, C. (2013). People with learning disabilities experiences of a dialectical behaviour therapy skills group: A thematic analysis. *Clinical Psychology & People with Learning Disabilities*, **11**(1–2), 7–11.

Hardoon, S., Hayes, J., Viding, E., et al. (2022). Prescribing of antipsychotics among people with recorded personality disorder in primary care: A retrospective nationwide cohort study using The Health Improvement Network primary care database. *BMJ Open* **12**, e053943. https://doi.org/10.1136/bmjopen-2021-053943.

Harrison, P., Cowen, P., Burns, T., & Fazel, M. (2017). *Shorter Oxford textbook of psychiatry*. Oxford University Press.

Kiani, R., Biswas, A., Devapriam, J., et al. (2015). Clozapine use in personality disorder and intellectual disabilities. *Advances in Mental Health and Intellectual Disabilities*, **9**(6), 363–70. https://doi.org/10.1108/AMHID-02-2015-0009.

Lew, M., Matta, C., Tripp-Tebo, C., & Watts, D. (2006). Dialectical behavior therapy (DBT) for individuals with intellectual disabilities: A program description. *Mental Health Aspects of Developmental Disabilities*, **9**(1), 1.

Macneil, C. A., Hasty, M. K., Conus, P., & Berk, M. (2012). Is diagnosis enough to guide interventions in mental health? Using case formulation in clinical practice. *BMC Medicine*, **10**, 111. https://doi.org/10.1186/1741-7015-10-111.

Mavromatis, M. (2000). The diagnosis and treatment of borderline personality disorder in persons with developmental disability: Three case reports. *Mental Health Aspects of Developmental Disabilities*, **3**, 89–97.

Morris, D., & Gray, N. (2015). Increasing knowledge of personality disorders in detained women with an intellectual disability. *Journal of Intellectual Disabilities and Offending Behaviour*, **6**(1), 23–32.

Morrissey, C., & Ingamells, B. (2011). Adapted dialectical behaviour therapy for male offenders with learning disabilities in a high secure environment: Six years on. *Journal of Learning Disabilities and Offending Behaviour*, **2**(1), 8–15.

Morrissey, C., Taylor, J., & Bennett, C. (2012). Evaluation of a therapeutic community intervention for men with intellectual disability and personality disorder. *Journal of Learning Disabilities and Offending Behaviour*, **3**(1), 52–60.

Mulder, R. T. (2021). ICD-11 personality disorders: Utility and implications of the new model. *Frontiers in Psychiatry*, **12**, 655548.

Naik, B. I., Gangadharan, S., & Alexander, R. T. (2002). Personality disorders in learning disability – the clinical experience. *The British Journal of Development Disabilities*, **48**(95), 95–100.

National Institute for Health and Care Excellence (2009). Borderline personality disorder: recognition and management. Clinical guideline [CG78]. National Institute for Health and Care Excellence.

National Institute for Health and Care Excellence (2013). Antisocial personality disorder: prevention and management. Clinical guideline [CG77]. National Institute for Health and Care Excellence.

National Institute for Health and Care Excellence (2015). Personality disorders: borderline and antisocial. Quality standard [QS88]. National Institute for Health and Care Excellence.

NHS England (2016). Stopping over-medication of people with a learning disability (STOMP-LD) pledge. NHS England, London. www.england.nhs.uk/2016/06/over-medication-pledge.

Roscoe, P., Petalas, M., Hastings, R., & Thomas, C. (2016). Dialectical behaviour therapy in an inpatient unit for women with a learning disability: Service users' perspectives. *Journal of Intellectual Disabilities*, **20**(3), 263–80.

Sakdalan, J. A., Shaw, J., & Collier, V. (2010). Staying in the here-and-now: A pilot study on the use of dialectical behaviour therapy group skills training for forensic clients with intellectual disability. *Journal of Intellectual Disability Research*, **54**(6), 568–72.

Smith, A., Petty, M., Oughton, I., & Alexander, R. T. (2010). Establishing a work-based learning programme: Vocational rehabilitation in a forensic learning disability setting. *British Journal of Occupational Therapy*, **73**(9), 431–6.

Stoffers-Winterling, J. M., Storebø, O. J., Ribeiro, J. P., et al. (2022). Pharmacological interventions for people with borderline personality disorder. *Cochrane Database of Systematic Reviews*, (**11**).

Thalayasingam, S., Alexander, R. T., & Singh, I. (2004). The use of clozapine in adults with intellectual disability. *Journal of Intellectual Disability Research*, **48**(6), 572–9. https://doi.org/10.1111/j.1365-2788.2004.00626.x.

Völlm, B. A., Kongerslev, M. T., Mattivi, J. T., et al. (2020). Psychological therapies for people with borderline personality disorder. *Cochrane Database of Systematic Reviews*, (**5**).

Wieland, J., Van Den Brink, A., & Zitman, F.G. (2015). The prevalence of personality disorders in psychiatric outpatients with borderline intellectual functioning: Comparison with outpatients from regular mental health care and outpatients with mild intellectual disabilities. *Nordic Journal of Psychiatry*, **69**(8), 599–604.

Williams, E. M., & Rose, J. (2020). Nonpharmacological treatment for individuals with intellectual disability and 'personality disorder'. *Journal of Applied Research in Intellectual Disabilities*, **33**(4), 767–78.

Wilson, S. R. (2001). A four-stage model for management of borderline personality disorder in people with mental retardation. *Mental Health Aspects of Developmental Disabilities*, **4**, 68–76.

Wink, L. K., Erickson, C. A., Chambers, J. E., & McDougle, C. J. (2010). Co-morbid intellectual disability and borderline personality disorder: a case series. *Psychiatry: Interpersonal and Biological Processes*, **73**(3), 277–87.

Winsper, C., Bilgin, A., Thompson, A., et al. (2020). The prevalence of personality disorders in the community: A global systematic review and meta-analysis. *The British Journal of Psychiatry*, **216**(2), 69–78.

Withers, P., Boulton, N., Morrison, J., & Jones, A. (2012). Occupational therapy in a medium secure intellectual disability and personality disorder service. *Journal of Learning Disabilities and Offending Behaviour*, **3**(4), 206–18.

World Health Organization (WHO). (1993). The ICD-10 classification of mental and behavioural disorders. World Health Organization.

World Health Organization. (2019). International statistical classification of diseases and related health problems (11th ed.).

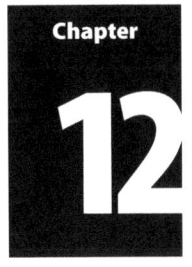

Chapter 12

Sexual Offences and Paraphilias

Stuart Banham, Gemma Lewin, and John Devapriam

Introduction

What Are Paraphilic Disorders?

Paraphilic disorders are a subgroup of sexual disorders (see Table 12.1). The International classification of diseases (ICD 11) describes paraphilic disorders as being characterised by persistent and intense patterns of atypical sexual arousal, manifested by sexual thoughts, fantasies, urges, or behaviours, the focus of which involves others whose age or status renders them unwilling or unable to consent, and on which the person has acted or by which he or she is markedly distressed.

Although the terms 'sexual offences' and 'paraphilias' are often used interchangeably, and there is overlap between them, there needs to be clarity about what each means. Sexual offences are marked by breaches of statute law, determined largely by the justice system (although an

Table 12.1 Paraphilic disorders in American Psychiatric Association's *Diagnostic and Statistical Manual of Mental Disorders* (DSM-V) and the International Classification of Diseases (ICD 11): disease classification systems

	American Psychiatric Association's *Diagnostic and Statistical Manual of Mental Disorders* DSM 5	International classification of diseases ICD 11
Exhibitionistic disorder	X	X
Voyeuristic disorder	X	X
Paedophilic disorder	X	X
Sexual sadism disorder	X	X
Frotteuristic disorder	X	X
Sexual masochism	X	
Transvestic	X	
Fetishistic	X	

individual's behaviour can place them at risk of law breaking). Only a proportion of sex offenders suffer from paraphilias, and not all individuals with a paraphilia are sex offenders.

Frequently, individuals suffering from paraphilias harbour extreme sexual fantasies and urges only, or their actions do not cross the threshold of involving a non-consenting individual or child. The treatment of paraphilias is not solely based on minimising risk, but also can include the aim of reducing the severe distress that an individual can feel about their extreme sexual urges.

Why Does Someone Develop a Paraphilic Disorder?

The development of a paraphilic disorder is complex and multifactorial in nature. Ward and Beech (2006; 2016) developed the Integrated Theory of Sexual Offending (ITSO), a broad aetiological framework that integrates previous theoretical models. Causal factors were highlighted, such as biological (evolution, genetic variations, neurobiology and brain development), ecological (social and cultural factors, personal circumstances, environment), core neuropsychological systems and personal agency. Empirical studies concerning paraphilias have shown an increased prevalence of a history of sexual abuse in childhood, attachment difficulties, social incompetence, emotional dysregulation and disinhibition caused by empathy deficits (Yakeley and Wood, 2014).

Testosterone, the main androgen produced by the testes, along with developing and maintaining male sexual characteristics, also controls sexuality, aggression, cognition and personality. Sexual fantasies, desire and behaviour are largely dependent on this hormone. The central serotonin metabolism also has a significant effect on sexual behaviour (Greenberg and Bradford, 1997).

How Are Paraphilic Disorders Different in People with Intellectual Disability?

The topic of paraphilic disorders in people with intellectual disability is controversial and difficult. Just as intellectual disability is a spectrum spanning a wide range of individual circumstances, so paraphilic disorders is a term covering a wide range of difficult circumstances. At one end of the spectrum are instances which clearly breach legal boundaries and place individuals at risk of prosecution and even imprisonment and at the other end circumstances which challenge the view of what constitutes 'normal' or acceptable behaviour. Viewed through the lens of intellectual disability, the definition of normal or acceptable becomes further distorted. Uppermost of any decisions regarding need for treatment, and which treatments are appropriate, should be a careful consideration of an individual's circumstances and the potential consequences of any behaviours.

Of note is the theory of 'counterfeit deviance' (Hingsburger et al, 2010), denoting a subgroup of people with intellectual disability whose behaviours presented as paraphilia-like but the function of the behaviour was not served by extreme sexual urges. This differentiation has clinical merit when considering an appropriate treatment pathway but should not exclude paraphilia as a diagnostic consideration. Factors are extensive in number but aim to further the understanding of both the individual with intellectual disability and the system in which they live (Griffiths et al, 2013). A lack of privacy, societal attitudes towards appropriate sexuality in people with intellectual disability, restricted access to appropriate sexual partners and 'peer-void', lack of educational access regarding appropriate sexual relations and inability to complete masturbation leading to a chronic state of sexual arousal have been described. Sexualised behaviours could also have a function of eliciting attention or care or avoiding an undesired situation.

In addition, people with intellectual disability experience higher rates of sexual abuse than the general population. A recent systematic review determined the combined prevalence of sexual abuse in adults with intellectual disability as 32.9% (95% CI: 22.7–43.0) (Tomsa et al, 2021). Sexual abuse can serve to influence future behaviour; which could include modelling of the behaviour or re-experiencing and communicating past traumatic experiences.

People with intellectual disability are more likely to live with a co-existing psychiatric condition (Hughes-McCormack et al, 2017). It is prudent to consider whether there is the potential for a differential diagnosis of another active psychiatric condition such as mania which could present with sexualised behaviour.

How Common Are Paraphilic Disorders in People with Intellectual Disability?

In the general population, the prevalence rates of any paraphilia have been recorded at rates between 0.4% and 15.9% (Joyal and Carpentier, 2016; Schöttle et al., 2017). When compared to the general population, a higher prevalence of paraphilic fantasies and behaviours in males with high functioning autism have been described (Schöttle et al., 2017).

Though sexual offending should not be used as a proxy for a paraphilia diagnosis, it remains that sexual offending comprises most of the available literature for people with intellectual disability. While many studies have highlighted a diagnosis of intellectual disability as more prevalent among those who offend and those who offend sexually, no definitive figure is available. A large population-based cohort study in Sweden (Latvala et al., 2021) observed the association of people with intellectual disability and sexual offending, and in addition observed the impact of a co-existing attention deficit hyperactivity disorder (ADHD) or autism diagnosis. The relative risks of both sexual offending and sexual victimisation were elevated in people with intellectual disability compared to the general population, with the highest risk of sexual offending in men being related to a diagnosis of intellectual disability and comorbid ADHD. Similarly, both sexual offending and sexual victimisation were increased in people with intellectual disability in a study by Nixon et al. (2017). In contrast, Callahan et al found that in an incarcerated population sample, people with intellectual disability were no more likely to commit sexual offences when compared to the general population (2022).

It should be noted that studies conducted in different settings have produced differing prevalence rates of offenders and types of offending. Due to differences in methodology and inclusion criteria of these studies, it has been difficult to reach a consensus on the prevalence of intellectual disability in sexual offenders (Lindsay et al., 2007).

Treatments: The Evidence Base

General Population

The remit of this chapter is pharmacological treatment, and it is suggested that readers refer to appropriate texts on psychological therapies for sexual offenders with intellectual disability. The different modalities utilised in this group include cognitive behavioural therapy (social skills training, cognitive restructuring, development of victim empathy, and imaginal desensitisation) and relapse prevention therapy (focused on dynamic factors such as intimacy, attachment, emotion regulation, and impulsivity). A Cochrane systematic review (Dennis et al., 2012) determined a need for further randomised controlled trials due to a lack of available evidence that such interventions were able to reduce recidivism significantly. Since this time outcomes have been variable, and no consensus has been upheld.

In men, sexual development and sexual drive are linked to testosterone production and activity. Central control of testosterone production emanates from the hypothalamus and anterior pituitary and involves the production of gonadotropin releasing hormone (GnRH), luteinising hormone (LH), and follicle stimulating hormone (FSH). Production and secretion of testosterone in the testes is stimulated by the action of luteinising hormone. When pharmacological therapies are considered, these are either hormonal or non-hormonal anti-ibido agents used with the intention of either temporarily or permanently diminishing or eradicating sexual desire and capacity.

Hormonal Treatments

This approach seeks to reduce testosterone production by either direct antiandrogen effects (antiandrogens such as cyproterone) or by increasing the level of gonadotrophin releasing hormone (GnRH analogues such as triptorelin), which in turn suppresses testosterone production via a negative feedback mechanism on the hypothalamus/anterior pituitary. A range of antiandrogens have been used in the management of paraphilias, including specific use in people with intellectual disability. With some of these agents there is the added advantage of long-acting injection formulations being available which can be beneficial in managing treatment adherence. Clinical trial evidence supporting the use of these agents is lacking, however. A 2015 Cochrane review of drug treatments for sexual offenders, or those at risk of offending, found only seven studies which could be considered, none of which involved the use of gonadotrophin-releasing-hormone analogues. With many of the studies included having methodological concerns, particularly being underpowered, the authors were unable to draw firm conclusions. They did, however, comment that the tolerability of these agents was uncertain and raise concerns about mandated treatment given the relative lack of efficacy evidence (Khan et al., 2015).

Non-Hormonal Treatments

Selective Serotonin Reuptake Inhibitors (SSRIs)

SSRIs are reported to reduce libido and delay orgasm in 60–70% of individuals who take them. The precise mechanism by which this effect is achieved is unclear but may involve central serotonergic regulation of mesolimbic dopamine pathways, which are involved in activation of sexual arousal. It is worth remembering that the predominant indication of SSRIs being the management of depression could increase the reported rate of reduced libido associated with this drug class; depression has an impact upon sexual desire. SSRIs may reduce paraphilic behaviours by reducing overall sexual interest, impulsiveness, and obsessive-compulsive symptoms. Small studies, with inevitable methodological limitations, have demonstrated the efficacy of SSRIs (including fluoxetine, sertraline, and citalopram) in treating a range of paraphilias. Sertraline has been reported to reduce deviant sexual behaviours, but it does not affect, and sometimes even improves, normal sexuality. (Bradford et al., 1995; Bradford, 2000). SSRIs prescribed between 12 and 18 years could prevent acting-out of deviant fantasies and behaviour (Bradford and Federoff, 2006). SSRIs have also been recommended in mild paraphilias, in cases that have comorbidity with obsessive-compulsive disorder and depression and in maintenance treatment (Bradford, 2000; Bradford and Federoff, 2006). It is worth noting that there is a lack of robust clinical trials in these fields.

Antipsychotics
The central activation of sexual arousal via mesolimbic dopamine pathways may account for the perceived action of antipsychotics on paraphilic disorders. This could also be attributed to antipsychotic-induced prolactin elevation (or even sedation), both of which reduce sexual desire and libido. Historically, a number of first-generation antipsychotics, such as chlorpromazine and haloperidol, have been used in the treatment of paraphilic disorders for people with intellectual disability. Benperidol, a butyrophenone antipsychotic like haloperidol, was licenced for the management of paraphilic disorders, although this should not be taken to indicate a superior efficacy. Recent supply issues with benperidol have further limited the usefulness of this treatment. Regarding second-generation antipsychotics, there is most experience with risperidone, but there are no robust studies to support its use. Overall, apart from in rare cases, where paraphilic behaviours have been associated with delusional beliefs of schizophrenia or similar conditions, no clear efficacy has been found with the use of antipsychotics. Although mood stabilisers such as lithium or valproate have historically been used for the treatment of paraphilic disorders, there is no evidence to support this in the absence of concurrent bipolar disorder. With both classes of non-hormonal agents considered (SSRIs and antipsychotics), the therapeutic aim is produced by what is principally a side-effect of the medication. This results in using medicines outside the terms of their principal product licence (although this does not mean they are ineffective). Using medicines for unlicenced indications poses issues when considering consent – issues made more challenging when considering individuals who have limited or impaired mental capacity.

People with Intellectual Disability
Most of the evidence associated with treatment of paraphilic disorders is centred upon the management of sexual offenders and is not directly related to management of paraphilic disorders in people with intellectual disability.

People with Intellectual Disability: Non-Medication Treatments
Adapted psychological programmes exist, which are predominantly adapted from the Sex Offender Treatment Programme (SOTP) utilised in the general population. The general content of interventions targets sex education (knowledge, law, consent), cognitive distortions, victim empathy and awareness, relapse prevention, appropriate sexual outlets, and confronting minimisation and denial. Meta-analyses have found that cognitive distortions are improved on completion of treatment (Patterson, 2018; Heppell et al., 2020).

People with Intellectual Disability: Medication Treatments
A variety of medications have been used for the management of paraphilic disorders in people with intellectual disability. Overall, the evidence supporting this use is poor, with no recent studies undertaken. Treatment guidelines for the management of paraphilic disorders among offenders have been constructed and these can be applied to people with intellectual disability. Selection of drug therapies should be based upon a stepwise approach, with better-tolerated agents being considered ahead of those agents with more concerning side effects. Before treatment is considered it should be clear what the desired outcomes are, and treatments should be reviewed against these individual treatment aims.

The Frith Treatment Guidelines for People with Intellectual Disability

Assessment

- A detailed diagnostic assessment (Alexander et al., 2010; Chester et al., 2023), as set out in Chapter 4, should be carried out. This will cover the degree of intellectual disability, cause of intellectual disability, and any behaviour phenotypes, autism spectrum disorder, other developmental disorders, mental illnesses, personality disorders, substance misuse, physical health conditions, experience of trauma, and types of challenging behaviour.
- A psychological formulation using the 5-P model of the presenting problem, predisposing, precipitating, perpetuating and protective factors (Macneil et al., 2012) or equivalent should be completed along with using the HELP framework of Health, Environment, Lived experience and Psychiatric problems (Green et al., 2018)

Non-Medication Treatments

Though not covered within this chapter, psychoeducation and adapted cognitive behavioural therapy-based programmes such as the adapted sex offender treatment programme should be considered. Please refer to appropriate texts on psychological therapies for sexual offenders with intellectual disability for further information.

Medication Treatments

- Assessment and treatment of paraphilic disorders in intellectual disability must always be conducted within the context of a robust biopsychosocial understanding of illness and formulation.
- Careful medication history, including any use of over-the-counter remedies and self-medication with alcohol and/or drugs.
- Check for potential drug interactions and history of sensitivity to side effects.
- Detailed discussion with the patient and/or carers and family, as appropriate, about the target symptoms, the rationale for prescribing, and the monitoring and review arrangements.

Table 12.2 summarises medication choice for the treatment of paraphilia in Intellectual disability.

Table 12.2 Medication choice for the treatment of paraphilia in Intellectual disability

First line	Second line	Third line	Fourth line	Fifth line	Sixth line
Cognitive behavioural therapy; other psychosocial and environmental interventions	Add selective serotonin reuptake inhibitor	Add low dose antiandrogen e.g., cyproterone acetate (CPA)	Increase cyproterone acetate, or alternatively use medroxyprogesterone acetate	Triptorelin every 3 months (GnRH agonist)	Add cyproterone acetate or medroxyprogesterone to GnRH agonist

Length of Treatment and Related Issues
- Paraphilia is a chronic disorder and a minimal duration of treatment of 3–5 years is highly recommended for severe paraphilia with a high risk of sexual violence (Garcia & Thibaut, 2011).

Algorithm
In 2016, Florence Thibaut et al. published *The World Federation of Societies of Biological Psychiatry (WFSBP) Guidelines for the Biological Treatment of Paraphilias*. This evaluated the role of pharmacotherapy in the treatment and management of paraphilic disorders in the treatment of adult males. The authors used an extensive literature search in the English language on MEDLINE/PubMed and used other published reviews. Though these guidelines are not specific for people with intellectual disability, they can be used for people with intellectual disability and cognitive deficits. With the usual clinical considerations and cautions they can provide valuable clinical options in addition to psychological therapy. A treatment algorithm derived from these guidelines is presented in Figure 12.1.

The Frith Prescribing Guidelines Editors' Expert Group Consensus Statements

Statements of High Confidence
- People with intellectual disability are more likely to be a victim of a sexual offences when compared to the general population.
- Careful diagnostic evaluation and a psychological formulation is a prerequisite for appropriate treatment.
- Both testosterone and serotonin have been implicated in sexual behaviour and are targets for pharmacological management of paraphilia.

Statements of Medium Confidence
- If medication is considered, the six-step treatment approach adapted from Thibaut et al. (2016) provides a stepwise approach to management

Statements of Low Confidence
- Adapted cognitive behavioural therapy may be a feasible and effective approach for the treatment of paraphilia and sexual offending in people with intellectual disability.

Resource Box

Resources for Sexual Behaviour, Education, and Relationships

Difficult sexual behaviour leaflet: The Challenging Behaviour Foundation

www.challengingbehaviour.org.uk/wp-content/uploads/2021/02/008-Difficult-sexual-behaviour-.pdf

A rich collection of resources on sexuality and relationships: Choice Support

www.choicesupport.org.uk/about-us/what-we-do/supported-loving/for-staff-supporters-and-family-members

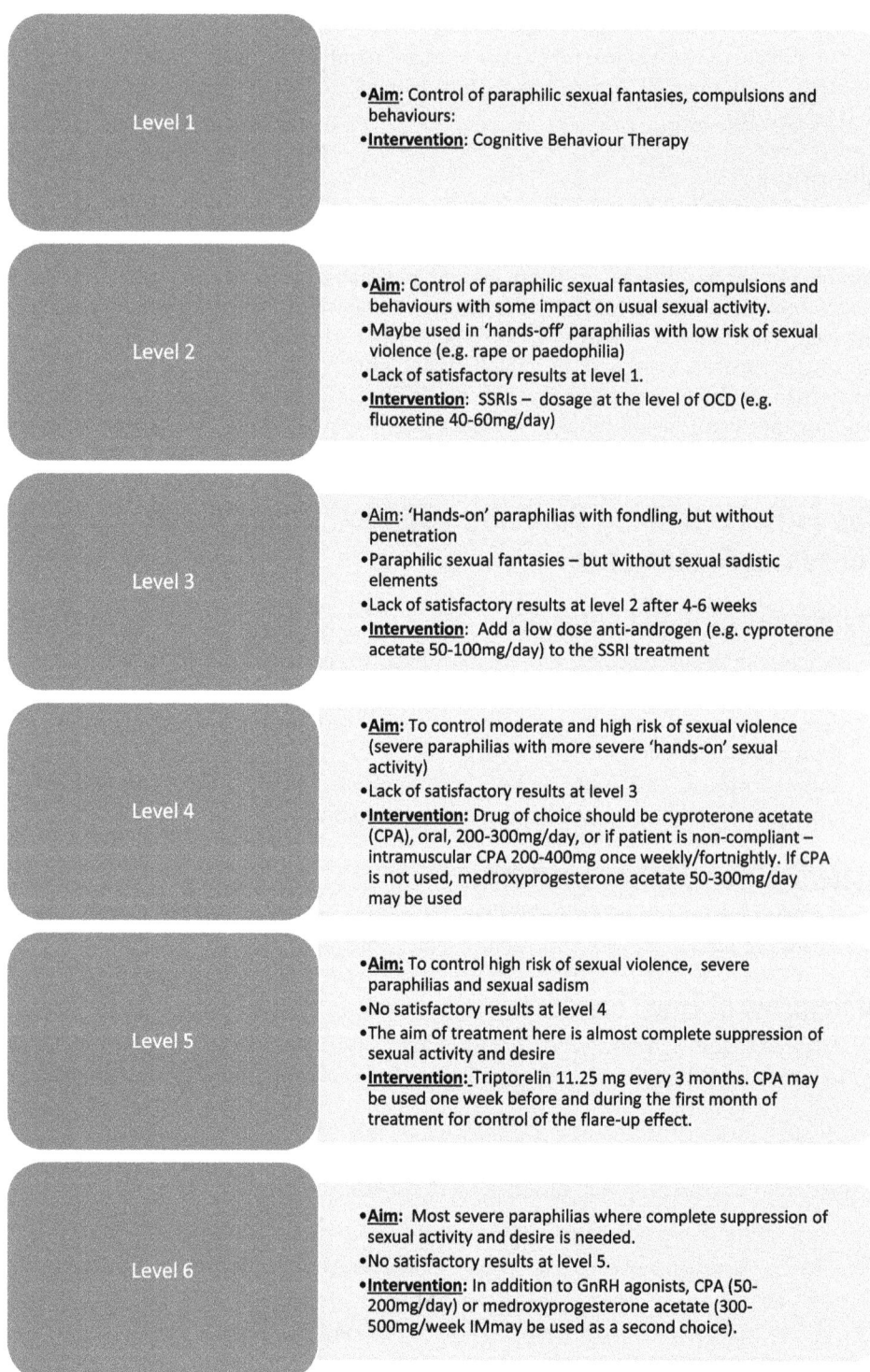

Figure 12.1 Algorithm of pharmacological treatment of paraphilias (adapted from Thibaut et al., 2016)

Easy-Read Documents for Medications
Choice & Medication
An information site (available through several NHS trusts or individual subscriptions) which offers patient information about mental health conditions and the treatments available to help make informed decisions about choosing the right medicine. Options include Very Easy Read Leaflets (VERAs), designed for people with an intellectual disability.
www.choiceandmedication.org/

SPECTROM Easy read medication
https://spectrom.wixsite.com/project/easy-read-medication-leaflets

Other Key Clinical Guidelines Referenced in This Chapter

Treatment algorithm for pharmacological treatment of paraphilia, adapted from: Thibaut, F., Bradford, J. M. W., Brikens P., et al. (2016). The World Federation of Societies of Biological Psychiatry (WFSBP) Guidelines for the treatment of adolescent sexual offenders with paraphilic disorders. *The World Journal of Biological Psychiatry*, 2010(17), 2–38.

References

Alexander, R.T., Green, F.N., O'Mahony, B., et al. (2010). Personality disorders in offenders with intellectual disability: A comparison of clinical, forensic and outcome variables and implications for service provision. *Journal of Intellectual Disability Research*, 54(7), 650–8.

Bradford, J. M. W. (1985). Organic treatments for the male sexual offender. *Behavioural Sciences and the Law*, 3, 355–75.

Bradford, J. M. W. (2000). The treatment of sexual deviation using a pharmacological approach. *Journal of Sex Research*, 3, 248–257.

Bradford, J., Greenberg, D. M., Gojer, J. J., Martindale, J. J., & Goldberg, M. (1995). Sertraline in the treatment of pedophilia – An open labelled study. Paper presented at the Annual American Psychiatric Association Congress, Miami, FL, May.

Bradford, J. M. W., & Fedoroff, P. (2006). Pharmacological treatment of the juvenile sex offender. In H. E. Barbaree & W. L. Marshall (Eds.), *The Juvenile Sex Offender* (2nd ed.) (pp. 358–83). New York, NY: Guilford.

Bradford, J. M. W. & Kaye, N. S. (1999). Pharmacological treatment of sexual offenders. *American Academy of Psychiatry and Law Newsletter*, 24, 16–17.

Callahan, P. A., Jeglic, E. L., & Calkins, C. (2021). Sexual offenders with intellectual disabilities: An exploratory comparison study in an incarcerated US sample. *International Journal of Offender Therapy and Comparative Criminology*. Advance online publication. https://doi.org/10.1177/0306624X211066825.

Chester, V., Tharian, P., Slinger, M., Varughese, A., & Alexander, R. T. (2023). Overview of offenders with intellectual disability. In J. M. McCarthy, R. T. Alexander, & E. Chaplin. (Eds.), *Forensic Aspects of Neurodevelopmental Disorders: A Clinician's Guide* (pp. 24–33). Cambridge University Press. https://doi.org/10.1017/9781108955522.003.

Clarke, D. (1989). Antilibidinal drugs and mental retardation: A review. *Medicine, Science and the Law*, 29(2), 136–46.

Craig, L. A., Lindsay, W. R., & Browne, K.D. (2010). *Assessment and treatment of sexual offenders with intellectual disabilities: A handbook*. John Wiley & Sons Ltd.

Dennis, J. A., Khan, O., Ferriter, M., et al. (2012). Psychological interventions for adults who have sexually offended or are at risk of offending. *Cochrane Database of Systematic Reviews*, **12**: CD007507. http://dx.doi.org/10.1002/14651858.CD007507.pub2.

Garcia, F. D. & Thibaut, F. (2011). Current concepts in the pharmacotherapy of paraphilias. *Drugs*, **71**(6), 771–90.

Greenberg, D. M., & Bradford, J. M. W. (1997). Treatment of the Paraphilic Disorders: A Review of the Role of the Selective Serotonin Reuptake Inhibitors. *Sexual Abuse*, 9(4), 349–360. https://doi.org/10.1177/107906329700900407.

Green, L., McNeil, K., Korossy, M., et al. A. (2018). HELP for behaviours that challenge in adults with intellectual and developmental disabilities. *Canadian Family Physician*, 64(Suppl 2), S23–S31.

Griffiths, D., Hingsburger, D., Hoath, J., & Ioannou, S. (2013). 'Counterfeit Deviance' Revisited. *Journal of Applied Research in Intellectual Disabilities*, 26(5), 471–80.

Gordon, H., & Grubin, D. (2004). Psychiatric aspects of the assessment and treatment of sex offenders. *Advances in Psychiatric Treatment*, 10, 73–80.

Heppell, S., Jones, C., & Rose, J. (2020). The effectiveness of cognitive-behavioural therapy group-based interventions for men with intellectual disabilities and sexual offending histories: A meta-analysis. *International Journal of Developmental Disabilities*, pp. 1–14. https://pubmed.ncbi.nlm.nih.gov/35937162/p.

Hingsburger, D., Dalla Nora, M., & Tough, S. (2010). The *key: A community approach to assessment, treatment and support for people with intellectual disabilities who sexually offend*. Diverse City Press and Vita Community Services.

Holland, S., & Persson, P. (2010). Intellectual disability in the Victorian prison system: Characteristics of prisoners with an intellectual disability released from prison in 2003–2006. *Psychology, Crime and Law*, 17(1), 25–41.

Hogue, T., Steptoe, L., Taylor, J. L., et al. (2006). A comparison of offenders with intellectual disability across three levels of security. *Criminal Behaviour and Mental Health*, **16**, 13–28.

Hughes-McCormack, L. A., Rydzewska, E., Henderson, A., et al. (2017). Prevalence of mental health conditions and relationship with general health in a whole-country population of people with intellectual disabilities compared with the general population. *BJPsych Open*, 3(5), 243–8.

Joyal, C. C., & Carpentier, J. (2016). The prevalence of paraphilic interests and behaviors in the general population: A provincial survey. *The Journal of Sex Research*, 54(2), 161–71.

Khan O, Ferriter M, Huband N, et al. (2015). Pharmacological interventions for those who have sexually offended or are at risk of offending. *Cochrane Database of Systematic Reviews*, 2, CD007989. https://doi.org/10.1002/14651858.CD007989.pub2.

Latvala, A., Tideman, M., Søndenaa, E., et al. (2022). Association of intellectual disability with violent and sexual crime and victimization: A population-based cohort study. *Psychological Medicine*, **53**, 3817–25. https://doi.org/10.1017/S0033291722000460.

Lindsay, W. R., Hastings, R. P., Griffiths, D. M. & Hayes, S. C. (2007). Trends and challenges in forensic research on offenders with intellectual disability. *Journal of Intellectual and Developmental Disabilities*, 32, 55–61.

Lindsay, W. R. (2009). The *treatment of sex offenders with developmental disabilities: A practice workbook*. John Wiley & Sons.

Lindsay, W. R., Hastings, R. P., & Beech, A. R. (2011). Forensic research in offenders with intellectual & developmental disabilities 1: Prevalence and risk assessment. Special Issue: Forensic research in offenders with intellectual & developmental disabilities Part 1. *Psychology, Crime & Law*, 17(1), 3–7.

Macneil, C. A., Hasty, M. K., Conus, P., & Berk, M. (2012). Is diagnosis enough to guide interventions in mental health? Using case formulation in clinical practice. *BMC Medicine*, **10**, 111. https://doi.org/10.1186/1741-7015-10-111.

Nixon, M., Thomas, S. D. M., Daffern, M., & Ogloff, J. R. P. (2017). Estimating the risk of crime and victimisation in people with intellectual disability: A data-linkage study. *Social Psychiatry and Psychiatric Epidemiology*, **52**(5), 617–26.

NHS England (2016). Stopping over-medication of people with a learning disability (STOMPLD) pledge. NHS England, London. www.england.nhs.uk/2016/06/over-medication-pledge.

Patterson, C. (2018). Does the adapted sex offender treatment programme reduce cognitive distortions? A meta-analysis. *Journal of Intellectual Disabilities and Offending Behaviour*, **9**(1), 9–21.

Rosler, A., & Witztum, E. (1998). Treatment of men with paraphilia with a long-acting analogue of gonatropin-releasing hormone. *New England Journal of Medicine*, **338**, 416–22

Schöttle, D., Briken, P., Tüscher, O., & Turner, D. (2017). Sexuality in autism: Hypersexual and paraphilic behavior in women and men with high-functioning autism spectrum disorder. *Dialogues in Clinical Neuroscience*, **19**(4), 381–93. www.ncbi.nlm.nih.gov/pmc/articles/PMC5789215/.

Thibaut, F., Bradford, J. M. W., Brikens P., et al. (2016). The World Federation of Societies of Biological Psychiatry (WFSBP) Guidelines for the treatment of adolescent sexual offenders with paraphilic disorders. *The World Journal of Biological Psychiatry*, **2010**(17), 2–38.

Tomsa, R., Gutu, S., Cojocaru, D., et al. (2021). Prevalence of sexual abuse in adults with intellectual disability: Systematic review and meta-analysis. *International Journal of Environmental Research and Public Health*, **18**(4), 1980.

Walker, N., & McCabe, S. (1973) Crime and Insanity in England (Vol. 2). Edinburgh University Press, Edinburgh.

Ward, T., & Beech, A. (2006). An Integrated Theory of Sexual Offending. *Aggression and Violent Behavior*, **11**(1), 44–63. https://doi.org/10.1016/j.avb.2005.05.002.

Ward, T., & Beech, A.R. (2016). The Integrated Theory of Sexual Offending-Revised. *The Wiley Handbook on the Theories, Assessment and Treatment of Sexual Offending*, [online], 123–37. https://doi.org/10.1002/9781118574003.wattso006.

Yakeley, J., & Wood, H. (2014). Paraphilias and paraphilic disorders: Diagnosis, assessment and management. *Advances in Psychiatric Treatment*, **20**(3), 202–13.

Chapter 13

Substance Use Disorders

Ayomipo J. Amiola, Sreeja Sahadevan, Saher Binnat Rafiq, and Regi T. Alexander

Introduction

What Are Substance Use Disorders?

According to the International Classification of Diseases (ICD-11) (World Health Organization, 2019), substance use disorders include disorders that result from a single occasion or repeated use of substances (both legal and illegal) that have psychoactive properties; all drugs that are taken in excess have in common direct activation of the brain reward system, which is involved in the reinforcement of behaviours and the production of memories. They produce such an intense activation of the reward system that normal activities may be neglected. Instead of achieving reward-system activation through adaptive behaviours, drugs of abuse directly activate the reward pathways. The pharmacological mechanisms by which each class of drugs produces reward are different, but the drugs typically activate the system and produce feelings of pleasure, often referred to as a 'high' (American Psychiatric Association, 2013).

The International Classification of Diseases (ICD-11) and American Psychiatric Association's Diagnostic and Statistical Manual of Mental Disorders (DSM-5) classify substance use disorders in a similar manner. In the American Psychiatric Association's *Diagnostic and Statistical Manual of Mental Disorders* (DSM-5), nine separate classes of substance are included; alcohol, caffeine, cannabis, hallucinogens, inhalants, opioids, sedatives and anxiolytics, stimulants and tobacco, including 'other' substances; the International Classification of Diseases (ICD-11) includes MDMA (methylene-dioxymethamphetamine), analogues such as MDA (methylene-dioxyamphetamine), and dissociative drugs (ketamine and phencyclidine), and subdivides psychostimulants into cocaine and other stimulants (including amphetamines, methamphetamine, or methcathinone) and synthetic compounds such as cannabinoids and cathinones.

Conceptually, the diagnostic syndromes are divided into those that represent the actual use of the substance (whether one-off or repeated) and its immediate effects, and those reflecting the complications of substance use, such as disease processes in the brain and the rest of the body (Saunders, 2017).

Substance use that has caused damage to one's health (through behaviour related to intoxication, direct or secondary toxic effects on body organs and systems, or a harmful route of administration) or has resulted in harm to the health of others is termed 'harmful use'. This could be a one-off (episodic) or repeated (harmful pattern) occurrence.

Dependence syndrome represents a disorder of regulation of substance use characterised by impaired control over substance use, often accompanied by a subjective sensation of urge or craving to use the substance, increasing priority of substance use over other activities, and persistence of use despite harm or negative consequences and physiological features indicative of neuroadaptation to the substance manifested by tolerance, withdrawal symptoms following cessation or reduction in use of that substance, or repeated use of the substance (or pharmacologically similar substance) to prevent or alleviate withdrawal symptoms (Saunders, 2017).

Intoxication describes a clinically significant transient condition that develops during or shortly after the consumption of a particular substance that is characterised by disturbances in consciousness, cognition, perception, affect, behaviour, or coordination. These disturbances are caused by the known pharmacological effects of the substance and their intensity is closely related to the amount consumed. They are time-limited and abate as the substance is cleared from the body. The specific features are substance specific.

Withdrawal is a clinically significant cluster of symptoms, behaviours, and/or physiological features, varying in degree of severity and duration, that occurs upon cessation or reduction of use of psychoactive substances in individuals who have developed dependence or have used the substance for a prolonged period or in large amounts. Like intoxication, the cluster of symptoms is specific to the substance used.

The complications of substance use are generally termed 'substance-induced disorders', and include substance-induced delirium, substance-induced psychotic disorder, substance-induced mood disorder, substance-induced anxiety disorder, substance-induced obsessive-compulsive or related disorder, and substance-induced impulse control disorder. The clinical presentation here is like the primary mental disorder but onset is temporally related to substance use and/or persists after cessation of substance use (see Table 13.1).

Why Does Someone Develop Substance Use Disorders?

Research suggests that substance use disorders result from a complex interaction of biological, psychological, and social factors. Risk factors for substance misuse are broadly similar in those with intellectual disability and the general population; hence, young age, male gender, higher cognitive functioning, and socioeconomic adversities such as poverty, living in deprived neighbourhoods, family discord, history of physical/sexual trauma, and comorbid mental health problems increase the risk of substance (mis)use. In addition, independent community living has been found to increase the risks of substance misuse among adults with intellectual disability (Swerts et al., 2017).

How Are Substance Use Disorders Different in People with Intellectual Disability?

Substance use in persons with intellectual disability can lead to more severe consequences than one may find in the general population. Among people with intellectual disability, substance use and misuse were associated with mental health problems, including mood dysregulation, suicidal thoughts, and more negative long-term consequences on their health, daily activity, and relationships, including being a risk factor for offending behaviour (To et al., 2014).

People with intellectual disability use and abuse all types of substances, as in the general population. The clinical features of the specific syndromes including the physiological and psychological sequelae of substance use among those with mild to moderate intellectual disability is comparable with the general population. Specific signs that may be found in individuals with intellectual disability include rapid development of organic substance-related conditions, worsening of previous cognitive and or neurological problems, and precipitation of acute psychopathological states (affective instability, anxiety/panic attacks, low mood, suicidality, paranoia including odd/bizarre behaviours). Common behavioural signs include hostility, aggression (verbal, physical), and other risky behaviours.

Many conditions present differently in people with intellectual disability, leading to underdiagnosis or misdiagnosis and, consequently, failure to access therapeutic interventions. However, in the case of substance use disorders, it is probable that applying the criteria in the international classification of diseases (ICD-11) and the American Psychiatric Association's *Diagnostic and Statistical Manual of Mental Disorders* (DSM-5) would be sufficient for individuals with mild to borderline intellectual disability, although it will be almost impossible to apply these to individuals with severe to profound intellectual disability and arrive at any meaningful diagnoses (Vannucchi et al., 2022).

Due to the presence of cognitive and linguistic difficulties, dependence on informants, comorbid conditions, diagnostic overshadowing, and atypical presentations in individuals with intellectual disability, assessment must be robust, with the clinician obtaining a good history of presenting problems, including the type of substance, quantity, route of use, and circumstances around and consequences (physiological, psychological, and social) after use; a psychiatric history will detect a comorbid mental illness if present. A full general physical examination and routine blood tests can help to identify pre-existing or substance-related physical health problems, and a toxicology screen will clarify exact substance consumed.

In the general population, several screening and diagnostic tools are available; however, this is not the case for the intellectual disability population. A useful adapted tool is the Substance Use and Misuse in Intellectual Disability Questionnaire (SumID-Q); it is easy to use, incorporates pictorial presentation of information to aid understanding, and assesses risk factors for substance use and their consequences. Other assessments typically used in the mainstream population have some potential for usefulness in intellectual disability service.

Table 13.1 Clinical presentation of substance use disorders in intellectual disability

Symptoms like the general population	<ul><li>Craving: strong desire or urge to use the substance provoked by environmental and inner stimuli</li><li>Increased period spent to obtain, use, or recover from effects of substance</li><li>Increasing precedence of substance use over other aspects of life, including maintenance of health, and daily activities and responsibilities.</li><li>Neglect of important social, occupational, and recreational activities</li><li>Tolerance: need to use increasing amounts of substance to achieve the same effect</li><li>Withdrawal symptoms following cessation or reduction in use of substance (symptoms differ for each class of substance)</li></ul>

Table 13.1 (cont.)

Behavioural symptoms (more common in intellectual disability)	• Challenging behaviour chronologically related to abstinence, stressful events, and places/moments of the day when/where they were used to consume the substance • Refusal to participate or reduced involvement in usual activities due to the search for or consumption of the substance • Repetitiveness and compulsivity with reduced involvement and focus on usual and pleasant activities
Symptoms unreliable in intellectual disability (especially severe to profound forms)	• Use in physically hazardous situations • Continued use or escalation in use despite knowledge of continuous or recurrent physical or psychological disturbances caused by the substance

How Common Are Substance Use Disorders in People with Intellectual Disability?

The use of psychoactive substances is highly prevalent around the world; about 52% of the world's population over 15 years of age have consumed alcohol in their lives, 21% of the world's population over the age of 15 are estimated to be tobacco smokers, and 5% of the world's adult population were estimated to have used other psychoactive drugs at least once in 2015 (Poznyak et al., 2018).

Historically, people with intellectual disability were considered to have lower rates of substance misuse compared with the general population. Subsequent research shows widely ranging prevalence rates due to various methodological issues, but generally suggests that those with intellectual disability are less likely to misuse substances than the general population, although with an increased risk of complications when they do (Bhaumik & Alexander, 2020; Vannucchi et al., 2022). In their systematic review, vanDuijvenbode and VanDerNagel (2019) reported lifetime prevalence rates ranging from 0.0% to 49.8% for tobacco use, 15.6–75.4% for alcohol use, 2.4–13.0% for cannabis use among children with mild to borderline intellectual disability, 6.0–98.4% for tobacco use, 2.5–97.3% for alcohol use, and 19.2–50% for stimulants.

Alcohol: This is perhaps the most frequently used substance among people with intellectual disability. Varying prevalence rates have been reported across studies; in a 2007 study, Cooper and colleagues reported a prevalence of alcohol-use disorder of 1.8% in those with mild intellectual disability and 0.5% in the moderate-to-profound intellectual disability group; in a cross-sectional multicentre study of 123 individuals with mild to moderate intellectual disability receiving support from independent living services, prevalence rates for hazardous drinking, harmful drinking, and alcohol dependence were found to be 17.8%, 4.4%, and 11.1% respectively (Swerts et al., 2017). However, other studies have reported rates of alcohol use as high as 77.9% among individuals with mild to severe intellectual disability (To et al., 2014).

Tobacco: There is limited data on the exact prevalence of tobacco use among individuals with intellectual disability; most of the studies showed a prevalence of between

15% and 30%. Higher rates have been detected in people with comorbid mental disorders (Vannucchi et al., 2022). Also, among individuals living independently, 20% were smokers, compared with 3.1% of those living with the assistance of family or friends and 5.2% of those living in community care facilities (Steinberg et al., 2009).

Cannabis: In the Netherlands, among 86 individuals with intellectual disability (which included 42 people with borderline intellectual functioning and 44 people with mild intellectual disability) aged 16–66, 34.8% used both alcohol and cannabis, while 8% used cannabis exclusively (Chapman & Wu, 2012). Rates as high as 51% were found in prisoners with intellectual disability (Vannucchi et al., 2022).

Cocaine: In a sample of 123 individuals with mild to moderate intellectual disability receiving support from independent living services in Flanders, in the northern region of Belgium, lifetime prevalence rate for cocaine use was 7.3% (Swerts et al., 2017). Among 88 adults with mild to severe intellectual disability receiving psychiatric treatment, file analysis revealed prevalence rate of 13.6% for cocaine use (vanDuijvenbode & VanDerNagel, 2019). In their study, To and colleagues (2014) identified 12.5% as cocaine (mis)users, suggesting that around 62% of cocaine users with intellectual disability develop cocaine misuse problems.

Opioids: Among 44 individuals with mild intellectual disability, a prevalence rate of 2.3% was reported (Chapman &Wu, 2012). In their own study, Swerts and colleagues (2017) reported a lifetime prevalence rate of 1.6% among people with mild to moderate intellectual disability. Among individuals living in the community, highest prevalence of heroin use was reported as 9.6% (To et al., 2014). Rates as high as 17.9% have been reported in intellectual disability offenders (Vannucchi et al., 2022).

Other Illicit Drugs: Data about amphetamines and derivatives, hallucinogens, and inhalants are limited, yet rates of drug use appear to be higher in those with mild to borderline intellectual disability compared with the general population (vanDuijvenbode & VanDerNagel 2019).

> **Case Study 13.1: Presentation**
>
> Saul, a 37-year-old man with a diagnosis of mild intellectual disability, was referred to the intellectual disability psychiatrist with complaints of poor sleep, unusual beliefs, and aggressive behaviours. Symptoms were noted to have been present for about two weeks, sleep had become dysregulated, and he had been verbally and physically aggressive towards carers and family members with little or no provocation. This included hitting staff and staring them down in an intimidating manner. He believed that he was a rock star, had a lot of money in the bank, and that there was a hit squad seeking to end his life. He denied hearing voices of people he could not see; however, he appeared distracted by abnormal perceptions.
>
> He acknowledged use of psychoactive substances; he started smoking cannabis at age 13 with 'friends' and by age 17 was regularly consuming it. Initially he spent about £10 per week on cannabis; this gradually increased to £25, but he was currently spending about £40 every week. He drinks alcohol occasionally but does not like its taste or effect and has stopped smoking tobacco. He has never used cocaine or heroin. Following a comprehensive assessment which included a mental state examination; a diagnosis of a cannabis-induced psychotic disorder was made.

Treatments: The Evidence Base
General Population
Alcohol: In the general population, the National Institute for Health, and Care Excellence (2011) has published guidance reviewing management of alcohol-use disorders. The general principles include:
- offering interventions to promote abstinence and prevent relapse as part of an intensive structured community-based intervention.
- interventions should be delivered by appropriately trained and competent staff.
- psychological interventions should be based on a relevant evidence-based treatment manual, which should guide the structure and duration of the intervention.
- pharmacological interventions should be administered by specialist and competent staff.

There is limited evidence concerning the interaction between psychosocial and pharmacological approaches or whether there is an optimal pharmacological–psychosocial combination. However, psychosocial approaches (cognitive behavioural therapies, behavioural therapies, or social network and environment-based therapies) focused specifically on alcohol-related cognitions, behaviour problems, and social networks are the mainstay of treatment for harmful use, while pharmacological interventions for the substance use disorder itself are of most value in dependence and are targeted at withdrawal syndromes, relapse prevention and maintenance of abstinence, harm-reduction (e.g., by substitute prescribing), and prevention of complications (Lingford-Hughes et al., 2012) (see Table 13.2).

In acute alcohol withdrawal, benzodiazepines or carbamazepine are equally efficacious, with clomethiazole reserved for inpatient settings only after due consideration of its safety (NICE, 2010; Lingford-Hughes et al., 2012). For alcohol-related seizures, the European Foundation of Neurorehabilitation Societies recommends longer-acting benzodiazepines (e.g., diazepam or lorazepam) since they are efficacious for primary and secondary seizure prevention (Bråthen et al., 2005); anticonvulsants are equally efficacious in seizure prevention, but the British Association of Psychopharmacology consensus guidelines suggest there is no advantage when combined (Lingford-Hughes et al., 2012). They also recommend benzodiazepines for alcohol-induced delirium (Lingford-Hughes et al., 2012). For alcohol-related brain disorder (Wernicke–Korsakoff syndrome), thiamine is the mainstay of treatment. The dose and route of administration is dependent on the risk of developing Wernicke–Korsakoff syndrome. In healthy uncomplicated alcohol-dependent/heavy drinkers (low risk) oral prophylactic thiamine (>300 mg/day) should be given during detoxification. For high-risk patients, prophylactic parenteral treatment (250 mg once daily for 3–5 days) should be given. If Wernicke–Korsakoff syndrome is suspected or established, parenteral thiamine of >500 mg should be given for 3–5 days, followed by 250 mg once daily for a further 3–5 days depending on response (NICE, 2010; Lingford-Hughes et al., 2012).

After a successful withdrawal for people with moderate and severe alcohol dependence, consider offering acamprosate or oral naltrexone in combination with an individual psychological intervention (cognitive behavioural therapies, behavioural therapies, or social network and environment-based therapies) focused specifically on alcohol misuse (NICE, 2011). Disulfiram is effective if intake is witnessed. It can be offered as a treatment option for patients who intend to maintain abstinence, and for whom there are no contraindications (Lingford-Hughes et al., 2012).

Tobacco: NICE (2023) recommends ensuring that the following are accessible to adults who smoke: behavioural interventions (such as individual and group behavioural support, very brief advice), medicinally licenced products (bupropion, nicotine replacement therapy, varenicline), nicotine-containing e-cigarettes, and Allen Carr's Easyway in-person group seminar.

The British Association of Psychopharmacology (Lingford-Hughes et al., 2012) recommends that:

- all smokers should also be encouraged to use behavioural support where this is available, although refusal to use behavioural support should not prevent prescribing pharmacotherapy.
- Nicotine replacement therapy, varenicline, bupropion, nortriptyline, and cytisine are all effective in aiding smoking cessation. Prescriptions for one of these should be offered to all smokers.
- Either varenicline or combination nicotine replacement therapy (long-acting patch plus a faster-acting nicotine replacement therapy) give optimal results.

In a review by Jahagirdar and Kaunelis (2017), four of five meta-analyses comparing varenicline to placebo found a significantly higher likelihood of abstinence or smoking cessation in the varenicline group. Varenicline was found to be well tolerated and effective for abstinence at the end of treatment in two randomised controlled trials of varenicline or placebo added to brief individual behavioural support. Similarly, the two bupropion plus nicotine replacement therapy studies also had positive findings, with bupropion treatment plus nicotine replacement therapy groups (with and without home visits) showing significantly greater reduction in cigarettes per day and expired carbon monoxide level compared to treatment as usual with any first-line medication.

In a 2013 Cochrane review by Cahill and colleagues, both nicotine replacement therapy and bupropion were superior to placebo. Varenicline increased the odds of quitting compared with placebo. Head-to-head comparisons between bupropion and nicotine replacement therapy showed equal efficacy. Varenicline was superior to single forms of nicotine replacement therapy, and to bupropion. Varenicline was more effective than single formulation nicotine replacement therapy patch, nicotine gum, inhaler, spray, tablets, or lozenges, but was not more effective than combination nicotine replacement therapy. Combination nicotine replacement therapy also outperformed single formulations.

Howes and colleagues, in a 2020 Cochrane review, demonstrated that there was high-certainty evidence that bupropion increased long-term smoking cessation rates; there was insufficient evidence to establish whether combination bupropion and nicotine replacement therapy resulted in superior quit rates to nicotine replacement therapy alone or whether combination bupropion and varenicline resulted in superior quit rates to varenicline alone. Bupropion and nicotine replacement therapy still showed equal efficacy, and bupropion was still inferior to varenicline in smoking cessation rates to varenicline.

Cannabis: Pharmacological treatment of cannabis abuse and dependence focuses mainly on alleviation of withdrawal symptoms to aid quit attempts. Although there were several placebo-controlled trials of various pharmacological agents (oral tetrahydrocannabinol, sodium valproate, bupropion, fluoxetine, and mirtazapine), open-label studies of lithium carbonate, and laboratory studies of lofexidine, baclofen, and extended-release zolpidem, at present there is no clear evidence base for pharmacological treatment of cannabis withdrawal and no pharmacological treatment is recommended (Lingford-Hughes et al., 2012).

Cocaine: Information about self-help groups (Cocaine Anonymous) based on a system called the 12-step programme should be given. If in close contact with a partner who does not misuse drugs, behavioural family and/or couples therapy should be offered. Cognitive behavioural therapy is not ordinarily offered except in the presence of comorbid anxiety or depression (National Institute for Health and Care Excellence (NICE) 2007).

Medications such as psychostimulants, antidepressants, antipsychotics, dopamine agonists, and anticonvulsants have been investigated for treating cocaine dependence or problematic use, but there is no convincing evidence supporting the use of pharmacological treatment for amphetamine and cocaine abuse and dependence (Lingford-Hughes et al., 2012).

Opioids: Opioid maintenance therapy is used to treat opioid dependence. Methadone and buprenorphine maintenance treatments are appropriate treatment options for opioid-dependent patients. Methadone is effective in reducing heroin use, injecting, and sharing of injecting equipment (Lingford-Hughes et al., 2012). For the management of opioid withdrawal, three approaches to detoxification have a robust evidence base: methadone at tapered doses, buprenorphine, or an α2 adrenergic agonist (usually lofexidine). The choice of agent will depend on what treatment patients are already receiving and individual preference. However, if short duration of treatment is desirable, or in patients with mild or uncertain dependence, α2 adrenergic agonists may be preferable (Lingford-Hughes et al., 2012). For formerly dependent people who are highly motivated to remain abstinent, oral naltrexone treatment should be considered (Lingford-Hughes et al., 2012).

Table 13.2 Medication use in the general population

SYNDROME	TREATMENT	REFERENCES
Alcohol		
Acute alcohol withdrawal	First line: benzodiazepines or carbamazepine Second line: clomethiazole	NICE, 2010; Lingford-Hughes et al., 2012
Alcohol-related seizures	First line: diazepam Second line: lorazepam	Bråthen et al., 2005
Alcohol-induced delirium	Longer-acting benzodiazepines	Lingford-Hughes et al., 2012
Wernicke–Korsakoff syndrome	Oral/parenteral thiamine	Lingford-Hughes et al., 2012
Maintaining abstinence	First line: acamprosate, naltrexone Second line: disulfiram	Lingford-Hughes et al., 2012
Tobacco		
Dependence	Bupropion, nicotine replacement therapy, varenicline	NICE, 2023; Lingford-Hughes et al., 2012
Cannabis		
Withdrawal/dependence	No clear evidence base for pharmacological treatment	
Cocaine		
Dependence/problematic use	No clear evidence base for pharmacological treatment	

Table 13.2 (cont.)

SYNDROME	TREATMENT	REFERENCES
Opioids		
Dependence	Methadone/buprenorphine maintenance treatment	Lingford-Hughes et al., 2012
Withdrawal	Methadone, buprenorphine, or lofexidine	Lingford-Hughes et al., 2012
Maintaining abstinence	Oral Naltrexone	Lingford-Hughes et al., 2012

People with Intellectual Disability

The evidence base for the treatment of substance use-related disorders in people with intellectual disability is quite limited. Few studies met the inclusion criteria as an alcohol and tobacco intervention study in a systematic review (Kerr et al 2013), and we are lacking data on treatments for other drugs of abuse. Effective interventions reported include psychotherapy (psychoeducation, motivational interviewing, and cognitive behavioural therapy techniques) and pharmacotherapy, with psychological interventions being first line. The choice of treatment is determined by the intensity, duration, and severity of symptoms, associated distress and impairment, the presence of comorbid physical/psychological disorders, patient characteristics and preferences, clinician experience, and the availability of proposed interventions, including features such as a good response to, or poor tolerability of previous treatments (Baldwin et al., 2014).

People with Intellectual Disability: Non-Medication Treatments

There is a paucity of data to support the effectiveness of psychological approaches used in the mainstream population for people with intellectual disability. Adaptations of such programmes with visual aids, easy-to-read materials, video vignettes, role plays of demonstration of inappropriate behaviours and helpful behaviours, and rehearsals have been found useful for people with intellectual disability.

In a Cochrane review of psychosocial interventions for people with both severe mental illness and substance misuse, findings revealed no compelling evidence to support any one psychosocial treatment to reduce substance use or to improve mental state for people with severe mental illnesses, although there were various methodological difficulties. This does not mean that treatments do not help, but that data is limited and the supportive evidence found in these studies need further replication through more methodologically sound studies (Hunt et al., 2019) (see Table 13.3).

People with Intellectual Disability: Medication Treatments

There are no studies evaluating medication use in people with intellectual disability. Hence, guidance follows good practice as in the general population, with reasonable adjustments made to ensure compliance.

Table 13.3 Evidence base for non-medication treatments in intellectual disability

Psychosocial treatment	Evidence in intellectual disability
Motivational interviewing	In a 2002 pilot study of motivational interviewing among seven adult offenders with alcohol-use disorder and mild to borderline intellectual disability admitted to a medium secure setting, the intervention showed positive effects on the readiness to change and self-efficacy of participants (Mendel and Hipkins, 2002) Following an evaluation of a motivational pre-treatment intervention delivered to 6 adults with mild to borderline intellectual disability and substance use receiving intellectual disability care, participants reported a significant increase in overall need satisfaction and autonomy satisfaction and a significant decrease of overall need frustration (Frielink et al, 2015)
Psychoeducation	A case report exploring the potential of a psycho-educational approach to increase knowledge and motivation (Steel & Ritchie 2004) A pilot study of an alcohol awareness group for adults with intellectual disability resident in a medium secure unit. Increase in alcohol-related knowledge for all participants following intervention (Forbat, 1999) McGillicuddy and Blane [1999] developed and evaluated two distinct 10-week interventions to educate those with intellectual disability about the consequences of psychoactive substance use and to provide participants with a behavioural repertoire they could use when confronted with risky situations involving substance use. Each programme improved at least short-term substance knowledge and enhanced skills, although substance use did not reduce Pilot of a smoking education course for people with intellectual disability (n=11), with encouraging results: 55% either quit smoking or cut down their intake significantly, 73% expressed a desire to stop smoking at the completion of the course, and 100% expressed an increased concern and knowledge about the effects of smoking on their health after completing the course (Tracy & Hosken 1997) In an audit to describe the effectiveness of a smoking cessation programme for people with intellectual disability resident in forensic settings, the authors concluded that simple smoking cessation programme with an emphasis on health education and nicotine replacement therapies appeared to be effective in cutting down smoking rates and tobacco consumption (Chester et al., 2011)
Mindfulness-based Therapies	Thirty-one-year-old male smoker with intellectual disability following a mindfulness-based smoking cessation programme successfully reduced and eventually stopped smoking; also, the results were maintained at a three-year follow-up (Singh et al., 2011)

Table 13.3 (cont.)

Psychosocial treatment	Evidence in intellectual disability
	Three men with mild intellectual disability who had smoked for many years were able to achieve abstinence for three years following the intervention, thus suggesting that mindfulness-based smoking cessation programme may be effective with other individuals with mild intellectual disabilities (Singh et al., 2013)
	In a two-group randomised controlled trial, 51 participants were randomly assigned to either mindfulness-based intervention or the control group (treatment as usual). The results suggest mindfulness-based interventions may be effective treatments for smoking cessation in individuals with mild intellectual disability (Singh et al., 2014)
Cognitive behaviour therapy (CBT)	The feasibility of an adapted cognitive behavioural therapy programme (CBT+) was evaluated; treatment acceptability was moderate, with high participant satisfaction. All participants showed post-treatment reduction in substance use, thus demonstrating the feasibility of CBT+ in treating persons with intellectual disability and substance use problems (Kiewik et al., 2020)
	Extended brief interventions were compared with treatment as usual for alcohol misuse in adults with mild to moderate intellectual disability. Results suggest extended brief interventions may provide an effective low-intensity treatment for this population (Kouimtsidis et al., 2017)
	The effectiveness of 'Take it personal!', a prevention programme (based on cognitive behavioural therapy and motivational interview principles) for individuals with mild intellectual disability to borderline intellectual functioning (MID-BIF) and substance use (SU) was assessed; the programme helped participants decrease substance use frequency and binge drinking (Schijven et al., 2021)

Treatment Guideline and Algorithm in Intellectual Disability

Assessment
- A detailed diagnostic assessment (Alexander et al., 2010; Chester et al., 2023), as set out in Chapter 4, should be carried out. This will cover the degree of intellectual disability, cause of intellectual disability and any behaviour phenotypes, autism, other developmental disorders, mental illnesses including anxiety disorders, personality disorders, substance misuse, physical health conditions, the experience of trauma, and types of challenging behaviour.

- A psychological formulation using the 5-P model of the presenting problem, predisposing, precipitating, perpetuating and protective factors (Macneil et al., 2012) or equivalent should be completed along with using the HELP framework of Health, Environment, Lived experience and Psychiatric problems (Green et al., 2018).

Non-Medication and Medication Treatments
- Alcohol
    - Regarding alcohol abuse, interventions mainly focus on the psychosocial therapies and medication as in the general population.
    - The first step will be to provide brief verbal support, following which further evaluation and follow-up should be in an integrated service with both intellectual disability and substance misuse expertise.
    - Motivational interviewing sessions and group interventions should adapt to the needs of the person with intellectual disability. It is recommended that the individual sessions should be longer and more frequent, and well-structured to allow the adaptation required for the person in need.
    - Individual sessions on top of group sessions are found to be beneficial. However, one-to-one sessions are preferred to address substance-related issues in people with intellectual disability, and this would aid in overall communication, understanding, and adaptations to novel ideas.
    - Skill-building sessions are recommended to address issues which would contribute to alcohol intake, such as assertiveness skills, coping skills, reduce alcohol-seeking behaviour, and social support for managing adverse life events and isolation.
    - The use of easy-to-read materials, video vignettes, role plays of demonstration of inappropriate behaviours and helpful behaviours, and rehearsals can consolidate the learning and memory. Positive reinforcements, such as rewards and encouragement/praise, could enhance the learning of the skill. Exposing to real-life situations – for instance, a visit to a pub and saying 'no' to alcohol – for assertiveness training are helpful.
    - Carer support and involvement is pivotal in the management of substance abuse, as lack of carer involvement could affect the compliance and engagement of the person with the therapy.
    - Medication use: the management of withdrawal symptoms for alcohol in persons with intellectual disability is like in the general population. The treatment should be explained in a way suitable for the person with intellectual disability, and close monitoring is advised during the withdrawal period as people with intellectual disability may not be able to communicate their difficulties effectively.
    - Benzodiazepines are first line, and the choice of benzodiazepine depends on the individual profile; thiamine should be supplemented as per NICE guidelines.
    - For people with increased risks of developing seizures during the withdrawal phase, use of carbamazepine is indicated as an adjunct to benzodiazepines.
    - Other preparations, such as beta-blockers and clonidine, also reduce symptoms of withdrawal but have no effect on seizures and can be used as adjuncts to benzodiazepines.

- Neuroleptics should be used to treat agitation and delirium, but with caution as they may reduce the seizure threshold during the withdrawal phase, hence first-generation antipsychotics (haloperidol and the phenothiazines) are preferred (Bhaumik & Alexander, 2020).
- Long-term medications used in the management of alcohol abuse in people with intellectual disability are acamprosate and naltrexone (see Table 13.4).
- The decision to prescribe disulfiram should only be made after a careful risk–benefit analysis, with input from specialised addiction services and with continued monitoring and close joint working between intellectual disability and addiction services as the person with intellectual disability might not understand the deterrent effect of disulfiram, or understand that all alcohol must be avoided, including that found in medications and food (Williams, Kouimtsidis, & Baldacchino, 2018); however, close supervision provided by a carer may be protective (Vanucchi et al., 2022).
- People with intellectual disability may have problems related to remembering the medication timings and dose. Service providers can help patients in various ways to ensure medication compliance: for instance, by giving a recovery-oriented ritual around taking medication, setting a watch alarm, wearing a reminder bracelet, and provision of a weekly blister card pack or special pill box.

- Tobacco
  - Due to the paucity of evidence to guide interventions for people with intellectual disability who wish to cut down or quit smoking, generic smoking cessation support should be offered.
  - As in the mainstream population and people with severe mental disorders, people with intellectual disability who smoke should be offered combined pharmacological and non-pharmacological interventions, such as tailored directive and supportive behavioural interventions (Das-Munshi et al., 2020).

Table 13.4 Medication use for alcohol-use disorder in intellectual disability

Medication	Usual dose	Advantages	Disadvantages
Acamprosate	666mg three times daily. Recommended for up to 6 months to 1 year depending on the response	Minimal side-effect profile, especially on liver. Minimal drug interaction. No withdrawal effects, so no need to taper the dose on discontinuation	Medication compliance due to thrice daily dosing
Naltrexone	25mg on day one, then 50mg once daily	Once daily dose	Cannot use in liver disease, kidney disease, or comorbid opioid dependence

- As highlighted earlier, psychoeducational interventions appear useful in intellectual disability, especially with adaptations such as visual aids, group discussions, short information giving segments, videos, role playing, et cetera.
- Behavioural smoking cessation interventions for those with severe mental disorders have employed a range of treatment strategies, including psychoeducational, motivational enhancement, and cognitive behavioural elements; however, the optimal frequency, duration, and format (individual vs group) of psychosocial treatments and the active ingredients of these multi-component interventions remain unclear (Evins et al., 2015).
- Medication use: available pharmacological interventions work by reducing nicotine withdrawal. The main medications found to be effective are nicotine replacement therapy, varenicline, and bupropion. Nicotine replacement therapy comes in various forms (transdermal patches, lozenges, gum, sublingual tablets, inhalator, nasal spray, mouth spray, and oral strips). Varenicline is a selective nicotinic acetylcholine receptor partial agonist and bupropion is believed to act by enhancing noradrenergic and dopaminergic release; also, it is an antagonist at the nicotinic acetylcholine receptor.
- Although combination nicotine replacement therapy is first line pharmacotherapy for smokers in the general population, there is no published research on the efficacy of nicotine replacement therapy in intellectual disability.

- Cannabis
    - In the mainstream population, psychosocial treatments for cannabis use disorder have demonstrated effectiveness over control conditions. High-intensity interventions of more than four sessions and those delivered over longer than one month – for example, cognitive-behavioural therapy, motivational enhancement therapy, a combination of both – including contingency management adjunct treatments, were most effective.
    - Other useful psychosocial interventions include social support, mindfulness-based meditation, and drug education and counselling. The psychosocial treatments are more effective than treatment as usual in reducing the frequency of cannabis use, quantity used per occasion and severity of dependence. However, treatment was not likely to be more effective than no treatment in improving cannabis-related problems, motivation to quit, or mental health (Gates et al., 2016).
    - Medication use: there are currently no accepted pharmacotherapies for the treatment of cannabis dependence, although various options have been proposed as possible interventions, such as preparations containing tetrahydrocannabinol, antidepressants (fluoxetine, escitalopram, vilazodone, nefazodone, mirtazapine, venlafaxine), mood stabilisers (divalproex sodium, gabapentin, lithium, topiramate), and other medications (bupropion, buspirone, atomoxetine, N-acetylcysteine, and oxytocin). Studies undertaken to date on pharmacotherapies for cannabis dependence are insufficient to guide clinical practice (Nielsen et al., 2019).
    - For cannabis-induced mental disorders, cessation of cannabis use and treatment as for the primary mental disorder should be instituted.

Table 13.5 Recommendations by Substance Abuse and Mental Health Services Administration (SAMHSA) for addiction service providers for people with intellectual disability

Ask simple questions and repeat them if necessary.

Teach refusal skills.

Avoid generalising (i.e., explain that the same refusal skills that are used at a party can also be used at a bar).

Have the individual repeat back a concept to make sure they understand.

Utilise role playing.

Have the individual focus on specific goals.

Address trauma in psychotherapy if it is an issue.

Medication-assisted treatment.

Modified Alcoholics Anonymous (AA) groups.

- Opioids
    - Alongside psychosocial interventions, useful pharmacological treatments for heroin dependence include the opioid agonist methadone and the partial agonist buprenorphine (with or without the addition of naloxone, an opioid receptor antagonist that can reverse opioid overdose).

Table 13.5 lists the key recommendations by Substance Misuse and Mental Health Services Administration (SAMHSA) for addiction service providers for people with intellectual disability.

Case Study 13.2: Treatment

Saul was admitted, and his treatment plan followed the 10-point treatment programme as outlined here:

1. **Diagnostic clarification:** This was confirmed as having three elements: mild intellectual disability, dissocial personality disorder with several emotionally unstable traits, and cannabis-induced psychosis.
2. **Medication:** Saul was started on oral risperidone and was compliant. It brought about an improvement in his mental state and behaviour. The oral medication was changed to a depot preparation to improve future compliance.
3. **Psychological formulation:** The predisposing, precipitating, and maintaining factors for his current violent behaviours and psychotic episode were examined and a formulation completed.
4. **Positive Behaviour Support (PBS):** A PBS plan has been formulated in line with the psychological formulation. A patient-friendly (easy-read) version was provided for him and there is a full version for staff who support him.
5. **Other psychological treatments:** As the key precipitating factor for the admission was substance misuse, Saul went through a 10-session brief intervention for substance misuse which incorporated motivational interviewing, psychoeducation, screening, and relapse prevention strategies. This was supplemented by supportive psychotherapy sessions that touched on appropriate assertiveness skills, low self-esteem, and problem solving.

6. **Offence specific treatments**: Although not convicted, his presentation was characterised by inter-personal violence. This was explored in psychology sessions and a co-produced relapse prevention plan is in place now.
7. **Structured programme of daily activities**: Saul was offered a structured timetable of sessions through nursing and occupational therapy. This will continue in the community.
8. **Risk assessments**: A detailed risk assessment and management plan was developed and is in place.
9. **Community participation**: Graded community leaves)including escorted, unescorted, and overnight leaves) commenced soon after his mental state stabilised. These have gone very well, with no untoward events or significant concerns.
10. **Discharge**: Following admission to hospital, Saul's mental state did not show any active psychotic or major affective features. His insight, although limited initially, improved with time, and his tendency to minimise adverse effects of illicit substances has also improved. With the involvement of a supportive community intellectual disability team, he was discharged to the community.

Frith Guidelines Editors' Expert Group Consensus Statements

Statements of High Confidence

- Prevalence rates of substance (mis)use in people with intellectual disability vary; although they may be less likely to misuse substances than the general population, there is an increased risk of complications when they do.
- People with intellectual disability (mis)use all types of substances as in the general population, and the clinical features of the specific syndromes among those with mild to moderate intellectual disability is comparable to the general population.
- Guidelines propose that treatment for drug misuse should always involve a psychosocial component.

Statements of Medium Confidence

- Psychoeducation, motivational interviewing, cognitive behavioural therapy and mindfulness-based techniques are effective.
- As in people without intellectual disability, benzodiazepines are first-line in alcohol withdrawal; long-term medications used in the management of alcohol abuse are acamprosate and naltrexone.
- There is no published research on the efficacy of nicotine replacement therapy in intellectual disability, although combination nicotine replacement therapy is first-line pharmacotherapy for smokers in the general population.
- Pharmacological treatments for heroin dependence include the opioid agonist methadone and the partial agonist buprenorphine.

Statements of Low Confidence

- Psychoeducational interventions appear useful in intellectual disability, especially with adaptations such as visual aids, group discussions, short information-giving segments, videos, role playing, et cetera.

> **Resource Box**
>
> Department of Health (England) and the devolved administrations (2007). Drug Misuse and Dependence: UK Guidelines on Clinical Management. London: Department of Health (England), the Scottish Government, Welsh Assembly Government and Northern Ireland Executive. https://webarchive.nationalarchives.gov.uk/ukgwa/20130123164248mp_/http://www.nta.nhs.uk/%2fuploads%2fclinical_guidelines_2007.pdf.
>
> National Institute for Clinical Excellence (2007). Drug misuse in over 16s: psychosocial interventions. National Institute for Health and Clinical Excellence. www.nice.org.uk/guidance/cg51.
>
> National Institute for Health and Care Excellence (2010). Alcohol-use disorders: diagnosis and management of physical complications. Clinical guideline [CG100]. National Institute for Clinical Excellence. www.nice.org.uk/guidance/cg100.
>
> National Institute for Health and Care Excellence (2011). Alcohol-use disorders: diagnosis, assessment and management of harmful drinking (high-risk drinking) and alcohol dependence. Clinical guideline [CG115]. National Institute for Clinical Excellence. www.nice.org.uk/guidance/CG115.
>
> National Institute for Health and Care Excellence (2023).Tobacco: Preventing uptake, promoting quitting and treating dependence [NG209]. National Institute for Clinical Excellence. https://www.nice.org.uk/guidance/ng209.
>
> Lingford-Hughes, A., Welch, S., Peters, L., & Nutt, D. (2012). BAP updated guidelines: Evidence-based guidelines for the pharmacological management of substance abuse, harmful use, addiction and comorbidity: Recommendations from BAP. *Journal of Psychopharmacology*, 26(7), 899–952. https://journals.sagepub.com/doi/10.1177/0269881112444324?url_ver=Z39.88-2003&rfr_id=ori:rid:crossref.org&rfr_dat=cr_pub%20%200pubmed#sec-6.
>
> Taylor, D. M., Barnes, T. R., & Young, A. H. (2021). The *Maudsley prescribing guidelines in psychiatry*. John Wiley & Sons.

References

American Psychiatric Association (2013). Substance-related and addictive disorders. In *Diagnostic and statistical manual of mental disorders* (5th ed.). American Psychiatric Publishing, Chapter 16.

Baldwin, D. S., Anderson, I. M., Nutt, D. J., et al. (2014). Evidence-based pharmacological treatment of anxiety disorders, post-traumatic stress disorder and obsessive-compulsive disorder: A revision of the 2005 guidelines from the British Association for Psychopharmacology. *Journal of Psychopharmacology*, 28(5), 403–39.

Bhaumik, S. & Alexander, R. (eds.) (2020). Oxford textbook of the psychiatry of intellectual *disability*. Oxford University Press.

Bråthen, G., Ben-Menachem, E., Brodtkorb, E., et al. (2005). EFNS guideline on the diagnosis and management of alcohol-related seizures: Report of an EFNS task force. *European Journal of Neurology*, 12(8), 575–81.

Cahill, K., Stevens, S., Perera, R., & Lancaster, T. (2013). Pharmacological interventions for smoking cessation: An overview and network meta-analysis. *Cochrane Database of Systematic Reviews*, (5).

Chapman, S. L. C. & Wu, L. T. (2012). Substance abuse among individuals with intellectual disabilities. *Research in Developmental Disabilities*, **33**(4), 1147–56.

Chester, V., Green, F. & Alexander, R. (2011). An audit of a smoking cessation programme for people with an intellectual disability resident in a forensic unit. *Advances in Mental Health and Intellectual Disabilities*, **5**(1), 33–41.

Cooper, S.A., Smiley, E., Morrison, J., Williamson, A. & Allan, L. (2007). Mental ill-health in adults with intellectual disabilities: Prevalence and associated factors. *The British Journal of Psychiatry*, **190**(1), 27–35.

Das-Munshi, J., Semrau, M., Barbui, C., et al. (2020). Gaps and challenges: WHO treatment recommendations for tobacco cessation and management of substance use disorders in people with severe mental illness. *BMC Psychiatry*, **20**(1), 1–13.

Evins, A. E., Cather, C. & Laffer, A. (2015). Treatment of tobacco use disorders in smokers with serious mental illness: Toward clinical best practices. *Harvard Review of Psychiatry*, **23**(2), 90.

Forbat, L. (1999).Developing an alcohol awareness course for clients with a learning disability. *British Journal of Learning Disabilities*, **27**(1), 16–19.

Frielink, N., Schuengel, C., Kroon, A. & Embregts, P.J.C.M. (2015). Pretreatment for substance-abusing people with intellectual disabilities: intervening on autonomous motivation for treatment entry. *Journal of Intellectual Disability Research*, **59**(12), 1168–1182.

Gates, P. J., Sabioni, P., Copeland, J., Le Foll, B. & Gowing, L. (2016). Psychosocial interventions for cannabis use disorder. *Cochrane Database of Systematic Reviews*, (5).

Howes, S., Hartmann-Boyce, J., Livingstone-Banks, J., Hong, B. & Lindson, N. (2020). Antidepressants for smoking cessation. *Cochrane Database of Systematic Reviews*, (**4**).

Hunt, G. E., Siegfried, N., Morley, K., Brooke-Sumner, C. & Cleary, M. (2019). Psychosocial interventions for people with both severe mental illness and substance misuse. *Cochrane Database of Systematic Reviews*, (**12**).

Jahagirdar, D. & Kaunelis, D. (2017). Smoking cessation interventions for patients with severe mental illnesses: A review of clinical effectiveness and guidelines. Canadian Agency for Drugs and Technologies in Health; Aug 24. www.ncbi.nlm.nih.gov/books/NBK525600/.

Kerr, S., Lawrence, M., Darbyshire, C., Middleton, A. R. & Fitzsimmons, L. (2013). Tobacco and alcohol-related interventions for people with mild/moderate intellectual disabilities: a systematic review of the literature. *Journal of Intellectual Disability Research*, **57**(5), 393–408.

Kiewik, M., VanderNagel, J., Engels, R. & de Jong, C. (2020). Cognitive behaviour therapy for adults with mild to borderline intellectual disabilities and substance use disorders: A feasibility study. *Prevention and Intervention of Substance Use and Misuse among Persons with Intellectual Disabilities*, **91**.

Kouimtsidis, C., Bosco, A., Scior, K., et al. (2017). A feasibility randomised controlled trial of extended brief intervention for alcohol misuse in adults with mild to moderate intellectual disabilities living in the community: The EBI-LD study. *Trials*, **18**(1), 1–12.

McGillicuddy, N. B. & Blane, H. T. (1999). Substance use in individuals with mental retardation. *Addictive Behaviors*, **24**(6), 869–78. https://doi.org/10.1016/S0306-4603(99)00055-6.

Mendel, E. & Hipkins, J. (2002). Motivating learning disabled offenders with alcohol-related problems: A pilot study. *British Journal of Learning Disabilities*, **30**(4), 153–8.

Nielsen, S., Gowing, L., Sabioni, P. & Le Foll, B., 2019. Pharmacotherapies for cannabis dependence. *Cochrane Database of Systematic Reviews*, (1).

Poznyak, V., Reed, G. M. and Medina-Mora, M. E. (2018). Aligning the ICD-11 classification of disorders due to substance use with global service needs. *Epidemiology and Psychiatric Sciences*, **27**(3), 212–18.

Saunders, J. B. (2017). Substance use and addictive disorders in DSM-5 and ICD 10 and the draft ICD 11. *Current Opinion in Psychiatry*, **30**(4), 227–37.

Schijven, E. P., Hulsmans, D. H., VanDerNagel, J. E., et al. (2021). The effectiveness of an indicated prevention programme for substance use in individuals with mild intellectual disabilities and borderline intellectual functioning: Results of a quasi-experimental study. *Addiction*, **116**(2), 373–81.

Singh, N. N., Lancioni, G. E., Winton, A. S., et al. (2011).Effects of a mindfulness-based smoking cessation program for an adult with mild intellectual disability. *Research in Developmental Disabilities*, **32**(3), 1180–5.

Singh, N. N., Lancioni, G. E., Winton, A. S., et al. (2013). A mindfulness-based smoking cessation program for individuals with mild intellectual disability. *Mindfulness*, **4**, 148–57.

Singh, N. N., Lancioni, G. E., Myers, R. E., et al. (2014). A randomized controlled trial of a mindfulness-based smoking cessation program for individuals with mild intellectual disability. *International Journal of Mental Health and Addiction*, **12**, 153–68.

Steel, A. & Ritchie, G. (2004). Psycho-educational approach to addiction – a case study. *Drugs and Alcohol Today*, **4**(4), 30–3.

Steinberg, M. L., Heimlich, L. & Williams, J. M. (2009). Tobacco use among individuals with intellectual or developmental disabilities: A brief review. *Intellectual and Developmental Disabilities*, **47**(3), 197–207.

Swerts, C., Vandevelde, S., VanDerNagel, J. E., et al. (2017). Substance use among individuals with intellectual disabilities living independently in Flanders. *Research in Developmental Disabilities*, **63**, 107–17.

To, W. T., Neirynck, S., Vanderplasschen, W., Vanheule, S. & Vandevelde, S. (2014). Substance use and misuse in persons with intellectual disabilities (ID): Results of a survey in ID and addiction services in Flanders. *Research in Developmental Disabilities*, **35**(1), 1–9.

Tracy, J. & Hosken, R. (1997). The importance of smoking education and preventative health strategies for people with intellectual disability. *Journal of Intellectual Disability Research*, **41**(5), 416–21.

van Duijvenbode, N. & VanDerNagel, J. E. (2019). A systematic review of substance use (disorder) in individuals with mild to borderline intellectual disability. *European Addiction Research*, **25**(6), 263–82.

Vannucchi, G., Ramella Cravaro, V. & Bertelli, M. O. (2022). Substance-related and addictive disorders in intellectual disability. In Textbook of Psychiatry for Intellectual Disability and Autism Spectrum Disorder (pp. 783–805). Springer International Publishing.

Williams, F., Kouimtsidis, C. & Baldacchino, A. (2018). Alcohol use disorders in people with intellectual disability. *BJPsych Advances*, **24**(4), 264–72.

World Health Organization (2019). International statistical classification of diseases and related health problems (11th ed.).

Chapter 14

Attention Deficit Hyperactivity Disorder

Bhathika Perera

Introduction

By the end of this chapter, the reader will have a better understanding of the diagnosis of Attention Deficit Hyperactivity Disorder (ADHD) and how it manifests in people with intellectual disability. There will be emphasis on how ADHD symptoms can be manifested differently in people with intellectual disability compared to the non-intellectual disability population and how this creates various challenges when making a diagnosis. Case examples are used to illustrate such differences. The American Psychiatric Association's *Diagnostic and Statistical Manual of Mental Disorders* (DSM-V) and the International Classification of Diseases (ICD-11) criteria for ADHD will be briefly discussed in relation to people with intellectual disability. This chapter will then discuss the management of ADHD in people with intellectual disability and how treatments need to be adapted for people with intellectual disability. Practical tips will be discussed when using pharmacological treatments to manage ADHD in people with intellectual disability and common pitfalls. These will be further illustrated by case studies.

Definition

Attention Deficit Hyperactivity Disorder (ADHD) is a neurodevelopmental disorder with onset during childhood. It is characterised by a persistent pattern of inattention and/or hyperactivity and impulsivity in more than one setting causing significant functional impairment. Functional impairment can be manifested in academic, occupational, or social domains (American Psychiatric Association 2013; ICD-11: International classification of diseases (11th revision) 2022). The degree of inattention and/or hyperactivity and impulsivity is beyond what is expected for the person's age or level of intellectual ability and can't be better explained by another mental disorder.

Prevalence

The worldwide prevalence of Attention Deficit Hyperactivity Disorder (ADHD) is estimated to be around 5% in children and 2.5% in adults (Faraone et al., 2021). Studying the prevalence rate of ADHD in people with intellectual disability is challenging due to extreme underdiagnosis. Current studies suggest the prevalence of ADHD in people with intellectual disability to be around 20% (La Malfa et al., 2008). This fits in with the understanding that neurodevelopmental disorders often coexist (Francés et al., 2022). Prevalence rates of ADHD in people with intellectual disability can be even higher in certain genetic syndromes. Smaller studies have shown the prevalence rate of ADHD to be around 34% in adults with Down syndrome (Oxelgren et al., 2017). Similarly, higher rates of ADHD have been shown in people with Fragile X syndrome, Velocardiofacial syndrome, Smith–Magenis syndrome, and Williams syndrome.

Diagnosis, and How It Is Different in Intellectual Disability from the General Population

Attention Deficit Hyperactivity Disorder (ADHD) can present with inattentive symptoms (predominantly inattentive type) or hyperactivity and impulsivity symptoms (predominantly hyperactive type). or a combination of both (combined type). Inattentive symptoms include difficulties with paying and sustaining attention and distractibility. Hyperactive symptoms include fidgetiness, difficulty sitting in one place for long periods, inner restless, and having a 'high level of energy' most of the time. Impulsivity symptoms include difficulty waiting for their turn and impatience. International Classification of Diseases (ICD-11) or the American Psychiatric Association *Diagnostic and Statistical Manual of Mental Disorders* (DSM-V) criteria are used to diagnose ADHD (Table 14.1). Both ICD-11 and DSM-V use the term 'ADHD' and employ broadly similar criteria, but there are some differences between the two classificatory systems. DSM-V requires five or more symptoms under the domains of inattention and/or hyperactivity and impulsivity in an adult or six or more in a child to diagnose Attention Deficit Hyperactivity Disorder. ICD-11 requires several symptoms from the clusters of inattention or hyperactivity/impulsivity.

Table 14.1 Diagnostic classifications of Attention Deficit Hyperactivity Disorder

International Classification of Diseases (ICD-11).	American Psychiatric Association *Diagnostic and Statistical Manual of Mental Disorders* (DSM-V)
• Difficulty sustaining attention to tasks that do not provide a high level of stimulation or reward or require sustained mental effort; lacking attention to detail; making careless mistakes in school or work assignments; not completing tasks. • Easily distracted by extraneous stimuli or thoughts not related to the task at hand; often does not seem to listen when spoken to directly; **frequently appears to be daydreaming or to have mind elsewhere**. • Loses things; is forgetful in daily activities; has difficulty remembering to complete upcoming daily tasks or activities; difficulty planning, managing and organising schoolwork, tasks, and other activities.	• Often fails to give close attention to detail or makes careless mistakes in schoolwork, at work, or with other activities. • Often has trouble holding attention on tasks or play activities. • Often does not follow through on instructions and fails to finish schoolwork, chores, or duties in the workplace (e.g., loses focus, side-tracked). • Often does not seem to listen when spoken to directly. • Often has trouble organising tasks and activities. • **Often avoids, dislikes, or is reluctant to do tasks that require mental effort over a long period of time** • Often loses things necessary for tasks and activities. • Is often easily distracted. • Is often forgetful in daily activities.

Table 14.1 (cont.)

• Excessive motor activity: leaves seat when expected to sit still; often runs about; has difficulty sitting still without fidgeting (younger children); feelings of physical restlessness, a sense of discomfort with being quiet or sitting still (adolescents and adults). • Difficulty engaging in activities quietly; talks too much. • Blurts out answers in school, comments at work; difficulty waiting turn in conversation, games, or activities; interrupts or intrudes on others conversations or games. • **A tendency to act in response to immediate stimuli without deliberation or consideration of risks and consequences.**	• Often fidgets with or taps hands or feet, or squirms in seat • Often leaves seat in situations when remaining seated is expected • Often runs about or climbs in situations where it is not appropriate (adolescents or adults may be limited to feeling restless) • Often unable to play or take part in leisure activities quietly • Is often 'on the go', acting as if 'driven by a motor' • Often talks excessively • Often blurts out an answer before a question has been completed • Often has trouble waiting their turn • Often interrupts or intrudes on others (e.g., butts into conversations or games)

* Criteria in bold are not found in the other diagnostic classification

Even though the core symptoms are the same, ADHD can manifest differently in people with intellectual disability compared to the general population. Severity of intellectual disability, communication difficulties, different life experiences, intellectual impairment, concurrent neurodevelopmental disorders such as autism, and physical health conditions such as epilepsy can affect the presentation of ADHD symptoms in people with intellectual disability. This makes the application of diagnostic criteria challenging in people with intellectual disability. For example, diagnostic criteria that rely on a person's ability to communicate (often talks excessively or often blurts out an answer before a question has been completed) cannot be applied in people with intellectual disability who have communication difficulties. There are often clinical challenges when trying to ascertain whether inattentive symptoms are due to attention deficit hyperactivity disorder or related to the person's intellectual disability itself. Therefore, it has been suggested that while application of diagnostic criteria is important, overall impression of the severity and pervasiveness of core symptoms ADHD symptoms within the context of the severity of intellectual disability is important when diagnosing ADHD in people with intellectual disability (Perera et al., 2020). Table 14.2 summarises the key points related to the clinical presentation of ADHD in people with Intellectual Disability.

Clinical diagnosis of ADHD in intellectual disability is based on history and mental state examination. Symptoms are determined by taking a detailed history focusing on three core symptom domains, their impact/functional impairment, and their presence during childhood. People with intellectual disability may struggle to describe these symptoms, so observations from carers are often used in the history to make the diagnosis. As a result, assessment can be mainly focused on hyperactivity and impulsivity as these are behavioural

Table 14.2 Clinical presentation of attention deficit hyperactivity disorder in people with intellectual disability

Inattentive symptoms	• Easily distracted • Jumping from one task to another even if they like those tasks • Not being able to stay focused when having meals and distracted by what happens around them • Getting bored easily
Hyperactivity/impulsivity symptoms	• 'On the go' • Can't sit in one place for long even for tasks that the person enjoys • Fidgety • Moves around a lot • Difficulty waiting • Getting angry/upset if they have to wait

manifestations. Inattention can manifest as being easily distracted, but it is often challenging to assess unless the person is able to describe it.

> **Case Study 14.1: Presentation of Attention Deficit Hyperactivity Disorder in a Person with Intellectual Disability**
>
> Mark is a 21-year-old man with moderate intellectual disability, autism, and behaviour seen as challenging going back to his childhood. He was known to children's services due to the nature of his behaviour seen as challenging, which includes physical and verbal aggression towards his parents, self-harm, and damage to property on a regular basis.
>
> A detailed history from his family carers found that Mark has been very active since early childhood. They described him as having lot of energy and wanting to be outside home most of the time. He found it hard to sit and have his meals or watch a tv programme that he likes without getting distracted. He struggled at college and day centres in the past and needed 1:1 support to redirect him when he tried to get up and walk around. Staff at day centres and college reported that he gets easily distracted, especially compared to other students of similar intellectual abilities. He often struggles to settle to sleep at night. He is also very impatient. One of the triggers for his behavioural challenges is when he is asked to wait or his demands are not met straight away. Following comprehensive assessment, a diagnosis of Attention Deficit Hyperactivity Disorder was made.

The Evidence Base to Support Treatments for Attention Deficit Hyperactivity Disorder in People with Intellectual Disability

Medication Treatments for Attention Deficit Hyperactivity Disorder in Intellectual Disability

Medications used to treat Attention Deficit Hyperactivity Disorder (ADHD) can be divided into stimulant and non-stimulant. Table 14.3 lists the main ADHD medications available in the United Kingdom. ADHD medication preparations can vary from one country to

Table 14.3 Attention Deficit Hyperactivity Disorder medications (available in the United Kingdom)

Stimulant	Non-stimulant
Methylphenidate immediate release (IR)	Atomoxetine
Methylphenidate modified release (MR) • Concerta XL • Medikinet XL • Equasym XL	Guanfacine
Dexamfetamine IR	Clonidine
Lisdexamfetamine	

another, so it is important to understand their mechanism of action, duration of action, and side effects profile prior to using them.

Immediate release methylphenidate can last up to 4 hours. Therefore, it may need dosing up to 3 times a day to get symptom control during the day. Concerta XL lasts up to 8–10 hours. Medikinet XL and Equasym XL can last up to 6–8 hours. Dexamfetamine lasts up to 4–6 hours. Lisdexamfetamine has the longest duration: up to 14 hours per day. Timing of ADHD medication needs to be decided based on the duration of action and when symptom control and improved functional impairment is needed.

Non-stimulant medications, mainly atomoxetine and guanfacine, have 24-hour symptom control. Guanfacine is given at night due to its sedative properties. Atomoxetine can be given at any of the day.

Concerta XL is a tablet and cannot be chewed. Medikinet XL and Lisdexamfetamine come in capsules, so the content can be mixed with food if the person with intellectual disability struggles to swallow medications or chew them. Atomoxetine comes as a liquid if a person struggles with tablets/capsules.

The evidence base for pharmacological treatments for ADHD in general population is well established. The National Institute for Health and Care Excellence (NICE) recommends medications for adults with ADHD if their symptoms are still causing a significant impairment in at least one domain after environmental modifications have been implemented (NICE, 2018). Stimulant medications are listed as first-line ADHD medication. Non-stimulants are recommended as second-line. A national audit looking at prescribing practices in the United Kingdom in people with intellectual disability showed that methylphenidate was the most commonly used ADHD medication (54%), followed by atomoxetine (37%) (Perera et al., 2021).

Studies looking at ADHD medications in people with intellectual disability are limited in number and sample size (Courtenay and Elstner, 2016; Miller et al., 2020); however, the effectiveness of ADHD medications in people with intellectual disability appears to be lower compared to the general population. Authors of some studies concluded that using low doses in people with intellectual disability was a possible reason for lower response rate; however, further studies are needed to understand the reasons for reduced effectiveness.

Evidence for Attention Deficit Hyperactivity Disorder Medications in Intellectual Disability

Methylphenidate

- A single blind randomised controlled trial (RCT) comparing methylphenidate with risperidone over 4 weeks in 46 children with intellectual disability and Attention Deficit Hyperactivity Disorder (ADHD) did not find a significant difference (Correia Filho et al., 2005).
- A double-blind randomised controlled trial comparing methylphenidate with placebo in 90 children with intellectual disability and ADHD showed methylphenidate was superior to placebo (Simonoff et al., 2013).
- A double-blind randomised controlled trial comparing methylphenidate with placebo in 24 children with intellectual disability and ADHD showed that methylphenidate was superior to placebo (Pearson et al., 2003).
- A retrospective open-label observational study looking at 18 children with intellectual disability, refractory epilepsy, and ADHD showed improvement with methylphenidate (Fosi et al., 2013).

Atomoxetine

- A prospective observational study looking at 48 children with intellectual disability, ADHD, and chromosomal disorders showed atomoxetine to be effective in improving ADHD symptoms (Fernández-Jaén et al., 2010).
- A retrospective observational study looking at 37 children with intellectual disability, ADHD, and autism spectrum disorder showed that atomoxetine was effective in improving ADHD symptoms (Kilincaslan et al., 2016).

Guanfacine

- A prospective observational study looking at 23 children with ADHD and Down syndrome showed that guanfacine is effective in improving attention deficit hyperactivity disorder symptoms (Capone et al., 2016).

Clonidine

- A double-blind placebo-controlled randomised controlled trial looking at 10 children with intellectual disability and attention deficit hyperactivity disorder (hyperkinetic disorder) showed clonidine to be effective in reducing attention deficit hyperactivity disorder symptoms (Agarwal et al., 2001).

The Evidence for Psychological Interventions for Attention Deficit Hyperactivity Disorder in People with Intellectual Disability

Evidence to support the use of psychological interventions is very limited in Attention Deficit Hyperactivity Disorder (ADHD) (Osugo and Cooper, 2016). A Cochrane review looking at use of cognitive behavioural therapy for ADHD found low-quality evidence for some potential benefits (Lopez et al. 2018). In people with intellectual disability, positive behaviour support (PBS) has become the main behavioural and psychological strategy to manage behaviours seen as challenging, despite limited evidence (Strydom et al., 2020). However, the use of behavioural support along with environmental changes can be helpful in people with intellectual disability and ADHD (Ageranioti-Bélanger et al., 2012). For example, a person with hyperactive symptoms of ADHD will find it beneficial to have regular activities to keep them active. Clear communication, along with a structured timetable, can be helpful to manage impatience and impulsivity. Psychoeducation is useful for people with intellectual disability, especially for their carers to understand symptoms and manifestations of ADHD, so they can support the person to manage the functional impairments associated with ADHD.

Case Study 14.2: Management

Management of Mark's Attention Deficit Hyperactivity Disorder (ADHD) included improving the understanding of symptoms of ADHD that Mark experiences, its manifestations, and the associated functional impairments. The diagnosis of ADHD helped support the development of a behaviour management plan, introducing various activities to reduce the functional impairment caused by core symptoms of ADHD. ADHD medication was started after discussion of benefits and side effects. Specific markers of effectiveness of medication were agreed with carers, with close monitoring to assess benefits of medication. Blood pressure, heart rate, and weight were checked prior to starting treatment and monitored every time the dose was increased.

Mark was started on a low dose and this gradually increased until there were clear benefits with minimal side effects. Carers described how Mark's overall wellbeing improved with ADHD treatment. These included Mark being able to sit in one place and engage in activities without getting distracted often, running around less than he used to, and being less impatient. A clear improvement was noted in his challenging behaviour, which was a functional impairment of his ADHD. This helped his carers to refine the PBS plan to further support him.

How Long Should Treatment Continue?

Duration of Attention Deficit Hyperactivity Disorder (ADHD) treatment needs to be agreed on a case-by-case basis. Continuing clear benefits with minimal side effects are reasons to continue the use of ADHD medications. If the benefit of ADHD treatment is not clear, medication free periods can be implemented to investigate the need for an ongoing benefit of medication (van de Loo-Neus et al., 2011).

Stopping Attention Deficit Hyperactivity Disorder Medications

Stimulant medications (methylphenidate and dexamfetamine preparations) can be stopped abruptly without any need for gradual withdrawal. Non-stimulant medications (atomoxetine, guanfacine, and clonidine) need to be gradually reduced. However, studies have shown no clinically meaningful withdrawal effects when atomoxetine was abruptly discontinued in a clinical trial (Camporeale et al., 2013). There is a risk of rebound hypertension if clonidine or guanfacine is withdrawn suddenly due to their action through alpha receptors.

The Frith Prescribing Guidelines Editors' Expert Group Consensus Statements

Statements of High Confidence

The evidence base for the treatment of Attention Deficit Hyperactivity Disorder (ADHD) in people with intellectual disability is limited to smaller studies showing some benefits; however, it is not strong enough to make specific recommendations, hence the recommendations given here are based on a strong evidence base in the non-intellectual disability population.

Stimulant ADHD medications are the first choice in both in the general population and those with intellectual disability; however, studies show that non-stimulants are widely used for treatment of ADHD in people with intellectual disability as well.

Most ADHD guidelines propose:

- Offering pharmacotherapy for treatment of ADHD symptoms along with behavioural interventions.
- For those that do not respond to the initial choice of therapy after 4–6 weeks, switch to a different ADHD medication.

Statements of Medium Confidence

The prevalence of ADHD is higher in the intellectual disability population compared to the general population.

Many people with intellectual disability, especially those with severe intellectual disability, may not meet the American Psychiatric Association's *Diagnostic and Statistical Manual of Mental Disorders* (DSM-V) criteria for ADHD. Therefore, applicability of certain criteria needs to be taken into consideration depending on the severity of intellectual disability and the presence of comorbid neurodevelopmental disorders.

Statements of Low Confidence

Between 40% and 50% of patients with intellectual disability respond to ADHD medications. Behavioural, psychological, and environmental interventions can be helpful to reduce functional impairment caused by ADHD.

Resource Box

Key Guidelines
Evidence-based guidelines for the pharmacological management of attention deficit hyperactivity disorder: Update on recommendations from the British Association for Psychopharmacology (2014) www.bap.org.uk/pdfs/BAP_Guidelines-AdultADHD.pdf
National institute for Health and Care Excellence (NICE) (2018) Attention deficit hyperactivity disorder: diagnosis and management. NICE guideline [NG87]: www.nice.org.uk/guidance/ng87
Royal College of Psychiatrists – ADHD in ID College Report (CR230): www.rcpsych.ac.uk/improving-care/campaigning-for-better-mental-health-policy/college-reports/2021-college-reports/ADHD-in-adults-with-intellectual-disability-CR230

Royal College of Psychiatrists in Scotland (2017) ADHD in adults: good practice guidelines: www.rcpsych.ac.uk/docs/default-source/members/divisions/scotland/adhd_in_adultsfinal_guidelines_june2017.pdf?sfvrsn=40650449_2

Structured diagnostic tool for ADHD in people with Intellectual disability: www.divacenter.eu/DIVA.aspx?id=534

References

Agarwal, V., Sitholey, P., Kumar, S., & Prasad, M. (2001). Double-blind, placebo-controlled trial of clonidine in hyperactive children with mental retardation. *Mental Retardation*, **39**, 259–67. https://doi.org/10.1352/0047-6765(2001)039%3C0259:dbpcto%3E2.0.co;2.

Ageranioti-Bélanger, S., Brunet, S., D'Anjou, G., et al. (2012). Behaviour disorders in children with an intellectual disability. *Paediatrics & Child Health* **17**, 84–8. https://doi.org/10.1093/pch/17.2.84.

American Psychiatric Association. (2013). *Diagnostic and Statistical Manual of Mental Disorders*, Fifth Edition. ed. American Psychiatric Association. https://doi.org/10.1176/appi.books.9780890425596.

Camporeale, A., Upadhyaya, H., Ramos-Quiroga, J. A., et al. (2013). Safety and tolerability of atomoxetine hydrochloride in a long-term, placebo-controlled randomized withdrawal study in European and non-European adults with attention-deficit/hyperactivity disorder. *The European Journal of Psychiatry*, **27**, 206–24. https://doi.org/10.4321/S0213-61632013000300005.

Capone, G. T., Brecher, L., & Bay, M. (2016). Guanfacine use in children with Down syndrome and comorbid attention-deficit hyperactivity disorder (ADHD) with disruptive behaviors. *Journal of Child Neurology*, **31**, 957–64. https://doi.org/10.1177/0883073816634854.

Correia Filho, A. G., Bodanese, R., Silva, T. L., et al. (2005). Comparison of risperidone and methylphenidate for reducing ADHD symptoms in children and adolescents with moderate mental retardation. *Journal of the American Academy of Child and Adolescent Psychiatry*, **44**, 748–55. https://doi.org/10.1097/01.chi.0000166986.30592.67.

Courtenay, K., Elstner, S. (2016). Drug therapy in ADHD in people with intellectual disabilities. https://doi.org/10.1108/AMHID-06-2015-0032.

Faraone, S. V., Banaschewski, T., Coghill, D., et al. (2021). The World Federation of ADHD International Consensus Statement: 208 Evidence-based Conclusions about the Disorder. *Neuroscience & Biobehavioral Reviews*. https://doi.org/10.1016/j.neubiorev.2021.01.022.

Fernández-Jaén, A., Fernández-Mayoralas, D. M., Calleja Pérez, B., et al. (2010). Atomoxetine for attention deficit hyperactivity disorder in mental retardation. *Pediatric Neurology*, **43**, 341–7. https://doi.org/10.1016/j.pediatrneurol.2010.06.003.

Fosi, T., Lax-Pericall, M. T., Scott, R. C., Neville, B. G., & Aylett, S. E. (2013). Methylphenidate treatment of attention deficit hyperactivity disorder in young people with learning disability and difficult-to-treat epilepsy: Evidence of clinical benefit. *Epilepsia*, **54**, 2071–81. https://doi.org/10.1111/epi.12399.

Francés, L., Quintero, J., Fernández, A., et al. (2022). Current state of knowledge on the prevalence of neurodevelopmental disorders in childhood according to the DSM-5: a systematic review in accordance with the PRISMA criteria. *Child and Adolescent Psychiatry and Mental Health*, **16**, 27. https://doi.org/10.1186/s13034-022-00462-1

Kilincaslan, A., Mutluer, T. D., Pasabeyoglu, B., Tutkunkardas, M. D., & Mukaddes, N. M. (2016). Effects of atomoxetine in individuals with attention-deficit/hyperactivity disorder and low-functioning autism spectrum disorder. *Journal of Child and Adolescent Psychopharmacology*, **26**, 798–806. https://doi.org/10.1089/cap.2015.0179.

La Malfa, G., Lassi, S., Bertelli, M., Pallanti, S., & Albertini, G. (2008). Detecting attention-deficit/hyperactivity disorder (ADHD) in adults with intellectual disability: The use of Conners' Adult ADHD Rating Scales (CAARS). *Research in Developmental Disabilities*, 29, 158–64. https://doi.org/10.1016/j.ridd.2007.02.002.

Lopez, P. L., Torrente, F. M., Ciapponi, A., et al. (2018). Cognitive-behavioural interventions for attention deficit hyperactivity disorder (ADHD) in adults. *Cochrane Database of Systematic Reviews*. https://doi.org/10.1002/14651858.CD010840.pub2.

Miller, J., Perera, B., Shankar, R. (2020). Clinical guidance on pharmacotherapy for the treatment of attention-deficit hyperactivity disorder (ADHD) for people with intellectual disability. *Expert Opinion on Pharmacotherapy*, 21, 1897–913. https://doi.org/10.1080/14656566.2020.1790524.

National Institute for Health and Care Excellence (2018). Attention deficit hyperactivity disorder: diagnosis and management: NICE guideline [NG87]. www.nice.org.uk/guidance/ng87/chapter/Recommendations#maintenance-and-monitoring.

Osugo, M., & Cooper, S.-A. (2016). Interventions for adults with mild intellectual disabilities and mental ill-health: A systematic review. *Journal of Intellectual Disability Research*, 60, 615–22. https://doi.org/10.1111/jir.12285.

Oxelgren, U.W., Myrelid, Å., Annerén, G., et al. (2017). Prevalence of autism and attention-deficit–hyperactivity disorder in Down syndrome: A population-based study. *Developmental Medicine & Child Neurology*, 59, 276–83. https://doi.org/10.1111/dmcn.13217.

Pearson, D.A., Santos, C.W., Roache, J.D., et al. (2003). Treatment effects of methylphenidate on behavioral adjustment in children with mental retardation and ADHD. *Journal of the American Academy of Child & Adolescent Psychiatry*, 42, 209–16. https://doi.org/10.1097/00004583-200302000-00015.

Perera, B., Chen, J., Korb, L., et al. (2021). Patterns of comorbidity and psychopharmacology in adults with intellectual disability and attention deficit hyperactivity disorder: An UK national cross-sectional audit. *Expert Opinion on Pharmacotherapy*, 22, 1071–8. https://doi.org/10.1080/14656566.2021.1876028.

Perera, B., Courtenay, K., Solomou, S., Borakati, A., & Strydom, A. (2020). Diagnosis of attention deficit hyperactivity disorder in intellectual disability: *Diagnostic and Statistical Manual of Mental Disorder V* versus clinical impression. *Journal of Intellectual Disability Research*, 64, 251–7. https://doi.org/10.1111/jir.12705.

Simonoff, E., Taylor, E., Baird, G., et al. (2013). Randomized controlled double-blind trial of optimal dose methylphenidate in children and adolescents with severe attention deficit hyperactivity disorder and intellectual disability. *Journal of Child Psychology and Psychiatry*, 54, 527–35. https://doi.org/10.1111/j.1469-7610.2012.02569.x.

Strydom, A., Bosco, A., Vickerstaff, V., et al. (2020). Clinical and cost effectiveness of staff training in the delivery of Positive Behaviour Support (PBS) for adults with intellectual disabilities, autism spectrum disorder and challenging behaviour – randomised trial. *BMC Psychiatry*, 20, 161. https://doi.org/10.1186/s12888-020-02577-1.

van de Loo-Neus, G. H. H., Rommelse, N., & Buitelaar, J. K. (2011). To stop or not to stop? How long should medication treatment of attention-deficit hyperactivity disorder be extended? *European Neuropsychopharmacology*, 21, 584–99. https://doi.org/10.1016/j.euroneuro.2011.03.008.

World Health Organization. (2022). *ICD-11: International classification of diseases* (11th revision). https://icd.who.int/.

Chapter 15

Autism

Dolly Sud, Danielle Adams, Rohit Shankar, and Samuel Tromans

Introduction

What Is Autism?

Autism, referred to as 'autism spectrum disorder' in the 11th revision of the International Classification of Diseases (ICD-11), is a neurodevelopmental condition characterised by persistent deficits in social interaction and communication, as well as a range of restricted, repetitive behaviours (World Health Organization, 2018). The onset of autism is in the developmental period (0–18 years of age), though for some autistic persons the symptoms may manifest later in life, at a time of increased social demands (World Health Organization, 2018).

In addition to the aforementioned core autistic features, many autistic people have associated symptoms, including hypo- or hypersensitivities to sensory stimuli, difficulties describing their emotional state (alexithymia), and problems with gross motor co-ordination (Brugha, 2018).

Though many autistic people experience difficulties in relation to their autistic features, it is important to recognise that many autistic people have strengths and abilities associated with their condition (Frith & Happé, 1994). Furthermore, the outside world has generally been designed to meet the needs of non-autistic persons, and thus some of the difficulties autistic people experience are a consequence of this (Lai et al., 2020). Additionally, recent research findings (Crompton et al., 2020) suggest that autistic people can communicate effectively between each other (i.e., when an autistic person communicates with an autistic peer), suggesting that difficulties in communication principally arise when an autistic person communicates with a non-autistic peer.

As shown in Table 15.1, autistic people experience greater rates of a variety of co-occurring mental and physical health conditions compared to their non-autistic peers (Croen et al., 2015; Lai et al., 2019), including conditions such as anxiety and depression (Hollocks et al., 2019) and epilepsy (Pan et al., 2021). Additionally, autism is associated with an increased risk of both self-harm and suicidality (Blanchard et al., 2021). However, such studies tend to employ passive-case finding techniques, where autistic persons are defined as those who have a pre-existing autism diagnosis, rather than active-case finding approaches, where attempts are made to also identify previously undiagnosed autistic individuals (Tromans & Brugha, 2022). Thus, we know less about rates of co-occurring conditions in undiagnosed autistic persons compared to their diagnosed peers.

Table 15.1 Pooled prevalence estimates for co-occurring mental health and neurological conditions in the autistic population, reported in recent meta-analyses (Lai et al., 2019)

Condition	Pooled prevalence estimate	95% confidence interval
Attention deficit hyperactivity disorder (ADHD)	28%	25–32
Anxiety disorders	20%	17–23
Depressive disorders	11%	9–13
Bipolar and related disorders	5%	3–6
Schizophrenia spectrum and psychotic disorders	4%	3–5
Obsessive-compulsive and related disorders	9%	7–10
Disruptive, impulse control, and conduct disorders	12%	10–15
Sleep-wake disorders	13%	9–17
Epilepsy	14%	11–17
Cerebral palsy	3%	2–4

What Causes Autism?

There is no single cause of autism; rather, autism appears to be influenced by the interaction of multiple genetic and environmental factors (Hodges et al., 2020).

Several candidate genes have been identified that are associated with an increased likelihood of autism (Wei et al., 2021). Furthermore, autism is highly heritable, with family studies demonstrating that individuals are more likely to be autistic if they have an autistic family member (Bai et al., 2019). Additionally, there are several genetic syndromes associated with an increased likelihood of being autistic (as well as being associated with intellectual disability), including Fragile X, Down, tuberous sclerosis, neurofibromatosis, Angelman, Prader–Willi, and Williams syndromes (Zafeiriou et al., 2013).

In relation to environmental factors associated with autism, associations have been found with advanced parental age, as well as complications relating to both pregnancy (maternal obesity, maternal diabetes, and caesarean section) and birth (leading to trauma, ischaemia, and/or hypoxia) (Modabbernia et al., 2017). Additionally, low levels of vitamin D appear to be present in autistic people (Modabbernia et al., 2017).

How Is Autism Different in People with Intellectual Disability?

In people with intellectual disability who are autistic, the co-presence of their intellectual disability may present them with additional challenges. For instance, their intellectual disability will impact upon their ability to learn skills and perhaps adapt to some of the difficulties they may experience from being autistic (Barrett & Brugha, 2020). Additionally, while autism itself confers an increased risk of a wide range of forms of physical and mental illness, intellectual disability has a similar effect on illness risk, and thus autistic people with co-occurring intellectual disability experience a double disadvantage with respect to their general health (Dunn et al., 2019).

How Common Is Autism in People with Intellectual Disability?

Approximately 1% of the general population are autistic (Baxter et al., 2015). However, autism is more prevalent in persons with intellectual disability, particularly those with moderate to profound intellectual disability (Brugha et al., 2016). An England-based study reported adult autism prevalence estimates of 42.3% for men (95% CI 31.1–54.3) and 35.2% (95% CI 23.5–49.0) for women (Brugha et al., 2016).

Autism appears to be more prevalent among adults using mental health services, including both inpatient and community-based services (Brugha et al., 2020; Tromans et al., 2018). Autism was historically believed to be more common in men than women at a ratio of 4:1, though a more recent meta-analysis (Loomes et al., 2017) found that studies rated as being of higher quality (using a risk-of-bias tool) had a lower male-to-female odds ratio, reporting that the ratio appears closer to 3:1 and that women were at disproportionate risk of not receiving a clinical diagnosis. The male-to-female ratio for autism appears to be lower among both children and adults with intellectual disability compared to their peers (Posserud et al., 2021), though many intellectual disability specialists report reduced confidence in recognising autism in their female patients (Tromans et al., 2019). Autism identification also appears to be lower in minority ethnic groups, and where autistic people are identified in these groups they often have more severe difficulties (Tromans et al., 2020).

Prescriptions of psychotropic medication have significantly increased over recent decades (Aishworiya et al., 2022); studies report that approximately two-thirds of autistic adolescents have been treated with psychotropic medications, especially those with challenging behaviours and co-occurring conditions such as intellectual disability, medical and mental health diagnoses (Aishworiya et al., 2022).

Treatments: The Evidence Base

General Population

The National Institute for Health and Care Excellence (NICE) Guideline (CG170) for autistic children and young people (NICE, 2021), defined as people under the age of 19 years, predominantly recommends non-pharmacological interventions, including making appropriate environmental adjustments (e.g., consideration of sensory sensitivities) and psychosocial interventions (e.g., play-based strategies) for autistic features. The guidance does not recommend pharmacological interventions for core autistic features, including antipsychotics, antidepressants, and anticonvulsants. With respect to challenging behaviour, the guidelines recommend consideration of antipsychotic medication where there has either been an insufficient response to psychosocial interventions alone, or where 'psychosocial or other interventions could not be delivered because of the severity of the behaviour'. It is also essential to assess autistic people with challenging behaviour for the presence of co-occurring mental illness, physical illness, or environmental-related problems. For autistic children and young persons with co-occurring mental illness, the guidance recommends offering pharmacological treatments consistent with pre-existing NICE guidance for such conditions.

With respect to autistic adults, the NICE guidance (CG142) (NICE, 2012) principally recommends psychosocial interventions, for both the core features of autism (e.g., group-based social learning programmes) and further development of life skills (e.g., structured leisure activity programmes). The guidance explicitly recommends avoiding pharmacological interventions for management of core autistic features, including anticonvulsants, antipsychotics, antidepressants, cholinesterase inhibitors, oxytocin, secretin, testosterone, and hyperbaric oxygen therapy. The pharmacological guidance for challenging behaviour and treatment of co-occurring mental illness mirrors that described earlier for children and young people.

In relation to core autistic features, it is important to recognise that many autistic people view their autism as simply 'a different way of being', with no wish to change such aspects of themselves (Brugha, 2018). Instead, as Brugha (2018) suggests, their focus is instead on receiving support with 'the negative consequences of autism, including poor mental health, economic, and social exclusion' (p. 183).

This chapter is focused on treatment intervention for core and associated autistic features. While beyond the scope of this chapter, it is important to identify any co-occurring mental illness in autistic people with intellectual disability as they are at high risk of such conditions. Furthermore, it is essential to make appropriate adaptations to one's treatment approach to any identifiable mental illness, taking account of the person's coexisting neurodevelopmental conditions (Brugha, 2018). For example, for psychological therapies, it is important to consider how abstract concepts are worded, as autistic people can be prone to interpreting phrases literally (Brugha, 2018), as well as adjusting one's language according to the patient's level of intellectual disability.

People with Intellectual Disability

For autistic people with co-occurring intellectual disability, the NICE Guideline CG170 (2021) recommend consideration for genetic testing if the person has 'specific dysmorphic features, congenital anomalies and/or evidence of a learning (intellectual) disability'.

For autistic adults with a mild intellectual disability, NICE guidance CG142 (NICE, 2012) recommends consideration of a supported employment programme, much like for autistic adults without co-occurring intellectual disability. For autistic adults with a mild to moderate intellectual disability, the guideline recommends considering either an individual or group-based social learning programme. For all autistic adults, including those with intellectual disability of all levels of severity, the guideline recommend consideration of a training programme to provide support with activities of daily living; such a programme should be developed in accordance with behavioural principles.

People with Intellectual Disability: Non-Medication Treatments

There is a relative lack of evidence for non-medication treatments from study populations of autistic people with co-occurring intellectual disability; thus, much of the evidence underpinning such recommendations comes from general autistic populations.

Positive Behaviour Support (PBS) is described as 'a person-centred framework for providing long term support to people with intellectual disability and/or autism, including those with mental health conditions, who have, or may be at risk of developing, behaviours that challenge' (Health Education England, 2017). It endeavours to enhance understanding of such behaviour to help in formulating a personalised approach to treatment (Hassiotis et al., 2018). A multicentre randomised controlled trial (RCT) of whether staff training in PBS reduced challenging behaviours in adults with intellectual disability (of which 21% were also autistic) reported that it did not reduce such behaviours (Hassiotis et al., 2018). However, a subsequent systematic review by Beqiraj et al. (2022), focused on children and young people in special education settings, reported that 28 of the 30 included studies reported significant reduction in behaviours that challenge. For further information related to management of behaviour that challenges in people with intellectual disability, please refer to Chapter 10.

A meta-analysis of group-based social skills interventions for autistic youths (Gates et al., 2017) reported a medium overall effect size, with improvements in social skills reported by parents, youth, and observers, but not teachers. Walton and Ingersoll (2013) report a lack of social skills intervention research for autistic adolescents and adults with co-occurring severe to profound intellectual disability. They do, however, suggest that such interventions may have potential therapeutic value in this patient group, but current evidence is drawn from small studies that require replication on a larger scale to be recommended for wider use.

With respect to social skills interventions, it is important to note, as Brugha (2018) describes, that 'many patients on the autism spectrum describe learning to use these skills, but at a considerable cost in energy and effort' (p. 189). Thus, while social skills interventions should be considered, it is also important to consider the need for reasonable adjustments for autistic people rather than there being an expectation for them to conform to non-autistic norms. Some autistic people may benefit from a 'personal passport': a document developed in collaboration with professionals that would confirm their diagnosis and summarise their individual needs (Tromans et al., 2023).

Weld-Blundell and colleagues (2021) conducted a systematic review of employment-related interventions for people with autism and/or intellectual disability. Unfortunately, the authors could not identify a single RCT that included people with intellectual disability, although there was some evidence for specific interventions in autistic adults, such as Project SEARCH and Autistic Spectrum Disorder Supports. However, such interventions are based on the principles of applied behaviour analysis (Whittenburg et al., 2020), about which widespread concern has been expressed in the autistic community (Leaf et al., 2022). With respect to broader social and community participation, Giummarra et al. (2022) suggest that such interventions can be effective for autistic people and people with intellectual disability, but that it is important to adopt a personalised approach, with opportunities to apply what they have learnt in real-life settings.

People with Intellectual Disability: Medication Treatments

There is a lack of a substantial evidence base pertaining to research into pharmacological autism treatments in people with co-occurring intellectual disability, so there is a need to extrapolate from findings from the autistic population more generally. Table 15.2 summarises the evidence for the main pharmacological treatments for autism.

Table 15.2 Evidence base for pharmacological treatment of autism

Medication	Evidence
Antidepressants	Selective serotonin reuptake inhibitors (SSRIs) represent the most widely studied antidepressants for autism treatment. A Cochrane review assessed the evidence for selective serotonin reuptake inhibitors in treating core autistic features, associated features (e.g., self-injurious behaviours), and quality of life in autistic people (Williams et al., 2013). The included studies evaluated fluoxetine, fluvoxamine, fenfluramine, and citalopram. The authors concluded that there was no evidence to support the use of SSRIs in autistic children for such indications, that there was limited evidence to support their use in adults, particularly for repetitive behaviours, and that fluoxetine seems the best tolerated of the SSRIs. Subsequent consensus guidelines coordinated by the British Association for Pharmacology (Howes et al., 2018) contrast with those of the Cochrane review (Williams et al., 2013), stating that 'there is not sufficient data to support the recommendation for fluvoxamine or fluoxetine' for repetitive behaviours associated with autism. Since the publication of the previously mentioned reviews, a randomised, double-blind, placebo-controlled trial was conducted to evaluate impact on language development for autistic children aged 24–72 months, reporting no significant difference from placebo (Potter et al., 2019). Additionally, a RCT of fluoxetine for obsessive-compulsive behaviours in young autistic people (Reddihough et al., 2019) reported a significant improvement at 16 weeks relative to placebo, though the authors cited imprecise estimates from pre-specified analyses as a limitation of their study.
Antipsychotics	The most widely studied antipsychotics for autism treatment are risperidone and aripiprazole. A Cochrane review of risperidone as an autism treatment (Jesner et al., 2007) concluded that it may be of benefit for certain autistic features, such as irritability, hyperactivity, and repetitive behaviours. However, they cited a limited evidence base and the need to consider side effects of treatment, particularly weight gain. The more recent perspective provided by Howes and colleagues (2018) remains consistent with this viewpoint. A Cochrane review of aripiprazole as an autism treatment (Hirsch & Pringsheim 2016) reported that current evidence suggests it may have value as a short-term intervention for young people with behavioural features, such as irritability, hyperactivity, and repetitive behaviours. However, they emphasised the need to also consider the side-effect burden and that continuation of aripiprazole should be evaluated after a period of stability, as one study found that relapse rates did not differ between young people switched to placebo relative to those remaining on aripiprazole. No studies were identified for its use in autistic adults.

Table 15.2 (cont.)

	A meta-analysis of the safety and tolerability of antipsychotics in autistic people further demonstrates the high risk of side effects in this patient group, with a pooled prevalence of 50.5% (95% CI 33–67) for adverse events across studies satisfying inclusion criteria. Consensus guidelines (Howes et al., 2018) report that the current evidence base suggests that risperidone and aripiprazole 'may be beneficial for the treatment of repetitive behaviours in autistic spectrum disorders' (p. 9). However, when factoring in the risk of adverse effects, they do not recommend their routine use in this context. Where used, they advise of the need to start at a low dose, a clear and agreed treatment goal, a plan for measurement of treatment response, and frequent review to ensure the treatment is providing net benefit.
Glutaminergic agents	Memantine and D-cycloserine are among the most widely studied glutaminergic agents for autism. Memantine is a non-competitive NMDA antagonist (Howes et al., 2018), currently used for Alzheimer's disease (British National Formulary, 2023). A Cochrane review relating to use of memantine for treatment of core autistic features was conducted (Brignell et al., 2022), with the authors identifying three RCTs satisfying inclusion criteria, all of which had child and adolescent study populations. The authors reported that there was 'no clear evidence of a difference between memantine and placebo with respect to the core symptoms of autism' (p. 2), though they did express uncertainty related to the evidence. They also noted that none of the studies reported findings from autistic adults. Consistent with the findings of the Cochrane review, Howes and colleagues (2018) had similarly reported previously that 'the evidence does not support the routine use of memantine' (p. 8). D-cycloserine is 'a partial agonist at the glycine-b site on NMDA receptors' (Howes et al., 2018, p. 9). Rationale for its potential use in autistic people is based on the shared features between negative symptoms in schizophrenia and social withdrawal in autistic persons (Howes et al. 2018; Posey et al., 2004). While there are some promising findings with respect to social difficulties, further evidence is needed, and it cannot currently be considered for routine use (Doyle & McDougle, 2022; Howes et al., 2018).

The Frith Treatment Guidelines for People with Intellectual Disability

Assessment

- A comprehensive diagnostic assessment is essential for all people with intellectual disability, including those who are suspected to be or known to be autistic. Such an approach is described elsewhere in this textbook, as well as in other sources (Bhaumik

et al., 2020). The assessment should include determination of the level of intellectual disability and adaptive functioning, any change from the person's normative functioning, and consideration of potential co-occurring mental and physical illness, challenging behaviour, neurodevelopmental conditions, genetic syndromes, and sensory impairments.
- Particular considerations pertaining to autistic people with co-occurring intellectual disability include being mindful of possible sensory sensitivities (e.g., making sure the assessment environment is not too noisy or brightly lit), and of their comfort with physical contact (e.g., a handshake may be detrimental to rapport for some people) (Bhaumik et al., 2020). It may be also helpful to identify and discuss any special interests of the person (as this may help develop rapport) (Bhaumik et al., 2020).

Non-Medication Treatments
- For autistic people with intellectual disability where therapeutic intervention is considered appropriate for their autistic features, such as when a behaviour is having a detrimental impact on the patient's wellbeing, non-pharmacological approaches should usually be considered in the first instance (the exception being where the behaviour is so severe that non-pharmacological approaches cannot be delivered).
- Non-pharmacological approaches include behavioural, educational, and social interventions.
- It is also important to ensure autistic people with intellectual disability have reasonable adjustments made relating to their conditions, such as environmental adaptations.

Medication Treatments
- Fluoxetine (a selective serotonin reuptake inhibitor) may be helpful in treatment of repetitive behaviours associated with autism.
- Risperidone and aripiprazole (both second-generation antipsychotics) may also be beneficial in the treatment of repetitive behaviours, as well as other associated autistic features, such as irritability and hyperactivity.
- The current evidence base does not support routine use of glutaminergic agents, such as memantine and D-cycloserine, for the treatment of autistic features.

Figure 15.1 provides an algorithm that could be used by clinicians for a quick reference. Please read the relevant sections for further details.

Length of Treatment and Related Issues
The NHS England (Stopping Over-Medication of People with a Learning Disability, Autism, or Both) (STOMP) programme aims to ensure that psychotropic medication prescribing for people with intellectual disability and/or autism is undertaken in a rationalised, judicious manner, involving appropriate consideration of non-pharmacological approaches; active involvement of patients, their families, and their carers in decision-making; and promoting active medication monitoring (NHS England, 2023). Inappropriate psychotropic medication prescribing creates unnecessary risks, including medication-related side effects and potential interactions with other medications (NHS England, 2020).

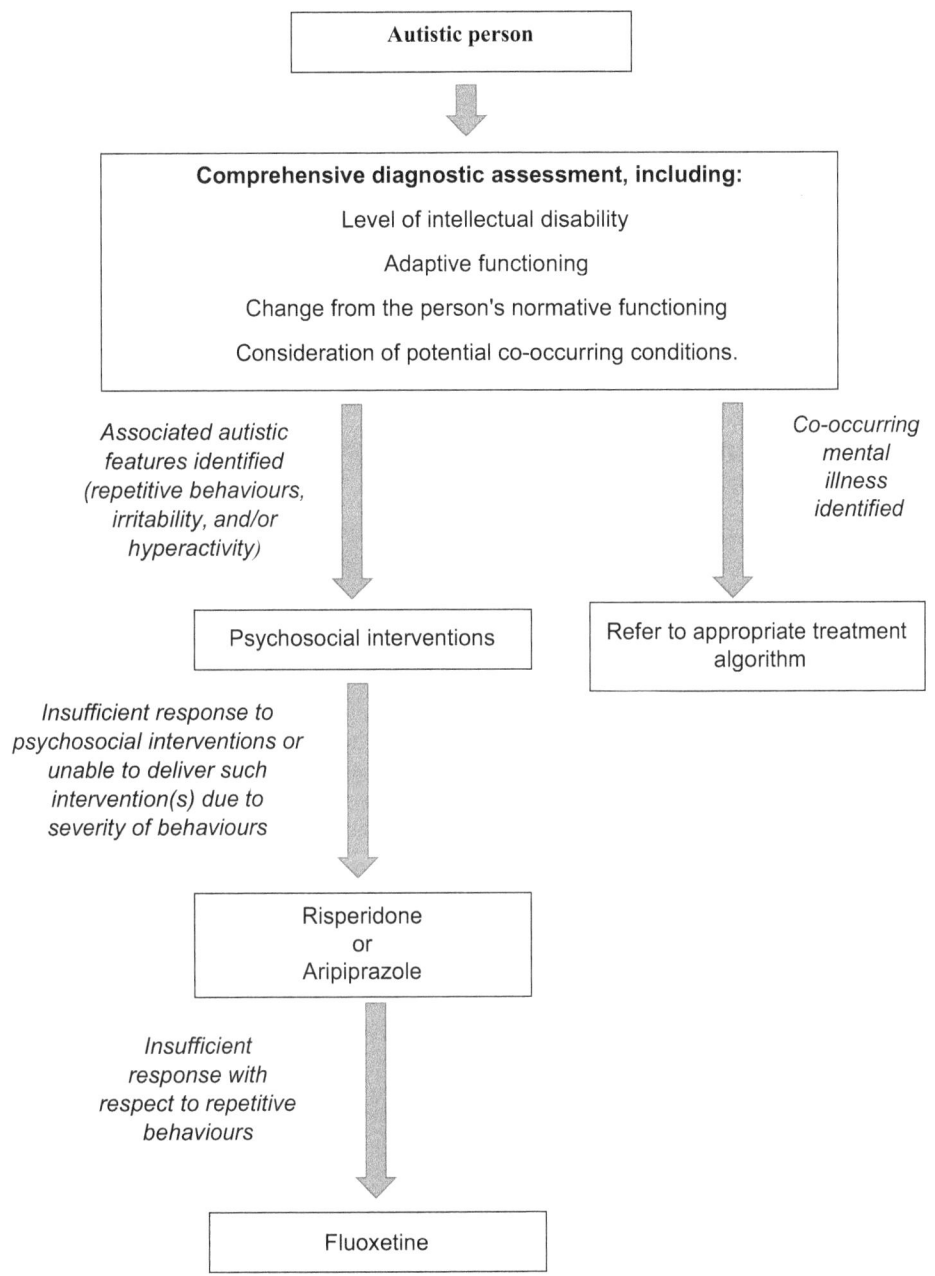

Figure 15.1 Assessment and treatment algorithm

Prescriptions of psychotropic medications for people with intellectual disability and/or autism need to be supported by clear evidence of patient benefit, and under most circumstances used in tandem with non-pharmacological interventions (Royal College of

Psychiatrists 2021). In the case of antipsychotic medications, the NICE Guideline, CG142 (NICE, 2012) recommends reviewing treatment response 3–4 weeks after commencement, and discontinuing the treatment if a clinically significant response has not been observed after 6 weeks. Regular medication review is important to assess for both treatment response as well as emergence of any side effects (Royal College of Psychiatrists, 2021). It is important to consider that autistic people with intellectual disability may have significant communication impairment, such that they may not always be able to report experiencing side effects themselves. Thus, collateral information from carers, as well as the clinician's own observational skills, are key.

Withdrawal of psychotropic medication frequently benefits from a multidisciplinary approach, with central involvement of the patient themselves, as well as their family and carers (Shankar et al., 2019). Under most circumstances, gradual withdrawal of psychotropic medication is preferable, as this can reduce the risk of discontinuation-related effects (NHS England, 2020).

The case study presented here illustrates the principles of assessment and management that are discussed in this chapter.

Case Study 15.1

Izabella is a 44-year-old autistic woman with co-occurring moderate intellectual disability. She lives in supported living accommodation, where she is supported by a consistent staffing team who have worked with her for many years. More recently, there has been an increase in the intensity and frequency of her long-standing behaviours that challenge, predominantly manifesting as self-harming (including skin-picking and head-banging) and physical aggression directed towards others (including hair-pulling, scratching, punching, and kicking). The increase in these behaviours has had a profound impact on Izabella's quality of life as she is no longer able to attend her regular day centre, which she greatly enjoyed, owing to the concerns of day centre staff about the risks to other attendees and themselves. A concerted multidisciplinary effort has been made to identify the cause of these behaviours, including primary care assessment for underlying physical health problems, intellectual disability psychiatrist-led assessment for underlying mental health problems, and direct observations made by the community intellectual disability team. Unfortunately, no clear precipitating factor has been identified. Furthermore, numerous non-pharmacological approaches have been undertaken, including reviewing her communication passport, use of positive behavioural support, and basic behavioural techniques (including distraction, diversion, and reassurance), all of which have failed to provide significant benefit. After much consideration, a trial of risperidone is considered. Despite making reasonable adjustments to support Izabella's understanding, she did not have capacity to consent to the use of risperidone and thus the medication was commenced as a best interest decision by her psychiatrist, after discussion with other members of the multidisciplinary team, her carer team, and her family. Related baseline and monitoring blood tests and electrocardiogram findings were reassuring. Commencement of risperidone led to a subsequent reduction in challenging behaviours, as well as a corresponding improvement in Izabella's wellbeing and quality of life. Following 12 months of sustained remission of these symptoms, it was considered appropriate to gradually reduce Izabella's risperidone dose while carefully monitoring for re-emergence of challenging behaviours, considering the metabolic risks and other side effects of long-term antipsychotic therapy. Izabella's risperidone was eventually discontinued without re-emergence of her challenging behaviours in the subsequent 12-month period.

The Frith Prescribing Guidelines Editors' Expert Group Consensus Statements

Statements of High Confidence
- Autism is substantially more prevalent among people with intellectual disability compared to the general population.
- Diagnosed autistic people are at heightened risk of a wide range of common mental illnesses compared to the general population, which require timely identification and treatment.
- Many autistic people with intellectual disability will not require pharmacological intervention for their autistic features; where such features are having a detrimental impact on their mental health and wellbeing one should usually first consider the role of non-pharmacological interventions.
- Pharmacological interventions should be considered when the patient has insufficiently responded to psychosocial interventions, or where the features are of such severity that such interventions cannot be delivered (NICE, 2021).

Statements of Medium Confidence
- Fluoxetine may be beneficial for treatment of repetitive behaviours associated with autism.
- Risperidone and aripiprazole may be beneficial in treatment of certain autistic features such as irritability, hyperactivity, and repetitive behaviours.

Statements of Low Confidence
- D-cycloserine, a glutaminergic agent, may be of benefit with respect to social difficulties associated with autism. However, the evidence base is currently limited, such that it cannot be recommended for routine use at this time.

> **Resource Box**
>
> Autism spectrum disorder in under 19s: Support and management. Clinical guideline [CG170] Published: 28 August 2013. Last updated: 14 June 2021 www.nice.org.uk/guidance/cg170/chapter/Recommendations.
>
> Autism spectrum disorder in adults: diagnosis and management. Clinical guideline [CG142] Published: 27 June 2012. Last updated: 14 June 2021 www.nice.org.uk/guidance/cg142.
>
> Cortese, S., Besag, F. M., Clark, B., et al. (2023). Common practical questions – and answers – at the British Association for Psychopharmacology child and adolescent psychopharmacology course. *Journal of Psychopharmacology*, 37(2), 119–34.
>
> Howes, O. D., Rogdaki, M., Findon, J. L., et al. (2018). Autism spectrum disorder: Consensus guidelines on assessment, treatment and research from the British Association for Psychopharmacology. *Journal of Psychopharmacology*, 32(1), 3–29.

References

Aishworiya, R., Valica, T., Hagerman, R., & Restrepo, B. (2022). An update on psychopharmacological treatment of autism spectrum disorder. *Neurotherapeutics*, **19**(1), 248–62.

Bai, D., Yip, B. H. K., Windham, G. C., et al. (2019). Association of genetic and environmental factors with autism in a 5-country cohort. *JAMA Psychiatry*, **76**(10), 1035–43.

Barrett, M., & Brugha, T. (2020). Autism spectrum disorder. In S Bhaumik, and R Alexander (eds.). *Oxford Textbook of the Psychiatry of Intellectual Disability*, Oxford University Press, 61–74.

Baxter, A. J., Brugha, T. S., Erskine, H. E., et al. (2015). The epidemiology and global burden of autism spectrum disorders. *Psychological Medicine*, **45**(3), 601–13.

Beqiraj, L., Denne, L. D., Hastings, R. P., & Paris, A. (2022). Positive behavioural support for children and young people with developmental disabilities in special education settings: A systematic review. *Journal of Applied Research in Intellectual Disabilities*, **35**(3), 719–35.

Bhaumik, S., Tromans, S., Gumber, R., & Gangavati, S. (2020). Clinical assessment including bedside diagnosis. In S. Bhaumik & R. Alexander (Eds.), *Oxford Textbook of the Psychiatry of Intellectual Disability*. Oxford University Press, 7–22.

Blanchard, A., Chihuri, S., DiGuiseppi, C. G., & Li, G. (2021). Risk of self-harm in children and adults with autism spectrum disorder: A systematic review and meta-analysis. *JAMA Network Open*, **4**(10), e2130272.

Brignell, A., Marraffa, C., Williams, K., & May, T. (2022). Memantine for autism spectrum disorder. *Cochrane Database of Systematic Reviews*, (8).

British National Formulary. (2023). Memantine hydrochloride. https://bnf.nice.org.uk/drugs/memantine-hydrochloride/#indications-and-dose.

Brugha, T. (2018). Approaches to treatment and care. In T. Brugha (Ed.), *The Psychiatry of Adult Autism and Asperger Syndrome*. Oxford University Press, pp. 183–93.

Brugha, T., Tyrer, F., Leaver, A., et al. (2020). Testing adults by questionnaire for social and communication disorders, including autism spectrum disorders, in an adult mental health service population. *International Journal of Methods in Psychiatric Research*, e1814.

Brugha, T. S. (2018). *The Psychiatry of Adult Autism and Asperger Syndrome: A Practical guide*. Oxford University Press.

Brugha, T. S., Spiers, N., Bankart, J., et al. (2016). Epidemiology of autism in adults across age groups and ability levels. *The British Journal of Psychiatry*, **209**(6), 498–503.

Croen, L. A., Zerbo, O., Qian, Y., et al. (2015). The health status of adults on the autism spectrum. *Autism*, **19**(7), 814–23.

Crompton, C. J., Ropar, D., Evans-Williams, C. V., Flynn, E. G., & Fletcher-Watson, S. (2020). Autistic peer-to-peer information transfer is highly effective. *Autism*, **24**(7), 1704–12.

Doyle, C. A., & McDougle, C. J. (2022). Pharmacologic treatments for the behavioral symptoms associated with autism spectrum disorders across the lifespan. *Dialogues in Clinical Neuroscience*, **14**(3), 263–79. https://doi.org/10.31887/DCNS.2012.14.3/cdoyle.

Dunn, K., Rydzewska, E., Macintyre, C., Rintoul, J., & Cooper, S. (2019). The prevalence and general health status of people with intellectual disabilities and autism co-occurring together: A total population study. *Journal of Intellectual Disability Research*, **63**(4), 277–85.

Frith, U., & Happé, F. (1994). Autism: Beyond 'theory of mind'. *Cognition*, **50**(1–3), 115–32.

Gates, J. A., Kang, E., & Lerner, M. D. (2017). Efficacy of group social skills interventions for youth with autism spectrum disorder: A systematic review and meta-analysis. *Clinical Psychology Review*, **52**, 164–81.

Giummarra, M. J., Randjelovic, I., & O'Brien, L. (2022). Interventions for social and community participation for adults with intellectual disability, psychosocial disability or on the autism spectrum: An umbrella systematic review. *Frontiers in Rehabilitation Sciences*, 3, 935473.

Hassiotis, A., Poppe, M., Strydom, A., et al. (2018). Clinical outcomes of staff training in positive behaviour support to reduce challenging behaviour in adults with intellectual disability: Cluster randomised controlled trial. *The British Journal of Psychiatry*, **212**(3), 161–8.

Health Education England (2017). The key messages about Positive Behaviour Support www.hee.nhs.uk/sites/default/files/docu ments/The%20key%20messages%20about% 20Positive%20Behaviour%20Support_0.pdf.

Hirsch, L. E., & Pringsheim, T. (2016). Aripiprazole for autism spectrum disorders (ASD). *Cochrane Database of Systematic Reviews*, (6).

Hodges, H., Fealko, C., & Soares, N. (2020). Autism spectrum disorder: Definition, epidemiology, causes, and clinical evaluation. *Translational Pediatrics*, **9** (Suppl 1), S55.

Hollocks, M. J., Lerh, J. W., Magiati, I., Meiser-Stedman, R., & Brugha, T. S. (2019). Anxiety and depression in adults with autism spectrum disorder: A systematic review and meta-analysis. *Psychological Medicine*, **49**(4), 559–72.

Jesner, O. S., Aref-Adib, M., & Coren, E. (2007). Risperidone for autism spectrum disorder. *Cochrane Database of Systematic Reviews*, (1).

Lai, M., Anagnostou, E., Wiznitzer, M., Allison, C., & Baron-Cohen, S. (2020). Evidence-based support for autistic people across the lifespan: Maximising potential, minimising barriers, and optimising the person–environment fit. *The Lancet Neurology*, **19**(5), 434—51.

Lai, M., Kassee, C., Besney, R., et al. (2019). Prevalence of co-occurring mental health diagnoses in the autism population: a systematic review and meta-analysis. *The Lancet Psychiatry*, **6**(10), 819–29.

Leaf, J. B., Cihon, J. H., Leaf, R., et al. (2022). Concerns about ABA-based intervention: An evaluation and recommendations. *Journal of Autism and Developmental Disorders*, **52**(6), 2838–53.

Loomes, R., Hull, L., & Mandy, W. P. L. (2017). What is the male-to-female ratio in autism spectrum disorder? A systematic review and meta-analysis. *Journal of the American Academy of Child and Adolescent Psychiatry*, **56**(6), 466–74.

Modabbernia, A., Velthorst, E., & Reichenberg, A. (2017). Environmental risk factors for autism: An evidence-based review of systematic reviews and meta-analyses. *Molecular Autism*, **8**(1), 1–16.

National Institute for Health and Care Excellence (2012). Autism spectrum disorder in adults: Diagnosis and management (CG142). www.nice.org.uk/guidance/cg142.

National Institute for Health and Care Excellence (2021). Autism spectrum disorder in under 19s: Support and management Clinical guideline [CG170]. https://www .nice.org.uk/guidance/cg170.

NHS England (2020). Stopping Over-Medication of People with a Learning Disability, Autism or Both. www.england .nhs.uk/wp-content/uploads/2017/07/stomp-gp-prescribing-v17.pdf.

NHS England (2023). Stopping over medication of people with a learning disability, autism or both (STOMP). https:// www.england.nhs.uk/learning-disabilities/ improving-health/stomp/.

Pan, P., Bölte, S., Kaur, P., Jamil, S., & Jonsson, U. (2021). Neurological disorders in autism: A systematic review and meta-analysis. *Autism*, **25**(3), 812–30.

Posey, D. J., Kem, D. L., Swiezy, N. B., et al. (2004). A pilot study of D-cycloserine in subjects with autistic disorder. *American Journal of Psychiatry*, **161**(11), 2115–17.

Posserud, M., Skretting Solberg, B., Engeland, A., Haavik, J., & Klungsøyr, K. (2021). Male to female ratios in autism spectrum disorders by age, intellectual disability and attention-deficit/hyperactivity disorder. *Acta Psychiatrica Scandinavica*, **144**(6), 635–46.

Potter, L. A., Scholze, D. A., Biag, H. M. B., et al. (2019). A randomized controlled trial of sertraline in young children with autism spectrum disorder. *Frontiers in Psychiatry*, **10**, 810.

Reddihough, D. S., Marraffa, C., Mouti, A., et al. (2019). Effect of fluoxetine on obsessive-compulsive behaviors in children and adolescents with autism spectrum disorders: A randomized clinical trial. *JAMA*, 322(16), 1561–9.

Royal College of Psychiatrists. (2021). Stopping the overmedication of people with intellectual disability, autism or both (STOMP) and supporting treatment and appropriate medication in paediatrics (STAMP): Position Statement. www.rcpsych.ac.uk/docs/default-source/improving-care/better-mh-policy/position-statements/position-statement-ps0521-stomp-stamp.pdf?sfvrsn=684d09b3_6

Shankar, R., Wilcock, M., Oak, K., McGowan, P., & Sheehan, R. (2019). Stopping, rationalising or optimising antipsychotic drug treatment in people with intellectual disability and/or autism. *Drug and Therapeutics Bulletin*, 57(1), 10–13.

Tromans, S., & Brugha, T. (2022). Autism epidemiology: Distinguishing between identification and prevalence. *Progress in Neurology and Psychiatry*, 26(1), 4–6.

Tromans, S., Chester, V., Gemegah, E., et al. (2020). Autism identification across ethnic groups: a narrative review. *Advances in Autism*, 7(3), 41–255. https://doi.org/10.1108/AIA-03-2020-0017.

Tromans, S., Chester, V., Kapugama, C., et al. (2019). The PAAFID project: Exploring the perspectives of autism in adult females among intellectual disability healthcare professionals. *Advances in Autism*, 5(3), 157–70.

Tromans, S., Chester, V., Kiani, R., Alexander, R., & Brugha, T. (2018). The prevalence of autism spectrum disorders in adult psychiatric inpatients: A systematic review. *Clinical Practice and Epidemiology in Mental Health: CP & EMH*, 14, 177.

Tromans, S., Stewart, Z., & Brugha, T. (2023). Autism: Social care, reasonable adjustments and the personal passport. *BJPsych Advances*, 29(5), 354–357.

Walton, K. M., & Ingersoll, B. R. (2013). Improving social skills in adolescents and adults with autism and severe to profound intellectual disability: A review of the literature. *Journal of Autism and Developmental Disorders*, 43, 594–615.

Wei, H., Zhu, Y., Wang, T., et al. (2021). Genetic risk factors for autism-spectrum disorders: A systematic review based on systematic reviews and meta-analysis. *Journal of Neural Transmission*, 128, 717–34.

Weld-Blundell, I., Shields, M., Devine, A., et al. (2021). Vocational interventions to improve employment participation of people with psychosocial disability, autism and/or intellectual disability: A systematic review. *International Journal of Environmental Research and Public Health*, 18(22), 12083.

Whittenburg, H. N., Schall, C. M., Wehman, P., McDonough, J., & DuBois, T. (2020). Helping high school-aged military dependents with autism gain employment through project SEARCH ASD supports. *Military Medicine*, 185(Supplement_1), 663–8.

Williams, K., Brignell, A., Randall, M., Silove, N., & Hazell, P. (2013). Selective serotonin reuptake inhibitors (SSRIs) for autism spectrum disorders (ASD). *Cochrane Database of Systematic Reviews*, (8).

World Health Organization (2018). *ICD-11 for Mortality and Morbidity Statistics*. Geneva: World Health Organization.

Zafeiriou, D. I., Ververi, A., Dafoulis, V., Kalyva, E., & Vargiami, E. (2013). Autism spectrum disorders: The quest for genetic syndromes. *American Journal of Medical Genetics Part B: Neuropsychiatric Genetics*, 162(4), 327–66.

Chapter 16

Sleep Disorders

Rebecca Dodds and Laura Korb

Introduction

Sleep is essential for life and health, having a vital role in brain function, metabolism, appetite regulation, and the functioning of the immune, hormonal, and cardiovascular systems (Medic et al., 2017). People with intellectual disability, with or without autism, experience sleep disorders at a higher rate than the general population (Esbensen et al., 2016).

What Are Sleep Disorders?

The *International Classification of Sleep Disorders, Third Edition* has classified sleep disorders into 7 categories (American Academy of Sleep Medicine 2014):

- Insomnias
- Sleep-Related Breathing Disorders
- Central Disorders of Hypersomnolence
- Circadian Rhythm Sleep-Wake Disorders
- Parasomnias
- Sleep-Related Movement Disorders
- Other sleep disorders

In this chapter we will focus on insomnia and its management. The International Statistical Classification of Diseases and Related Health Problems 11 (ICD-11) defines insomnia as the complaint of persistent difficulty with sleep initiation, duration, consolidation, or quality that occurs despite adequate opportunity and circumstances for sleep, and results in some form of daytime impairment (World Health Organization 2022). There must be daytime impairment and daytime symptoms including fatigue, depressed mood or irritability, general malaise, and cognitive impairment (British National Formulary 2021).

How Common Are Sleep Disorders in People with Intellectual Disability?

Sleep disorders are common in people with intellectual disability, with an estimated prevalence of significant sleep problems of 9.2%, and any sleep problems up to 34% (range 6–74%) (Shanahan et al., 2022). The higher rates of sleep difficulties encountered in the intellectual disability population may reflect higher rates of structural and functional abnormalities of the brain and associated factors such as severe locomotor disability, blindness, and active epilepsy, which are independent predictors of sleep disturbances

(Lindblom et al., 2001). Sleep disorders are commonly found in neurodevelopmental conditions and genetic syndromes associated with intellectual disability (Korb et al., 2021). There is an increased likelihood of people with intellectual disability having physical comorbidities, which in turn increase sleep problems (Esbensen et al., 2016). Sleep problems can be a risk factor for psychiatric illness in this population, as well as exacerbating current mental health issues (Korb et al., 2021).

How Are Sleep Disorders Different in People with Intellectual Disability?

Sleep disorders can be multifactorial and are often considered to be secondary rather than primary diagnoses (Korb et al., 2021). People with intellectual disability, with or without autism, can exhibit sleep difficulties due to circadian rhythm dysfunction and abnormal endogenous melatonin levels (Esbensen et al., 2016). Challenging behaviour could either be a cause or a result of sleep problems in this group (Van den Broek et al., 2022). Poor sleep can add to carer stress and family crises, which can increase service requirements (Wiggs 2001).

The causes of insomnia may be multifactorial; Table 16.1 provides a range of factors taken from several sources (Korb et al., 2021; Medic et al., 2017; National Institute for Health and Care Excellence 2022).

Table 16.1 Causes of sleep difficulties

Cause	Explanation	Examples
Physiological	Relating to bodily functions	Older age, hormonal changes including menarche, menopause, and pregnancy
Circadian	Lack of exposure to natural daylight	Lack of blackout blinds, less daytime structured activities, little exercise, heavy use of screens
Homeostatic	Not waking at the same time	Daycentre holidays, changing routines
Psychiatric	Relating to mental illness	Anxiety, delirium, dementia, affective or psychotic disorders
Stress	Adverse or demanding circumstances	Grief, change of room or placement
Medical symptoms	Often relating to pathology	Pruritis, pain, nocturia, or cough
Medical conditions	Relating to physical health diagnoses	Epilepsy, cardiac disease, respiratory disease, thyroid disorders, gastro-oesophageal reflux disease. Or neurogenerative diseases
Iatrogenic	Relating to treatments	Acetylcholinesterase inhibitors, dopamine agonists, selective serotonin reuptake inhibitors, ibuprofen, beta blockers, or paradoxical reaction to benzodiazepines
Lifestyle	Habits formed	Caffeine, alcohol, or illicit drugs
Environmental	Living conditions	Noise, temperature, regular carer checks, or other residents

Sleep disorders have short- and long-term consequences that can present differently in people with intellectual disability in comparison to the general adult population. Sleep disorders can lead to poor concentration and memory, impaired learning and communication skills, and behavioural problems, including irritability, stereotypies, aggression, and self-injurious behaviour (Van den Broek et al., 2022). In the long term, sleep disorders can contribute to hypertension, dyslipidaemia, cardiovascular disease, weight-related issues, metabolic syndrome, type 2 diabetes, and colorectal cancer.

Poor sleep patterns are associated with certain genetic syndromes, including Angelman syndrome, Williams syndrome, Fragile X syndrome, Prader–Willi syndrome, Sanfilippo syndrome, tuberous sclerosis, and Jacobsen syndrome (Surtees et al., 2018). Individuals with Smith–Magenis syndrome often show inverted melatonin cycles (Korb et al., 2021). Sleep problems are present for up to 80% of children with Rett syndrome (Gilbertson et al., 2021). Increased autistic symptomology predicts an increased likelihood of problems with sleep (Surtees et al., 2018).

Attention Deficit Hyperactivity Disorder (ADHD) is commonly associated with sleep disorders, including obstructive sleep apnoea (OSA), periodic limb movement disorder, restless legs syndrome, and circadian-rhythm sleep disorders (Hvolby, 2015). These can lead to poor quality of sleep and consequent daytime behavioural manifestations (Wiggs, 2001).

Epilepsy is common in people with intellectual disability and is associated with seizure-related sleep disruption. In addition, antiepileptic medications may impact sleep. Poor sleep can consequently worsen epilepsy control (Jain & Kothare 2015).

Due to the increased rates of obesity in people with intellectual disability, OSA occurs more commonly than in the general population (Lindblom et al., 2001). More than 50% of children with Down syndrome have sleep-related breathing disorders (Gilbertson et al., 2021). Individuals with Down syndrome have an increased prevalence of OSA due to the characteristic features of the condition, including obesity, short neck, hypotonia, and structural abnormalities of the upper respiratory tract (narrow airways, large adenoid and tonsils, large tongue, and small jaw) (Wiggs, 2001). Obstructive sleep apnoea occurs with an increased frequency in conditions such as Rubinstein–Taybi syndrome, Prader–Willi syndrome, Angelman syndrome, and Fragile X syndrome.

Identification of Sleep Disorders

In individuals with intellectual disability, communication difficulties can prevent the identification of sleep disorders and the likelihood of the individual or their family seeking help, therefore screening for sleep disorders is important (Van den Broek et al., 2022). Due to diagnostic overshadowing, carers or family members may accept sleep disturbance as part of the person with intellectual disability's usual presentation. Sleep-related breathing disorders, such as OSA, have an especially high prevalence in this group, which is often not reflected in carer reports.

For a general approach to the diagnosis and management, refer to Figure 16.1.

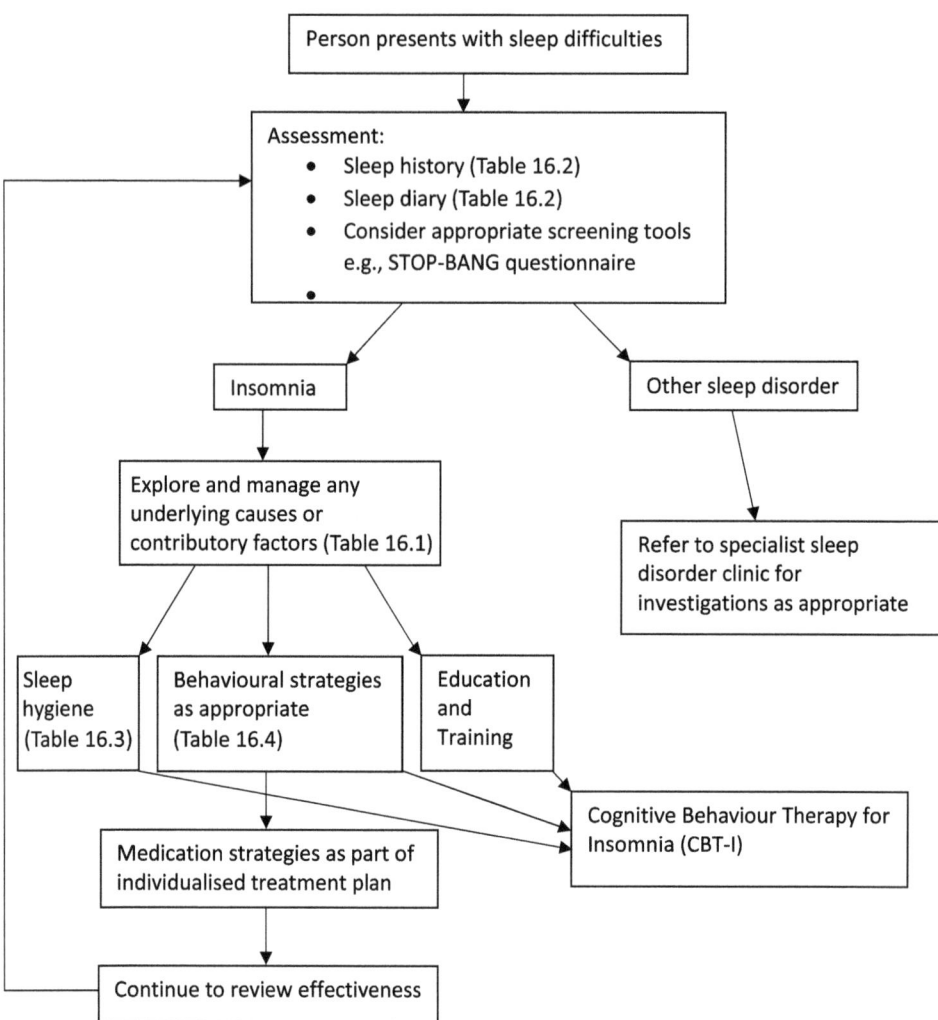

Figure 16.1 Algorithm: Factors to consider when a person with intellectual disability presents with sleep difficulties

Sleep History

It is important to take a thorough sleep history (Table 16.2) to diagnose a sleep disorder and to identify targets for treatment (Van den Broek et al., 2022).

Although many sleep questionnaires are not designed for individuals with intellectual disability and demonstrate poor reliability (Esbensen et al., 2016), it is often useful to use validated screening tools to identify sleep problems. Questionnaires such as the Insomnia Severity Index and the Karolinska Sleepiness Scale can give details on specific aspects of sleep and can be used to assess severity and treatment response (Korb et al., 2021). The STOP-BANG questionnaire is another simple and clinically useful screening tool to determine an individual's

Table 16.2 Taking a sleep history

- Onset, duration, and nature of the problem.
For example: difficulty falling asleep (initial insomnia), difficulty staying asleep (broken sleep), waking too early (late insomnia), daytime hypersomnolence, and unusual behaviours seen only in and around the sleep period (parasomnias)
- Information on sleep hygiene and routine
- Effect of insomnia on person and caregiver, particularly the daytime impact
- Past sleep difficulties and previous treatments
- Psychiatric and medical diagnosis
- Current medication regime
- Family history of sleep problems
- Illicit drug and alcohol misuse

risk for OSA. This information can be used to consider management options, including onward referral to respiratory physicians (Korb et al., 2021).

It is useful to complete a sleep diary as part of the assessment (Figure 16.2). This can be completed by the individual with intellectual disability, with support as required, or by carers.

Further Investigations

Objective investigations, such as actigraphy, ambulatory circadian monitoring, or polysomnography, can provide additional information but are not deemed necessary to diagnose insomnia (Van den Broek et al., 2022). They can be considered where insomnia is poorly responsive to conventional treatments or where there are symptoms (e.g., physical symptoms) which indicate sleep disturbances other than insomnias (see Clinical Knowledge Summary (CKS) by National Institute for Health and Care Excellence (NICE) 2022).

If the history is unreliable or monitoring sleep–wake timing is difficult, then actigraphy performed in the home setting is generally tolerated by individuals with intellectual disability (Esbensen et al., 2016). This can also be used to study treatment effects. It may not be possible or accessible in some people with intellectual disability, for instance where there is intolerance to wearing the device (Esbensen et al., 2016).

Polysomnography measures brain, muscle, and heart activity via electroencephalography, oculography, myography, cardiography, and pulse oximetry. This investigation can be successfully used to assess sleep in individuals with intellectual disability; however, this resource is not always available (Esbensen et al., 2016). There can be problems administering polysomnography to individuals with intellectual disability, such as in individuals with sensory sensitivity. The test is undertaken in a hospital environment and therefore presents the additional challenge of a new environment for sleep, which could interfere with the results (Esbensen et al., 2016). If indicated, it is possible to support the implementation of polysomnography through desensitisation techniques, social stories, and preparatory visits (Esbensen et al., 2016).

Case study 16.1 illustrates the presentation of insomnia in an individual with severe learning disability.

SLEEP DIARY

✓ – Went to sleep
x – Woke up
x✓ – Woke up then went back to sleep

TIME	MONDAY	TUESDAY	WEDNESDAY	THURSDAY	FRIDAY	SATURDAY	SUNDAY
Midnight							
1am							
2am							
3am							
4am							
5am							
6am							
7am							
8am							
9am							
10am							
11am							
Midday							
1pm							
2pm							
3pm							
4pm							
5pm							
6pm							
7pm							
8pm							
9pm							
10pm							
11pm							

Rating of sleep quality each night (from 1 to 5) where 1 = very poor

Figure 16.2 Information to be collected in a sleep diary (for two weeks)
It can be helpful to note time taken to fall asleep, times of meals, alcohol and caffeine, and significant daytime events such as exercise or stress.

Case Study 16.1

Marcus, a 20-year-old man with a severe intellectual disability, Down syndrome, autism, and ADHD, was referred to local intellectual disability services at age 19 by his college. His behaviour was becoming increasingly difficult to manage, with poor engagement and episodes of aggression directed at staff. The college highlighted environmental triggers, including the recent death of a grandparent and the breakdown of his parents' relationship.

Marcus was not able to join his first appointment in the clinic as he had not slept the night before the appointment. A detailed collateral was obtained from his mother. His mother described him as a 'happy sociable man with a bold personality'. He had experienced lifelong symptoms of ADHD, poor sleep, and oppositional behaviours. As a child he was prescribed medication, including a stimulant for ADHD, risperidone for anxiety in the context of autism, and melatonin for sleep regulation. Unfortunately, he experienced side effects on all these medications.

Marcus did not sleep at night, but instead fell asleep in the morning at around 6am, with broken sleep until the afternoon. He had previously been diagnosed with OSA, but he would not tolerate the CPAP machine. His mother's view was that if his sleep pattern could improve then his quality of life would improve, and his behaviour would be easier to manage during the day.

A discussion was had about optimising his environment for sleep, including limiting evening screen time, getting blackout blinds, and ensuring exposure to light during the day. Unfortunately, these were a challenge to implement, as Marcus and his mother were temporarily living in a cramped house with her extended family.

The cause of his sleep disorder was multifactorial: a poor environment for good quality sleep; a genetic disorder associated with sleep disordered breathing; the psychological sequelae of a recent bereavement; a transition to college; and the comorbid diagnoses of autism and ADHD, both neurodevelopmental disorders associated with sleep disorders.

The Frith Treatment Guideline for People with Intellectual Disability

Management

The management of sleep disorders in people with intellectual disability is complex given the heterogeneity of underlying causes. If sleep investigations are not tolerated, a pragmatic trial of treatment may be necessary (Korb et al., 2021). Initial management should be targeted to identify and address modifiable environmental, psychiatric, or physical health conditions. It is important to consider medication rationalisation, optimal control of epilepsy, and regular health checks to reduce other contributing factors (Shanahan et al., 2019).

Non-Medication Approaches

Non-medication management of sleep difficulties should always be considered first; however, if this is insufficient then the addition of medication could be considered. Although the interventions for the general population may not always be appropriate for individuals with intellectual disability, in general people with intellectual disability benefit from following these approaches (Shanahan et al., 2019).

It is important to ensure a comfortable sleeping environment and encourage healthy sleep habits (Wiggs, 2001). There is evidence that supports the use of sleep hygiene techniques (Table 16.3) (Hvolby, 2015) and behavioural strategies (Table 16.4) (Wiggs, 2001; Shanahan et al., 2019) being effective and tolerated in individuals with intellectual disability (Richdale et al., 2014).

Behavioural techniques should be implemented gradually, and the choice of technique must be guided by individual preference (Wiggs, 2001). Cognitive behaviour therapy for

Table 16.3 Sleep hygiene

Encourage daily exercise, except several hours prior to bedtime

Avoid daytime napping

Avoid large meals, large volumes of fluid, caffeine, tobacco, nicotine, and alcohol before bedtime

Eliminate factors that impede sleep (e.g., TV, games consoles or other devices with a screen before bed)

Use the bedroom just for sleep and intercourse

Set and maintain a regular routine of sleeping and waking at the same time every day and have a calm bedtime routine

Ensure sleeping environment is comfortable, quiet, dark, and at the right temperature

Support withdrawal from any illicit substances

Table 16.4 Behavioural strategies

Behavioural extinction and stimulus control: increasing the association between bed and sleep by reducing reinforcers that promote wakefulness in the sleeping environment and leaving the bedroom after 15 minutes if unable to sleep until feeling sleepy.

Chronotherapy for sleep phase disorders: progressive incremental adjustment of bedtime to reset the body clock.

Sleep restriction therapy: limiting the amount of time spent in bed to match the ability to fill this mostly with sleep.

Change in daily routine: activities at a more suitable time during the day, increasing the number or duration of daytime activities and ensuring more physical activities.

insomnia (CBT-I) is advised before medication in chronic insomnia (National Institute for Health and Care Excellence, 2022). CBT-I includes psychoeducation, behavioural strategies, cognitive therapy, and relaxation training (National Institute for Health and Care Excellence, 2022). Modified CBT-I can be useful for people with intellectual disability (Korb et al., 2021). Educational training for caregivers supporting adults with intellectual disability, both individualised instruction and educational booklets, has led to sleep improvement and reduced napping (Esbensen et al., 2016).

The Evidence Base for Treatments

People with Intellectual Disability: Medication Treatments

There is a limited evidence base around medication treatment of sleep for people with intellectual disability. A randomised double-blind placebo-controlled trial with 51 individuals with intellectual disability found that melatonin improved overall sleep by decreasing sleep latency, advancing sleep onset, and increasing total time of sleep (Braam et al., 2009).

There was a systematic review in 2019 where the majority of the 9 studies included were case series and case studies (Shanahan et al., 2019). Another review from 2016 included a randomised placebo-controlled trial for melatonin in Angelman syndrome; one in children with autism spectrum disorder, Fragile X syndrome, or autism spectrum disorder and Fragile X syndrome; and two others in children with autism spectrum disorder (Esbensen et al., 2016). However, the specificity of these studies affects their applicability for all individuals with intellectual disability.

People with Intellectual Disability: Non-Medication Treatments

There are very few studies of psycho-social treatments for sleep in intellectual disability. There was a systematic review of behavioural strategies (Esbensen et al., 2016). This included a few smaller studies in children with autism spectrum disorder, with one individual controlled trial; however, these findings would not be applicable to all people with intellectual disability. It also included case studies of children with intellectual disability.

When looking at the evidence base for sleep hygiene, one literature review (Wiggs, 2001) was primarily considered; however, this contained considerably older studies. There was also one systematic review, but this pertained to the application of sleep hygiene in just ADHD, and therefore is less applicable to all individuals with intellectual disability (Hvolby, 2015).

In terms of modified cognitive behavioural therapy-insomnia (CBT-I), there was one systematic review considered (Richdale et al., 2014) which included a positive randomised placebo-controlled trial of 160 children with autism, with melatonin MR used singly and combined with CBT-I. However, again this study will not be applicable to all individuals with intellectual disability.

One literature review included comment on educational training for caregivers supporting adults with intellectual disability, both individualised instruction and educational booklets; however, the evidence base was largely from multiple case studies.

Medication Strategies

The prescription of medication to aid sleep should be made as a shared decision with the service user or their support network, weighing the risks and benefits to the individual with intellectual disability. The medications used do not usually treat underlying causes of insomnia but are often used as a temporary adjunct, for crises or in refractory cases (see Clinical Knowledge Summary (CKS) by National Institute for Health and Care Excellence 2022).

Melatonin

This naturally occurring hormone has been successfully used in the management of sleep—wake cycle disturbances in people with intellectual disability, autism spectrum disorder, and visual impairment (Braam et al., 2009). Melatonin is used for insomnia in patients with intellectual disability, if initiated under specialist supervision. However, in the United Kingdom it is not licenced for this group and is only licenced for a maximum of 13 weeks for adults over 55 years with insomnia (Shanahan et al., 2019). The long-terms effects and safety of melatonin are still unknown (Braam et al., 2009).

For the unlicenced management of insomnia in patients with intellectual disability and behaviour that challenges, where sleep hygiene measures have been insufficient, the British

National Formulary advises prescribing oral modified-release tablets, starting 2 mg once daily and increased if necessary to 4–6 mg once daily, and maximum 10 mg per day. The advice is for the dose to be taken 30–60 minutes before bedtime (British National Formulary, 2021). It has a favourable side-effect profile (Korb et al., 2021). Common side effects are arthralgia, headaches, increased risk of infection, and pain (British National Formulary, 2021). It is not generally considered to produce tolerance, rebound insomnia, or dependency – problems often associated with other sedative hypnotics (National Institute for Health and Care Excellence, 2022). Immediate release melatonin if taken with food may have increased bioavailability and may impair blood glucose control (British National Formulary, 2021).

There are cautions with melatonin use in renal impairment and autoimmune disease and it is recommended to avoid in pregnancy, breastfeeding, and hepatic impairment (British National Formulary, 2021). There are increased risks, including falls, if used in the elderly, and there is no evidence found for the use of melatonin in dementia (National Institute for Health and Care Excellence, 2022). It is always important to be aware of drug interactions, particularly with other substances which have a central nervous system depressant effect, such as alcohol.

Hypnotics

A medication used to induce sleep is described as a 'hypnotic'. Hypnotics licenced to be used in insomnia in the United Kingdom include benzodiazepines (diazepam, lorazepam, nitrazepam, loprazolam, lormetazepam, and temazepam) and z-drugs (zopiclone, zolpidem, and zaleplon) (National Institute for Health and Care Excellence, 2004). Prescription of a hypnotic should only be considered in severe cases of insomnia when non-pharmacological alternatives have failed. If prescribed, this must be at the lowest effective dose for the shortest duration possible (maximum of 4 weeks). Ideally, use should be 'as required' rather than nightly due to risks of tolerance, dependency, withdrawal symptoms, and rebound insomnia. The individual must be made aware of the risks of taking the medication, including interactions with other sedative agents, including alcohol (British National Formulary, 2021).

Other Medication with Sedative Effects

In the United Kingdom, several antihistamines such as promethazine have been used to manage insomnia, either by prescription or over the counter; however, these are not recommended for treatment (British Medical Journal Best Practice, 2002). These medications have not demonstrated lasting benefits and have side effects such as their long half-life leading to morning 'hangover' sleepiness.

Antidepressants

If insomnia is secondary to a diagnosis of moderate to severe depression or anxiety, for which antidepressants are recommended, then these should be the medication of choice (Wilson et al., 2019). Insomnia is a core feature of depression and therefore treatment of depression will treat the sleep disruption. Mirtazapine or clomipramine prescribed at night for depression may also benefit sleep (National Institute for Health and Care Excellence, 2004).

Antipsychotics

Antipsychotics often cause sedation as a side effect but are not licenced for treatment of any specific sleep disorder. If individuals with intellectual disability require an antipsychotic for another indication and have difficulty with falling asleep at night or oversedation during the day, then the daily dose can be adjusted, taking into consideration the person's sleep pattern, on a case-by-case basis (Wilson et al., 2019).

Other Sleep Disorders

Other sleep disorders should always be considered for people with intellectual disability where presentation may be complex. If suspected, referral should be made to a sleep disorder centre for consideration of sleep neurology/specialist psychiatry assessment (Korb et al., 2021).

It is important to consider sleep disorders such as the Sleep-Related Movement Disorders (particularly restless leg syndrome), Central Disorders of Hypersomnolence (particularly narcolepsy), Parasomnias (particularly sleepwalking and sleep terrors) and Other Sleep Disorders (particularly sleep-related epilepsy). These should be differentiated from night-time epilepsy, where referral for 24-hour electroencephalograph (EEG) recording is indicated. Circadian Rhythm Sleep-Wake Disorders are particularly relevant as they have been found to be more common in autism spectrum disorder and visual impairment (Carr et al., 2007).

As mentioned, sleep-related breathing disorders are particularly important to consider in the intellectual disability population. Obstructive sleep apnoea may present with daytime sleepiness and a combination of loud frequent snoring with short periods of apnoea (a temporary cessation of breathing), identified by a third party. The gold standard for diagnosis is polysomnography in a sleep clinic. This is often impractical and difficult to obtain for many people with intellectual disability; however, referral to a Respiratory Clinic for investigation and advice is helpful (Korb et al., 2021). Management can include weight loss, continuous positive airway pressure, and, where appropriate, surgical correction of structural abnormalities.

Case study 16.2 is a continuation of Case Study 16.1, where focus was on clinical presentation of the sleep problem. In Case Study 16.2, management of this sleep problem is explored.

Case Study 16.2: Management

Marcus has a known diagnosis of sleep apnoea, which is not uncommon in those with Down syndrome; however, he was unable to tolerate specific interventions for this condition. Sleep hygiene measures, including adapting his environment, were unfortunately not practical in his situation. The recommendation was made for modified cognitive behavioural therapy for insomnia, including setting a fixed rising time and natural light exposure, relaxation before bed, and recommendation for engagement with regular exercise. These interventions were a challenge to implement for Marcus's family. We therefore considered the medication options. Melatonin had been helpful when he was a child, but he did not tolerate this medication and his mother did not feel that it was safe to try again.

Marcus was referred to the behavioural support specialist team with the aim of providing more support with behavioural strategies. His mother had started him on an over-the-counter antihistamine, so the decision was made to support her by prescribing 'as required' promethazine in the short-term.

Long-Term Management of Sleep Difficulties

It is important not to issue further prescriptions for hypnotics without review, and over-the-counter treatments for insomnia are not recommended (National Institute for Health and Care Excellence, 2022). A follow-up appointment should be made within four weeks of starting a hypnotic. If there is doubt about the diagnosis or treatment has failed, it may be helpful to refer to a specialist centre (National Institute for Health and Care Excellence, 2022).

Melatonin requires regular review with documentation of any benefits and side effects. It is recommended initially to start treatment for three weeks and then review the response (National Institute for Health and Care Excellence, 2022). If there is continued efficacy, such as improved quality or life and the benefits outweigh any side effects, then this should be clearly documented and melatonin can be continued. There should be continued review of the medication, and ongoing attempts to try to taper and stop or find the minimum effective dose.

Withdrawal of Medications

Review and withdrawal of hypnotics, especially benzodiazepines, is important and requires time for discussion with the individual and/or their support network (National Institute for Health and Care Excellence, 2022). They should be tapered and stopped gradually. Many individuals develop tolerance to the effects of hypnotics, with little long-term benefit if they continue. Individuals can also become physically and psychologically dependent, leading to withdrawal. The withdrawal symptoms can be prolonged, developing any time from a few hours up to three weeks after cessation. They can include anxiety, depression, nausea, and perceptual changes and rebound insomnia.

Case Study 16.3 illustrates the intertwining of various contributory factors in insomnia. This indicates the need for ongoing review of the management of insomnia even after a medication is started.

> **Case Study 16.3: Optimising Psycho-Social Interventions and Management of Comorbid Conditions**
>
> Marcus struggled with compliance with medication, including his medication for hypothyroidism. His living environment remained suboptimal, and his mother struggled with her own mental health. His college placement ended so he did not have regular daytime activities. Understandably, his sleep issues continued.
>
> A new carer started working with Marcus. She was experienced in managing behaviour seen as challenging in those with intellectual disability. As well as providing consistency, she informed his mother that his hyperactivity and inattention appeared to prevent him from engaging with daytime activities. He was started on a non-stimulant medication to target ADHD symptoms. On starting this medication, he was more engaged with activities, meaning he was more tired by the evening. His sleep pattern noticeably improved. This led to his mother making further applications for daytime opportunities, as she now felt he would be able to engage, resulting in a better routine.
>
> This case illustrates the complex aetiology of sleep disorders in those with intellectual disability, and the impact that management of sleep disorders can have on an individual's quality of life, and that of their support network.

The Frith Prescribing Guidelines Editors' Expert Group Consensus Statements

Statements of High Confidence

- There is high-quality evidence available for the general adult population. For people with intellectual disability the evidence base for diagnosis and treatment for sleep disorders has yet to be well established.
- There is high-quality evidence that poor sleep patterns are associated with genetic syndromes.
- There is good evidence that sleep-related breathing disorders are more prevalent for individuals with intellectual disability, with a particular association between OSA and Down syndrome.

Statements of Medium Confidence

- There is evidence for the use of sleep studies for people with intellectual disability.
- There is also evidence for the use of hypnotics if they are used according to licenced conditions.
- There is evidence that melatonin reduces sleep latency and night waking for individuals with intellectual disability. However, in the United Kingdom melatonin is not licenced for this group.

Statements of Low Confidence

- The overall quality of research, guidance, and evidence on the assessment and management of sleep disorders in adults with intellectual disability is low.
- Prevalence estimates vary widely as the criteria for insomnia in studies in people with intellectual disability is inconsistent (Van den Broek et al., 2022).
- Sleep disorders are thought to be linked to behavioural disturbances; however, whether this is cause, effect, or both is unclear.
- There is low-quality evidence for assessment tools, as well as for behavioural interventions, for this specific population.
- There is low-quality evidence on the long-term safety and efficacy of melatonin.

Resource Box

Easy Health: www.easyhealth.org.uk/resources/category/142-sleep

NSF Sleep Diary: www.thensf.org/wp-content/uploads/2021/02/NSF-Sleep-Diary-Rev-2-2021.pdf

STOP-Bang Questionnaire: www.sleepfoundation.org/sleep-apnea/stop-bang-score

Insomnia diagnosis and treatment, UK: https://cks.nice.org.uk/topics/insomnia/

Insomnia, Parasomnias and Circadian Rhythm Disorders treatment, UK: www.bap.org.uk/pdfs/BAP_Guidelines-Sleep.pdf

Insomnia diagnosis and treatment Europe: https://onlinelibrary.wiley.com/doi/epdf/10.1111/jsr.12594

Z-drugs for Insomnia, UK: www.nice.org.uk/guidance/ta77/resources/guidance-on-the-use-of-zaleplon-zolpidem-and-zopiclone-for-the-shortterm-management-of-insomnia-pdf-2294763557317

Medicines associated with dependence or withdrawal symptoms, UK: www.nice.org.uk/guidance/ng215/resources/medicines-associated-with-dependence-or-withdrawal-symptoms-safe-prescribing-and-withdrawal-management-for-adults-pdf-66143776880581

References

American Academy of Sleep Medicine (2014). International classification of sleep disorders, 3rd ed. Darien, IL. https://j2vjt3dnbra3ps71l1clb4q2-wpengine.netdna-ssl.com/wp-content/uploads/2019/05/ICSD3-TOC.pdf.

Braam, W., Smits, M. G., Didden, R., et al. (2009). Exogenous melatonin for sleep problems in individuals with intellectual disability: a meta-analysis. *Developmental Medicine & Child Neurology*, **51**(5), 340–9.

British Medical Journal Best Practice. (2002). *Insomnia*. https://bestpractice.bmj.com/topics/en-gb/227/pdf/227/Insomnia.pdf.

British National Formulary. (2021). BMJ Group and the Royal Pharmaceutical Society. Accessed via Medicines Complete, Royal Pharmaceutical Society 2022. https://bnf.nice.org.uk/.

Carr, R., Wasdell, M. B., Hamilton, D., et al. (2007). Long-term effectiveness outcome of melatonin therapy in children with treatment-resistant circadian rhythm sleep disorders. *Journal of Pineal Research*, **43**(4), 351–9.

Esbensen, A. J. & Schwichtenberg, A. J. (2016). Sleep in neurodevelopmental disorders. *International Review of Research in Developmental Disabilities*, **51**, 153–91. https://doi.org/10.1016/bs.irrdd.2016.07.005.

Gilbertson, M., Richardson, C., Eastwood, P., et al. (2021). Determinants of sleep problems in children with intellectual disability. *Journal of Sleep Research*, **30**(5), e13361.

Hvolby, A. (2015). Associations of sleep disturbance with ADHD: implications for treatment. *ADHD Attention Deficit and Hyperactivity Disorders*, **7**(1), 1–18.

Jain, S. V. & Kothare, S. V. (2015). Sleep and epilepsy. *Seminars in Pediatric Neurology*, **22**(2), 86–92. https://doi.org/10.1016/j.spen.2015.03.005.

Korb, L., O'Regan, D., Conley, J., et al. (2021). Sleep: The neglected life factor in adults with intellectual disabilities. *BJPsych Bulletin*, **47**(3), 139–45.

Lindblom, N., Heiskala, H., Kaski, M., et al. (2001). Neurological impairments and sleep-wake behaviour among the mentally retarded. *Journal of Sleep Research*, **10**(4), 309–18.

Medic, G., Wille, M. & Hemels, M. E. (2017). Short- and long-term health consequences of sleep disruption. *Nature and Science of Sleep*, **9**, 151.

National Institute for Health and Care Excellence (2004). Guidance on the use of zaleplon, zolpidem and zopiclone for the short-term management of insomnia. www.nice.org.uk/guidance/ta77/resources/guidance-on-the-use-of-zaleplon-zolpidem-and-zopiclone-for-the-shortterm-management-of-insomnia-pdf-2294763557317.

National Institute for Health and Care Excellence (2022). *Insomnia* (https://cks.nice.org.uk/topics/insomnia/ [cited 9.11.22])

National Institute for Health and Care Excellence (2022). Medicines associated with dependence or withdrawal symptoms: Safe prescribing and withdrawal management for adults. www.nice.org.uk/guidance/ng215/resources/medicines-associated-with-dependence-or-withdrawal-symptoms-safe-prescribing-and-withdrawal-management-for-adults-pdf-66143776880581.

Richdale, A. L. & Baker, E. K. (2014). Sleep in individuals with an intellectual or developmental disability: Recent research reports. *Current Developmental Disorders Reports*, **1**(2), 74–85.

Shanahan, P., Ahmad, S., Smith, K., Palod, S. & Fife-Schaw, C. (2022). The prevalence of sleep disorders in adults with learning disabilities: A systematic review. *British Journal of Learning Disabilities*, **53**(3), 344–67.

Shanahan, P. J., Palod, S., Smith, K. J., Fife-Schaw, C. & Mirza, N. (2019). Interventions for sleep difficulties in adults with an intellectual disability: A systematic review. *Journal of Intellectual Disability Research*, **63**(5), 372–85.

Surtees, A. D., Oliver, C., Jones, C. A., Evans, D. L. & Richards, C. (2018). *Sleep duration and sleep quality in people with and without intellectual disability: A meta-analysis.* Sleep Medicine Reviews, **40**, 135–50.

Wiggs, L. (2001). Sleep problems in children with developmental disorders. *Journal of the Royal Society of Medicine*, **94**(4), 177–9.

Wilson, S., Anderson, K., Baldwin, D., et al. (2019). British Association for Psychopharmacology consensus statement on evidence-based treatment of insomnia, parasomnias, and circadian rhythm disorders: An update. *Journal of Psychopharmacology*, **33**(8), 923–47.

World Health Organization (2022). International Classification of Diseases 11. https://icd.who.int.

Van den Broek, N., Festen, D., Tan, F., Overeem, S. & Pillen, S. (2022). What is in a name? Definitions of insomnia in people with intellectual disabilities. *Journal of Applied Research in Intellectual Disabilities*, **35**(2), 506–18.

Chapter 17

Epilepsy

Lance Watkins, Márie O'Dwyer, Reza Kiani, and Rohit Shankar

Introduction

What Is Epilepsy?

Epilepsy is a disease of the brain that is characterised by a predisposition to seizures. A seizure is the transient excessive or abnormal neuronal activity associated with a range of neurological symptoms that may be motor, sensory, or even emotional in quality. Epilepsy also has long-term neurological, psychological, and social impacts on a person, beyond the immediate direct effect of seizures. The criteria that define a clinical diagnosis of epilepsy by the International League Against Epilepsy (ILAE) are any of the following: two or more unprovoked seizures, more than 24 hours apart (unprovoked meaning no factors known to be associated with increased risk of seizures identified); one unprovoked seizure and a high probability of further seizures; identification of an epilepsy syndrome (Fisher et al. 2014).

How Common Is Epilepsy in People with Intellectual Disability?

Epilepsy is the number one comorbidity associated with intellectual disability. Identifying the prevalence rate has historically been challenging, owing to methodological challenges and discrete population samples. Overall, an estimated 1 in 5 people with intellectual disability have epilepsy; for context, this is more than 20 times higher than the general population prevalence. The prevalence rate increases with level of intellectual disability, with approximately 1 in 2 people with severe to profound intellectual disability having epilepsy. In addition, people with intellectual disability have a tendency towards greater complexity of seizure disorder, with 2 in 3 having treatment resistant epilepsy (having failed trials of two different antiseizure medications at adequate doses for an adequate duration). This complexity is associated with lower psychological functioning and increased rates of comorbid psychiatric illness, particularly anxiety disorders and depression.

There are higher levels of multi-morbidity and polypharmacy in people with intellectual disability and epilepsy (Sun et al., 2022, 2023). Associations with other psychotropic medication use is greater than for those with just epilepsy or intellectual disability without epilepsy. People with intellectual disability have five times higher rates of preventable emergency admissions. Those with intellectual disability and epilepsy account for 40% of these. Similarly, epilepsy is found comorbid in approximately 40% of all premature mortality in people with intellectual disability.

People with epilepsy and intellectual disability have higher rates of premature preventable deaths than people with intellectual disability or epilepsy alone. The standardised mortality ratio for people with epilepsy and intellectual disability is five times higher than for the general population. The Learning Disabilities Mortality Review Programme (LeDER) identified that people with epilepsy and intellectual disability are dying more than 10 years younger than those with other causes of death, such as pneumonia or sepsis. A significant proportion of the deaths reported were sudden unexpected death in epilepsy (SUDEP).

SUDEP, which is considered the second-most impactful neurological cause (after stroke) for human-years lost in those under 70 in developed countries, is 3-9 times more frequent in people with intellectual disability (Watkins et al., 2018a, Watkins et al., 2018b). The incidence of sudden unexpected death in people with epilepsy and intellectual disability is an estimated 20 times higher than in the general population. Intellectual disability in itself is a known risk factor for SUDEP. People with intellectual disability also have a number of identifiable risk factors for SUDEP, including early onset of seizures, chronic epilepsy, and treatment resistant seizures.

The Different Types of Epilepsy

The prevalence of epilepsy in the general population is an estimated 0.6%. There are two peaks in incidence: in the early years (associated with genetic epilepsy syndromes and neurological insults) and later in life (associated with degenerative neurological disorders and insults). Seizures can present in many different ways depending upon the origin and/or the route that the abnormal electric discharge travels through the brain. Considering the semiology of seizures (signs and symptoms) is not only useful for specialist surgical assessment but also helps us differentiate between seizures and other differential diagnoses. Seizures may present with motor, sensory, or a combination of symptoms. Seizures can be associated with auras (or warnings) that may precede subsequent sensory or motor symptoms. Seizures originating from certain parts of the brain can present with typical patterns of symptoms, which helps the epileptologist in the diagnostic process (Noachtar & Peters, 2009).

The ILAE Classification Framework identifies three stages (Table 17.1). The ILAE classification system is not only important for communication, it is also clinically relevant to identify seizure type in order to consider the most appropriate evidence-based interventions. Defining the epilepsy syndrome may provide access to restricted specialist medication prescriptions for people with treatment resistance.

Table 17.1 The International League against Epilepsy Classification Framework for the Epilepsies (Scheffer et al., 2017)

Stage 1	Seizure type (generalised, focal, unknown)
Stage 2	Epilepsy type (generalised, focal, multiple, unknown)
Stage 3	Epilepsy syndrome (based upon seizure type, epilepsy type, clinical characteristics, investigations, and aetiological considerations)

How Is Epilepsy Different in People with Intellectual Disability?

People with epilepsy and intellectual disability are a heterogeneous population; the aetiology of epilepsy and intellectual disability may be consistent for both, or there may be individual precipitating factors. There is a strong association between epilepsy and intellectual disability and other neurological disorders – for example, cerebral palsy, and other neurodevelopmental disorders (autism, attention deficit hyperactivity disorder). With advances in technology, we are now able to identify disease genes associated with both epilepsy and intellectual disability, often associated with a spectrum of phenotypes. Within the epilepsies there are a severe group classified as developmental and epileptic encephalopathies associated with declining cognition and function over time (Table 17.2). The complexity of epilepsy associated with intellectual disability and other neurodevelopmental disorders should be considered greater than the sum of the two conditions.

Considering the complexities we have discussed, making a diagnosis of epilepsy is not straight forward in people with intellectual disability. Around one in three people are misdiagnosed, and the challenge increases with severity of intellectual disability, communication impairment, and associated neurodevelopmental disorders such as autism. It is essential to be aware of physical health conditions that may 'mimic' epilepsy, particularly in this population. Common differential diagnoses include sleep disorders and cardiac syncope. It can also be challenging to distinguish between stereotyped repetitive behaviours

Table 17.2 Important epilepsy syndromes with a strong association with intellectual disability

Epilepsy syndrome	Aetiology	Clinical presentation	Key factors
Dravet syndrome (severe myoclonic epilepsy of infancy)	Associated with SCN1A mutation (>80%)	Febrile and non-febrile seizures in first 12 months of life. Focal (hemi-clonic) seizures and individual tonic-clinic seizures. Episodes of status epilepticus. Intellectual decline and multiple seizure types develop from second year with treatment resistance.	Seizures are typically exacerbated with the use of sodium channel blocking drugs (carbamazepine, oxcarbazepine, phenytoin, and lamotrigine)
Lennox–Gastaut syndrome	Range of aetiologies	Presence of (1) multiple seizure types (one of which must include tonic), onset in neurodevelopmental period, treatment resistant; (2) cognitive and often behavioural symptoms; (3) characteristic EEG changes.	MRI strongly recommended, commonly associated with structural abnormalities

and focal motor seizures, whether awareness is affected or not. Therefore, making a diagnosis may take longer and relies on detailed accurate history taking and reliable informant information.

Like diagnosing epilepsy in the general population, diagnosis of epilepsy in people with intellectual disability is mainly clinical, but more so reliant on eye-witness accounts and obtaining history thorough collateral information from carers and families capturing the details of presentation using a seizure diary.

In addition to differential diagnoses commonly reported in the general population, in people with intellectual disability, especially in those with severe intellectual disability and those who are non-verbal, there can be additional complexity making it challenging to make a confident diagnosis. Box 17.1 provides some examples of these associated conditions.

In comparison to the general population, presentation of epilepsy is also different in people with intellectual disability. For example, a subjective account of aura or postictal symptoms might be missing in those with communication difficulties or might be attributed to other accompanying psychological or physical health issues. Some other differences in presentation are summarised in Box 17.2.

Box 17.1 Examples of Differential Diagnoses or Accompanying Conditions Which Might Be Mistaken for Epilepsy in People with Intellectual Disability

- Autism stereotypies and rituals (vs automatism/complex partial seizures)
- Sensory processing disorders (sensory seeking and sensory avoiding behaviours)
- Behavioural and motor side effects of medications including antipsychotics (e.g., akathisia, acute dystonic reactions and Parkinsonian symptoms)
- Atypical presentation of psychiatric disorders in this population
- Attention deficit hyperactivity disorder symptoms: deficits in attention/concentration (vs absences) and hyperactivity
- Involuntary movements (e.g., dystonia in those with cerebral palsy) (vs tonic episodes)
- Psychogenic seizures, especially in those with mild to moderate intellectual disability
- Other comorbid conditions within the context of various genetic syndromes (e.g., cardiac arrhythmias) (vs drop attacks)
- Parasomnias/sleep difficulties (vs nighttime seizures)

Box 17.2 Differences in the Presentation of Epilepsy in People with Intellectual Disability Compared to the General Population

- Higher likelihood of an accompanying brain damage or rare genetic syndromes/epileptic encephalopathies (e.g., Dravet syndrome)
- Multiple types of epilepsies can be present in one person at any given time
- Other types of epilepsies can develop overtime as people grow older (e.g., myoclonic jerks in those with Down syndrome)
- The likelihood of refractory epilepsy is higher due to structural brain damage and accompanying genetic syndromes

(cont.)

- Polypharmacy and use of multiple antiseizure medications are more common in this population due to higher likelihood of various comorbidities adversely impacting on quality of life due to their side effects, medication interaction.
- Polypharmacy can exacerbate some types of epilepsies especially in the context of rare genetic syndromes (e.g., carbamazepine and myoclonic jerks)
- Atypical presentation of tonic-clonic seizures in those who might have spasticity (i.e., in those with cerebral palsy) or paralysis from childhood
- Higher risks of epilepsy-related morbidity and mortality including SUDEP
- Non-convulsive seizures/status presenting with drooling, confusion, unresponsiveness, and quietness (i.e., dementia-like picture)

Case Study 17.1

Tariq, a 25-year-old man with severe intellectual disability and autism living with his parents, presented with unprovoked tonic-clonic seizures. His history revealed that he had a similar episode five years previously, and, on further exploring the symptoms, his parents also described other accompanying episodes over the past few years which had been attributed to his visual impairment, autism, and challenging behaviour. These were happening a few times during the week and were short lived. The episodes were self-limiting but triggered and exacerbated by respiratory or urinary infections, perceived stressful situations, insomnia, extreme tiredness, and so forth. These cliché-like episodes consisted of pacing purposelessly, fumbling with his shirt, and unusual tongue and lip movements as if he was tasting food/drink. A few hours before each episode, he would present with self-injurious behaviours, including head banging, and looked pale.

The management included multidisciplinary involvement, especially input from the speech and language and occupational therapist colleagues. Further investigations, including brain MRI under general anaesthesia, using the Mental Capacity Act framework, were carried out. Mesial temporal sclerosis was reported in his brain scan, and as a result he was referred to the neurosurgical department. A referral was also sent to the clinical genetics team to explore the possibility of a genetic syndrome. Accessible information leaflets on epilepsy and epilepsy-related risks including SUDEP were shared with him and his family, and use of antiseizure medication (i.e., lamotrigine) was discussed for the pharmacological management of his epilepsy.

The Frith Treatment Guidelines for People with Intellectual Disability

Overview of Management

The mainstay to keep people with epilepsy safe is antiseizure medication (ASM). There are presently 34 licenced antiseizure medications, ranging from early medications such as phenobarbitone and phenytoin to modern designer treatment-resistant epilepsy medications such as perampanel, lacosamide, and brivaracetam. There are broad-spectrum well-established medications such as lamotrigine, levetiracetam, and sodium valproate, and modern medications focused on specific syndromes, such as cannabidiol, fenfluramine, and cenobamate.

However, little is understood or known about how these antiseizure medications work for people with intellectual disability given their vulnerabilities to treatment resistance and multimorbidity. This chapter focuses on outlining the current best evidence for the available antiseizure medications when prescribing in people with intellectual disability and epilepsy. The chapter also looks to highlight the strengths and weaknesses of these molecules individually and as a group, as applied to this vulnerable population.

The 2015 Cochrane review into the pharmacological treatment of people with epilepsy and intellectual disability identified 14 randomised controlled trials (RCTs) (1116 participants), with the quality of evidence deemed to be low to moderate (Jackson et al., 2015). This highlights the paucity of evidence to help guide treatment for people in this complex population.

The updated 2022 National Institute for Health and Care Excellence guidelines recommend the development of an individualised antiseizure medication treatment strategy with the person with epilepsy, and their carer/family, taking certain factors into account (Table 17.3).

Management of epilepsy in people with intellectual disability may vary from that of the general population in several ways: for example, there may be more reliance on carers/families and the multidisciplinary team for ensuring:

1. A holistic management of accompanying risks (e.g., aspiration pneumonia, falls and injuries, SUDEP).
2. Modification of treatment plan based on individual needs and legal frameworks (i.e., use of Mental Capacity Act/Deprivation of Liberty for gastrostomy feeding), covert administration of medications, change of medication formulations (i.e., granules or liquid to be mixed with food or drinks).

There are also challenges in implementing the management plan in the community – for example, training formal and informal carers, day-centre staff, educational institutions in basic epilepsy awareness, and use of rescue medication. Furthermore, and according to the latest National Institute for Health and Care Excellence epilepsy guidelines, people with

Table 17.3 National Institute for Health and Care Excellence (NICE) Clinical Guideline NG217 Factors to be considered when developing an individualised treatment strategy. (NG217, 2022)

Age
Gender (consider additional considerations for women of childbearing age?)
Seizure type
Type of epilepsy
Risks and benefits of antiseizure medications, including their importance in reducing epilepsy-related death
Interactions with other medicines
Comorbidities
How and when medicines need to be taken
The preferences of the person with epilepsy, their carers/family
Personal circumstances of the person: for example, driving, likelihood of pregnancy, alcohol use

> **Box 17.3 Alternatives to Medication Management of Epilepsy**
>
> - Ketogenic diet
> - Dietary regimes in certain genetic syndromes (e.g., glucose transporter deficiency type 1)
> - Environmental adaptations to manage risk and also those addressing seizure episodes related to photosensitivity, hot environment seen in rare genetic syndromes, etc.
> - Vagal nerve stimulation
> - Neurosurgery

intellectual disability and their carers should be proactively offered all non-pharmacological approaches for the long-term management of epilepsy, as for other population groups with epilepsy (Box 17.3) (NG217, 2022).

Non-Medication Approaches

Medication Approaches to Epilepsy Treatment

The ILAE classification of the epilepsies will help guide medication choice based upon seizures type, epilepsy syndrome, and aetiological factors (Scheffer et al., 2017). Therefore, establishing the most accurate diagnosis possible with supportive investigations will help guide which antiseizure medication has the best evidence base for outcomes, including efficacy and tolerability. In addition to person-related factors, it is important to consider medication-related factors and how these may impact upon a person with epilepsy. Some of these important effects of antiseizure medication are considered in Table 17.4.

The treatment of epilepsy for people with intellectual disability should be person-centred and consider individualised factors by working collaboratively with patients, their families, and care-givers. Some of the important factors that should influence prescribing practice include the antiseizure medication side-effect profile (effects of cognition, bone health, weight, and neuropsychiatric symptoms), medication-to-medication interactions (people with epilepsy and intellectual disability experience high rates of polypharmacy), medication preparation (maintaining consistent prescribing by brand may be necessary for certain antiseizure medications), comorbid psychiatric illness (consider the impact of concomitant psychotropic prescribing and impact upon seizure threshold), and gastrostomy tube administration (not all antiseizure medications available, may require monitoring of serum levels).

Antiseizure Medicine Polytherapy

Many people with intellectual disability may be exposed to antiseizure polytherapy due to the refractory nature of epilepsy. The 2022 National Institute for Health and Care Excellence guidelines recommend for all adults to use a single antiseizure medication (monotherapy) wherever possible. The National Institute for Health and Care Excellence guidelines recommend that if first- and second-line monotherapy are unsuccessful, consideration should be given to an add-on treatment, including monitoring for adverse effects and frequent treatment review. Many studies have shown that more than 40% of people receive two or more antiseizure medications, yet despite this many still experience seizures. A cross-sectional study

Table 17.4 Categories of adverse effects associated with antiseizure medications (Adapted from RCPsych CR206; Watkins et al, 2020)

Behavioural disturbances: Are often reported after initiation of a new antiseizure medication / increase in dose. Changes in behaviour are usually multifactorial, with other influences, in addition to the neuropsychiatric impact of antiseizure medications. A baseline assessment of behaviour is recommended before initiating an antiseizure medication.

Cognition: Older antiseizure medications such as phenobarbitone and phenytoin which affect cognition and also have high anticholinergic burden (associated with cognitive impairment, constipation, falls) should be avoided if possible. Some antiseizure medications such as lamotrigine have demonstrated some positive effects on cognition, and positive cognitive changes can be observed with improved seizure control.

Bone health: People with intellectual disability who take antiseizure medications are at increased risk of fragility fractures and osteoporosis. This risk is heightened by chronic antiseizure medication use, which may be worse with enzyme-inducing antiseizure medications. People with intellectual disability who have epilepsy will already have increased risk factors for lower bone density, such as immobility, sedentary behaviour, poor sunlight exposure (low vitamin D levels), early menopause, use of other medicines affecting density including antipsychotics, and proton pump inhibitors.

Weight change: Valproate, gabapentin, pregabalin, and levetiracetam are associated with weight gain and risk of metabolic syndrome. People with intellectual disability may already be predisposed to obesity due to lower activity or mobility levels, use of antipsychotics, and diet. Weight loss has been associated with topimirate and zonisamide.

of a nationally representative cohort of older adults with intellectual disability in Ireland found that more than 50% of those with epilepsy were taking two or more antiseizure drugs, but 40% of these were still experiencing monthly seizures (O'Dwyer et al., 2018). Concurrent exposure to antipsychotics that lower the seizure threshold (e.g., olanzapine) may also affect seizure frequency. A recent narrative review outlines that a history of epilepsy is seen as the primary prescribing reason; however, often it is a legacy and the indication is no longer clear (Branford et al., 2023). The proportion receiving antiseizure medications continues to rise with age and does not correlate well with seizure onset (Branford et al., 2023).

Specific Guidance for the Management of Epilepsy for People with Intellectual Disability

The evidence base to guide prescribing for epilepsy in people with intellectual disability is limited, with only a few individual double-blind controlled trials, with low numbers of participants, for a limited number of antiseizure medications. Therefore, we are often reliant upon extrapolating findings from robust investigations undertaken with participants without intellectual disability. However, although rigorous trials are important, they do not consider the complexities of people with both intellectual disability and epilepsy. Some of the challenges in developing investigations for this vulnerable population include recruitment, informed consent, and ethical considerations. The Royal College of Psychiatrists College Report CR206 (2017) 'Management of epilepsy in adults with intellectual disabilities' summarises the evidence base for antiseizure medication choice alongside expert clinical opinion. Antiseizure medications are individualised in a 'traffic light' system to guide prescribing choices with first-line options, second-line options (clinicians should

Table 17.5 Classification of commonly prescribed antiseizure medications (ASMs) based on evidence and expert opinion (RCPsych CR206, 2017, Watkins et al., 2020)

First line (GREEN)	Lamotrigine
Second line (AMBER)	Levetiracetam
	Topiramate
	Gabapentin
	Perampanel
	Lacosamide
Other second-line options with limited evidence base for people with intellectual disability	Eslicarbazepine
	Zonisamide
	Oxcarbazepine
	Ethosuximide
Drugs only used if essential (RED)	Phenobarbital
	Phenytoin
Specialist ASMs	Cenobamate
	Epidyolex (cannabidiol)
	Everolimus
	Fenfluramine
Sodium Valproate (MHRA Regulations)	

weigh up benefits and risk), and those antiseizure medication to avoid unless absolutely necessary due to acute and chronic adverse effects (Table 17.5).

RED: Only use in exceptional circumstances.

AMBER: Could be considered if benefits outweigh risks or as second-line

GREEN: Needs to be considered as first-line treatment.

Newer antiseizure medications are under investigation and likely to be more precisely targeted at specific genetic epilepsies. Some of the antiseizure medications for prescribing by an epilepsy specialist include cenobamate, targeted at treatment resistant focal epilepsy. The cannabidiol epidyolex is restricted to certain epilepsy syndromes based on the evidence available, currently limited to Dravet syndrome, Lennox–Gastaut Syndrome, and epilepsy associated with tuberous sclerosis complex (TSC). Everolimus is also now available for treatment of epilepsy specifically for people with TSC, and this medication targeted at a specific genetic syndrome starts to show us the potential future path for seizures treatments. There are numerous molecules under investigation targeted at specific genetic epilepsies. It is likely most of the newer antiseizure medications will be restricted to specialist supervision, as is the case with the adopted medication fenfluramine for Dravet syndrome.

Principles of Prescribing Antiseizure Medications for People with Intellectual Disability

1. Consider the seizure type and epilepsy syndrome in accordance with the ILAE classification.
2. 'Start low and go slow': prescribing at the lowest possible dose with slow titration will reduce the risk of adverse effects and increase the likelihood of tolerability. This is particularly important for a highly treatment resistant population.
3. Aim for monotherapy.
4. Make one change to antiseizure medications at a time, so the effect can be more readily identified.
5. Avoid older antiseizure medications unless clinically necessary. Phenobarbital and phenytoin are associated with significant adverse effects, particularly with long-term use, and have a narrow therapeutic window.
6. Consider the Medicines and Healthcare products Regulatory Agency (MHRA) guidance on ensuring consistent prescribing of branded medicines.
7. Formulation-swallowing challenges, gastrostomy administration, and sensory needs may influence choice.
8. Consider medication-to-medication interaction with other antiseizure medications and medications prescribed for other comorbidities. Reduce the burden of polypharmacy and anticholinergic effects, particularly as people get older.

Choice of Antiseizure Medications

Focal Seizures

1st Line Lamotrigine

2nd Line Levetiracetam

(Caution risk of behavioural (aggression) and psychiatric adverse effects, particularly of pre-existing psychiatric illness/neuropsychiatric symptoms)

Generalised Seizures

1st Line Lamotrigine

2nd Line Levetiracetam (caution as above), Carbamazepine, Topiramate

Consider for any seizure type based upon antiseizure medications previously trialled, person and medication profile:

Topiramate

Lacosamide

Perampanel (caution neuropsychiatric adverse effects)

Oxcarbazepine

Eslicarbazepine

Zonisamide

Sodium Valproate (MHRA regulations)

Pregabalin

Brivaracetam

To Avoid Unless Clinically Necessary Due to Side-Effect Profile
Phenobarbital, phenytoin

Specialist Prescription for Specific Epilepsy Syndromes
Dravet syndrome/Lennox–Gastaut Syndrome/Tuberous Sclerosis Complex epilepsy: Epidyolex (with Clobazam) (*liver function monitoring*)

Dravet syndrome: Fenfluramine (*echocardiogram monitoring*)

Treatment-resistant focal seizure syndrome: Cenobamate (*medication interactions, caution with carbamazepine, benzodiazepines (clobazam), phenytoin*)

Case Study 17.2

Sam is a 40-year-old man with mild intellectual disability, epilepsy, and emotionally unstable personality disorder. He developed epilepsy in childhood but has been stable on a combination of lamotrigine and sodium valproate (one or two tonic-clonic seizures every few months) for many years. He was referred to the epilepsy clinic with a recent exacerbation of seizure episodes, including attendances to accident and emergency departments. At first this was thought to be prolonged psychogenic seizures brought on following breakdown in his care support and the referral requested psychological input for the management of accompanying psychogenic seizures, given the patient had a diagnosis of personality disorder. Initial blood investigations were reported normal in A & E and acute infections were ruled out; however, Sam continued presenting with more tonic-clonic seizures.

A brain MRI scan was therefore subsequently requested, which revealed a frontal meningioma. The meningioma was thought to have been caused by exposure to radiotherapy during childhood for the management of lymphoma. This was operated and incised by the neurosurgical team upon referral. Which led to return of epilepsy presentation to baseline. Sam continued on the same dosage of his antiseizure medication given further attempts post-op to reduce any of them resulted in worsening of his epilepsy control.

How Long Should Treatment Continue?
There is no evidenced best practice for this population to define treatment duration with antiseizure medications. There are multiple considerations for both withdrawal of antiseizure medications and in support of their continuity.

Since the launch of the STOMP (Stopping Over Medication of People with a learning disability, autism or both) programme (2015 to current), there has been additional focus on providing clarity about how long treatments should continue. The STOMP programme, while focused on suitable and rationale prescribing of psychotropics to people with intellectual disability, was principally involved in wanting to reduce the antipsychotic burden in this population (Branford & Shankar, 2022). It was recognised that around 17% of people with intellectual disability were prescribed antipsychotics while the indication to do so was around 3% (Branford & Shankar, 2022). Over the last eight years there has been some improvements in reducing the national antipsychotic burden to approximately 15%. However, in that time period there has been an increased prescribing of antidepressants and/or antiseizure medications for non-licenced indications in this vulnerable population (Branford & Shankar, 2022; Branford et al., 2023). There are also higher rates of polypharmacy of different genres of psychotropics, particularly involving antidepressants and antiseizure medications. Specific to the licenced use of antiseizure medications in people with intellectual disability, there is recognition that the amount of prescribed antiseizure medications continues to rise with age. This pattern of use is not well correlated with when the seizures commenced or their patterns. It highlights a legacy of antiseizure medications as people age with no clear indication for its continued utility (Branford et al., 2023). Alongside this, it needs to be considered that 70% or more of people with intellectual disability and epilepsy are treatment resistant and likely have an increasing year-on-year SUDEP risk (Young et al., 2015). An additional issue is having a good grasp of the past history of seizures; history of any previous attempts to stop treatment; the outcome of those efforts, in particular if they failed to understand probable causes of failure (was the antiseizure medication reduced too fast, the person developed other problems like behaviours seen as challenging, etc.); and resultant harm (paramedic callout, hospital admissions, psychotropic addition, etc.). Other matters, such as anticholinergic burden of polypharmacy, bone harm, and other related iatrogenic considerations, need to be factored in, to inform when and if to discontinue.

Withdrawal of Medications

There is no high-quality evidence on withdrawing antiseizure medications in general, or specifically in people with intellectual disability (Branford et al., 2023). It is advised that, given the lack of any best practice evidence, a pragmatic common-sense approach be taken.

Given the practical challenges outlined in the previous section, for non-urgent situations the decision to withdraw and how to do so needs to be taken at a person-centred level, involving all key stakeholders (particularly the patient and/or their families/carers), ensuring there is good visualisation of the potential risks and benefits of the planned intervention. Following the Mental Capacity Act 2005 principles of ensuring informed decision making, or, in in its absence, having a suitable empowered best interest process, is absolutely necessary. Adequate attention needs to be paid to safety (i.e., mitigating the risk of SUDEP or withdrawal seizures). This requires building the individual, family, and other stakeholders' confidence by providing suitable understanding of past history, good communication of the relevant factors and decisions, and epilepsy awareness training (Tittensor et al., 2021). Focus on environmental and community safety is paramount. There should be an awareness of the onset of dangerous seizures during withdrawal. Likewise, the availability of nocturnal monitoring and trained rescue medication administrators are equally important factors (Tittensor et al., 2021).

Once agreed, dose reduction should be 'low and slow'. For example, if reducing lamotrigine from 500 mg/day, consider withdrawing it in 25 mg steps every 3 months. It is strongly advised there be regular reviews, preferably 8–12 weeks post dose-reduction. Maintaining seizure diaries and other records is imperative to identify change. Based on response and confidence, the gradient of reduction could be modified to be steeper (i.e., 25 mgs taken off every 6–8 weeks) or more gradual (25 mgs to be taken off every 6 months). The first principles remain listening and reacting to the feedback of individuals and their families/carers to facilitate a successful withdrawal.

> **Case Study 17.3**
>
> Ade, a 30-year-old man with severe intellectual disability and autism, was referred with significant self-injury in spite of multidisciplinary team input, and refractory tonic-clonic seizures on optimal dose of levetiracetam and valproate. There was a history of falls and arm fracture. The history also revealed exacerbation of self-injury with initiating levetiracetam and gradually increasing the dose. Levetiracetam was first crossed-tapered with brivaracetam at an equivalent dosage. Although the self-injury reduced in frequency and intensity, the improvements were not significant. Further agreement was reached with the family to replace brivaracetam with lamotrigine, which brought about significant improvement in his mental health but had little if no impact on epilepsy. Ade was then referred and subsequently accepted for vagal nerve stimulation, which contributed to a better seizure control. Vitamin D/calcium supplement were also initiated based on National Institute for Health and Care Excellence guidelines.

The Frith Prescribing Guidelines Editors' Expert Group Consensus Statements

Statements of High Confidence

An estimate 1 in 4 people with intellectual disability have epilepsy.

- The prevalence of epilepsy increases with severity of intellectual disability.
- Epilepsy is the most common chronic comorbid medical condition in intellectual disability.
- The majority of people with intellectual disability who have epilepsy have treatment resistant epilepsy.
- People with epilepsy and intellectual disability die younger, and many of the deaths are considered premature and potentially preventable.
- Rates of SUDEP are significantly higher in people with intellectual disability and epilepsy.
- Lamotrigine is the best studied antiseizure medication in people with intellectual disability and should be considered a first-line treatment.
- Antiseizure medications are also increasingly used for non-seizure management reasons in this population.

Statements of Medium Confidence

- Valproate containing medicines have a good evidence base for the treatment of multiple seizure types, particularly in generalised epilepsies. However, this requires consideration of the MHRA regulations for women and girls of childbearing potential and men.
- Levetiracetam, lacosamide, perampanel, gabapentin, and topiramate have an evidence base for efficacy and safety in people with epilepsy and intellectual disability and should be considered second-line treatment options.

Regular specialist review, an accurate epilepsy care plan including individualised risk assessments, and appropriate levels of supervision (particularly at night) can reduce the risk of mortality.
- High rates of psychotropic medication use in people with intellectual disability and epilepsy adds on to the premature mortality risk.

Statements of Low Confidence
- There is limited evidence or national guidance to guide treatment choice specifically for people with epilepsy and intellectual disability. Extrapolation from the evidence for the general population with epilepsy is therefore recommended.

Resource Box

National guidance on management of epilepsy in children, young people and adults were updated by NICE in 2022 (NG217). For people with intellectual disability the NICE guidelines includes specific recommendations: www.nice.org.uk/guidance/ng217/resources/visual-summary-pdf-11067088285
Epilepsies in children, young people and adults (nice.org.uk)
- Access to a tertiary specialist's epilepsy service for people with suspected/confirmed epilepsy and intellectual disability who require additional specialist support.
- Provide support at appointments: including, but not limited to longer appointments, different formats for information as appropriate to the patient (e.g., easy read, audio, involve family members).
- Provide co-ordinated care through use of a multidisciplinary team.
- Arrange regular reviews and monitoring (at least annually).
- Consider whole genome sequencing for people with epilepsy of an unknown cause who have intellectual disability.
- Do not exclude people with intellectual disability from referral for surgery for epilepsy if indicated.
- Begin the process of transition early for young people with intellectual disability who have epilepsy.

The Royal College of Psychiatrists, College Report CR203, Good Psychiatric Practice, Management of Epilepsy in Adults with Intellectual Disability (2017): college-report-cr203.pdf (rcpsych.ac.uk).
The 2017 Royal College Report CR203 outlines a framework for a tiered competency model (bronze, silver, gold). The professional competencies at each level are aligned to the NICE outcome indicators and SIGN 143 Guidance (Scottish Intercollegiate Guideline Network Diagnosis and Management of Epilepsy in Adults, National Clinical Guidance, SIGN 143 (2018)) (www.sign.ac.uk/media/1079/sign143_2018.pdf). Bronze-level competency is the minimum expected standard for any psychiatrist working with people with intellectual disability. The competency levels also consider service provision.
NICE outcome indicators associated with bronze level:
- Adults with epilepsy have an agreed and comprehensive written care plan
- Adults with a history of prolonged or repeated seizures have an agreed written emergency care plan
- Adults with epilepsy who have medical or lifestyle issues that need review are referred to specialist epilepsy services

– Young people with epilepsy have an agreed transition period during which their continuing epilepsy care is reviewed jointly by paediatric and adult services

The Royal College of Psychiatrists College Report CR206, Good Psychiatric Practice, Prescribing Anti-epileptic Drugs or Adults with Epilepsy and Intellectual Disability (2017): college-report-cr206.pdf (rcpsych.ac.uk).

This guidance was developed by consensus of expert opinion based upon the available evidence and clinical experience. It provides psychiatrists tailored advice to approaching assessment and treatment for people with intellectual disability and $^$epilepsy in the context of multi-morbidity and polypharmacy. This includes specific guidance on choosing the most appropriate antiseizure medication.

Resource Documents

Harden C, Tomson T, Gloss D, et al. Practice guideline summary: Sudden unexpected death in epilepsy incidence rates and risk factors: Report of the Guideline Development, Dissemination, and Implementation Subcommittee of the American Academy of Neurology and the American Epilepsy Society. *Neurology*. 2017 Apr 25;88(17):1674-1680. https://doi.org/10.1212/WNL.0000000000003685. Erratum in: *Neurology*. 2019 Nov 26;93(22):982. Erratum in: *Neurology*. 2020 Mar 3;94(9):414. PMID: 28438841.

National Institute for Health and Care Excellence (NICE), Clinical Guidelines (NG217). Epilepsies in children, young people and adults. Apr 2022. www.nice.org.uk/guidance/ng217.

Royal College of Psychiatrists, College Report CR203. Management of epilepsy in adults with intellectual disability. 2017. www.rcpsych.ac.uk/improving-care/campaigning-for-better-mental-health-policy/college-reports/2017-college-reports/management-of-epilepsy-in-adults-with-intellectual-disability-cr203-may-2017.

Royal College of Psychiatrists, College Report CR206. Prescribing antiepileptic drugs for people with epilepsy and intellectual disability. 2017. www.rcpsych.ac.uk/improving-care/campaigning-for-better-mental-health-policy/college-reports/2017-college-reports/prescribing-anti-epileptic-drugs-for-people-with-epilepsy-and-intellectual-disability-cr206-oct-2017.

Scottish Intercollegiate Guidelines Network (SIGN). Diagnosis and management of epilepsy in adults. Edinburgh: SIGN; 2015. (SIGN publication no. 143). May 2015 Rev. Sep 2018. www.sign.ac.uk.

References

Branford, D., & Shankar, R. (2022). Antidepressant prescribing for adult people with an intellectual disability living in England. *The British Journal of Psychiatry: The Journal of Mental Science*, **221**(2), 488–93. https://doi.org/10.1192/bjp.2022.34.

Branford, D., Sun, J. J., & Shankar, R. (2023). Antiseizure medications prescribing for behavioural and psychiatric concerns in adults with an intellectual disability living in England. *The British Journal of Psychiatry*, **22**(5), 191–5. http://doi.org/10.1192/bjp.2022.182.

Branford, D., Sun, J. J., Burrows L & Shankar, R. (2023). Patterns of anti-seizure medications prescribing in people with intellectual disability and epilepsy: a narrative review and analysis. *The British Journal of Clinical Pharmacology*, **89**(7), 2028–38.

Fisher, R. S., Acevedo, C., Arzimanoglou, A., et al. (2014). ILAE official report: A practical clinical definition of epilepsy. *Epilepsia*, 55(4), 475–82.

Jackson, C. F., Makin, S. M., Marson, A. G., & Kerr, M. (2015). Pharmacological interventions for epilepsy in people with intellectual disabilities. *Cochrane Database of Systematic Reviews*, 9, CD005399. https://doi.org/10.1002/14651858.CD005399.pub3.

Noachtar, S., & Peters, A. S. (2009. Semiology of epileptic seizures: A critical review. *Epilepsy & Behavior*. May 1; 15(1), 2–9.

O'Dwyer, M., Peklar, J., Mulryan, N., et al. (2018). Prevalence and patterns of antiepileptic medication prescribing in the treatment of epilepsy in older adults with intellectual disabilities. *Journal of Intellectual Disability Research*. Mar; 62(3), 245–61.

Scheffer, I. E., Berkovic, S., Capovilla, G., et al. (2017). ILAE classification of the epilepsies: Position paper of the ILAE Commission for Classification and Terminology. *Epilepsia*. Apr; 58(4), 512–21.

Sun, J. J., Perera, B., Henley, W., et al. (2022). Epilepsy related multimorbidity, polypharmacy and risks in adults with intellectual disabilities: A national study [published correction appears in J Neurol. 2022 Mar 5]. *Journal of Neurology* 269(5), 2750–60. https://doi.org/10.1007/s00415-021-10938-3.

Sun, J. J., Watkins, L., Henley, W., et al. (2023). Mortality risk in adults with intellectual disabilities and epilepsy: An England and Wales case-control study. *Journal of Neurology*, 270, 3527–36. https://doi.org/10.1007/s00415-023-11701-6.

Tittensor, P., Tittensor, S., Chisanga, E., et al. (2021). UK framework for basic epilepsy training and oromucosal midazolam administration. *Epilepsy & Behavior*, 122, 108180. https://doi.org/10.1016/j.yebeh.2021.108180.

Watkins, L., Shankar, R., & Sander, J. W. (2018). Identifying and mitigating Sudden Unexpected Death in Epilepsy (SUDEP) risk factors. *Expert Reviews in Neurotherapy*, 18(4), 265–74. https://doi.org/10.1080/14737175.2018.1439738.

Watkins, L. & Shankar, R. (2018). Reducing the risk of sudden unexpected death in epilepsy (SUDEP). *Current Treatment Options in Neurology*, 20(10), 40. https://doi.org/10.1007/s11940-018-0527-0.

Watkins, L. V., Linehan, C., Brandt, C., et al. (2022). Epilepsy in adults with neurodevelopmental disability: What every neurologist should know. *Epileptic Disorders*. Feb; 24(1), 9–25.

Watkins, L., O'Dwyer, M., Kerr, M., et al. (2020). Quality improvement in the management of people with epilepsy and intellectual disability: The development of clinical guidance. *Expert Opinion on Pharmacotherapy*, 21(2),173–81.

Young, C., Shankar, R., Palmer, J., et al. (2015). Does intellectual disability increase sudden unexpected death in epilepsy (SUDEP) risk? *Seizure*, 25, 112–16. https://doi.org/10.1016/j.seizure.2014.10.001.

Chapter 18

Dementia

Shweta Gangavati, Elizabeta Mukaetova-Ladinska, Satheesh K. Gangadharan, and Remon Mosaad

Introduction

What Is Dementia?

Dementia is a syndrome of a chronic or progressive nature that leads to deterioration in cognitive function beyond that seen in biological ageing. It affects memory, thinking, orientation, comprehension, calculation, learning new information, language, and judgement, in the absence of altered consciousness. The impairment in cognitive function is commonly accompanied, and occasionally preceded, by changes in mood, emotional control, behaviour, or motivation. Dementia affects people's ability to perform everyday activities, and thus has a significant impact on carers and family.

Although it is often seen in older people, dementia is neither an inevitable part of the normal ageing process nor is it a problem exclusively of the elderly. In fact, people with intellectual disability often develop dementia at a younger age than those without an intellectual disability.

Clinical Presentation of Dementia

In the current versions of both the International Classification Diseases (ICD11) (Carulla et al., 2011) and the *Diagnostic and Statistical Manual of Mental Disorders* (DSM-V) (American Psychiatric Association, 2013), the diagnosis of dementia requires evidence of marked change in two or more cognitive domain, such as the impairments in memory, language ability (aphasia), ability to perform complex tasks (apraxia), and orientation in time and place. The change should show a clear decline from the individual's previous level of functioning. The main features of dementia are summarised in Table 18.1.

Table 18.1 Main features of dementia

Cognitive	Decline in memory, aphasia, apraxia agnosia, executive dysfunction
Non-cognitive	Emotional lability, irritability, apathy coarsening of social behaviour
Social	Decline in self-care and daily living skills Interpersonal difficulties and behaviour problems

How Is Dementia Different in People with Intellectual Disability?

Memory loss can be a reliable early sign in people with mild intellectual disability and a small number of those with moderate intellectual disability (Cosgrave et al., 2000); however, overall evidence from studies indicates Behavioural and Psychological Symptoms of Dementia (BPSD) to be the best early indicators of dementia in people with intellectual disability in general and those with Down syndrome in particular. A typical presentation is general deterioration in functioning followed by behavioural and emotional changes. The frontal lobe symptoms that manifest in the later stages of dementia in the general population can appear early in people with Down syndrome (Deb et al., 2007) Behavioural and personality changes can appear along with executive dysfunction (Ball et al., 2008). Behavioural presentation could be in the form of behavioural excesses such as irritability, overactivity, or exaggeration of personality traits, or behavioural deficits such as apathy, social withdrawal, and a general lack of interests. Neurological symptoms such as myoclonus or generalised seizures are more common in people with intellectual disability in the initial stages of dementia compared to the general population (Robertson et al., 2015). Incontinence can also be seen earlier in people with intellectual disability and dementia compared to general population with dementia.

In the later stages of dementia, patients may present with loss of ability to speak, inability to walk, being unresponsive to the environment, incontinence, seizures, and strong Parkinsonian features (Cosgrave et al., 2000; Visser et al., 1997).

The objective measurement of cognitive function and the detection of any changes in people with moderate or severe intellectual disability remains a challenge for clinicians.

Challenges in Establishing the Features of Dementia in People with Intellectual Disability

- Difficulty for the person in providing a subjective account due to diminished ability to think abstractly and to communicate.
- Difficulties in recognising subtle clinical changes due to variable level of pre-existing impairment in cognitive functions and adaptive skills.
- Presence of other disabilities such as sensory impairments and autism masking or altering the presentation.
- Difficulties in co-operating with investigations such as blood tests, sensory screening, and neuroimaging.

Several clinical problems may mimic dementia in those with Down syndrome. These disorders may also co-exist with dementia and require treatment. Table 18.2 gives a list of other possible causes of dementia-like symptoms to consider before making a diagnosis of dementia.

Clinical Stages of Dementia in People with Intellectual Disability

It is difficult to identify the stages dementia in people with intellectual disability due to the variability in presentation as well as their heterogenous level of premorbid

Table 18.2 Clinical situations/problems that mimic dementia in people with intellectual disability

Causation	Details
Psychosocial	Bereavement, loss of contact with key individuals, changes in day activities, any significant stressful life events (e.g., sexual or physical abuse), etc.
Environment	Increased demand from a new environment, lack of adequate stimulation in the environment
Sensory Impairments	Hearing deficits, visual impairment (cataracts), etc.
Epilepsy	Uncontrolled epilepsy with frequent seizures
Pain	Abdominal pain, back ache, discomfort from severe constipation in the context of inability to communicate distress appropriately
Metabolic changes	Hypothyroidism, anaemia, vitamin B12 or folate deficiencies, hypoglycaemia or hyperglycaemia, electrolyte disturbances, etc.
Other brain conditions	Haematoma, ischaemia, infections affecting brain as well as brain tumours
Mental Health conditions	Depression, psychotic conditions, severe forms of anxiety, etc.
Medication	Raised levels of antiseizure medications, medications with anticholinergic side effects, polypharmacy, electrolyte disturbances such as hyponatraemia, etc.

cognitive functioning and adaptive skills. Figure 18.1 gives a general guideline in identifying the early, middle, and late stages of dementia in people with intellectual disability.

Use of antidementia medications is most likely to be effective at early stages and may show limited effectiveness in the middle and late stages.

How Common Is Dementia in People with Intellectual Disability?

People with intellectual disability have a higher risk of developing dementia when compared to the general population. Studies investigating the rates of clinical dementia in people with intellectual disability have reported variable prevalence rates depending on the diagnostic criteria used. In a study by Strydom and colleagues using DSM-IV criteria, prevalence rates for clinical dementia in intellectual disability were observed to be 13.1% in those over 60 years and 18.3% in those 65 years and over (Strydom et al., 2007). This is substantially higher than the dementia prevalence seen in the general population, which currently stands at 0.9% for those aged 60–64 years (Prince et al., 2014).

Down syndrome is the most frequent known cause of intellectual disability. Dementia presents early in people with Down syndrome and is commonly the dementia of

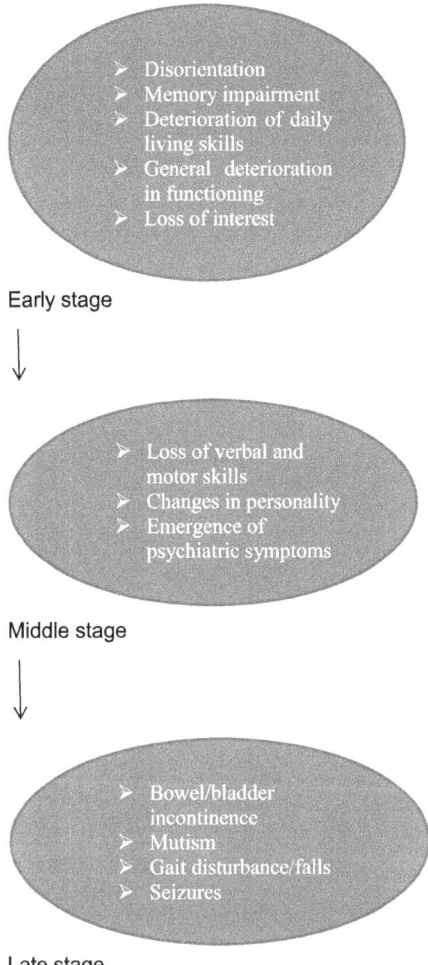

Figure 18.1 Clinical stages of dementia in people with intellectual disability

Alzheimer's type. Prevalence of clinical dementia in people with Down syndrome starts at less than 5% in the 30–39 years age group, increases dramatically to 50% in over the 50s, and ascends to 75% in people over the age of 60. The peak incidence is believed to be in the early fifties.

People with intellectual disability without Down syndrome also have a much higher prevalence rate when compared to the general population (Strydom et al., 2013) (see Figure 18.2). The cause for this higher prevalence rate is unknown due to lack of valid studies in this population; however, people with intellectual disability may be at increased risk due to their underlying physical health conditions and lifestyle (i.e., they are high risk for diabetes, obesity, sedentary lifestyle (inactivity) and depression, all known to be modifiable risk factors for dementia) (Montero-Odasso et al., 2020). The four most common causes of dementia among people with intellectual disability are Alzheimer's disease, Lewy body dementia, vascular dementia, and fronto-temporal dementia.

Assessment

The National Task Group on Intellectual Disabilities and Dementia Practices (Moran et al., 2013) recommends a nine-step approach. A detailed description of the assessment process is provided in the joint dementia guidance from Royal College of Psychiatrists and the British Psychological Society (Joint Standing Committee of the British Psychological Society and the Royal College of Psychiatrists, 2015). Joint dementia guidance recommends the use of structured tool to capture the changes in skills (e.g., the Dementia Scale for Learning Disability (DLD) supplemented by a direct assessment). Table 18.3 summarises the clinical approach for assessing dementia in people with intellectual disability.

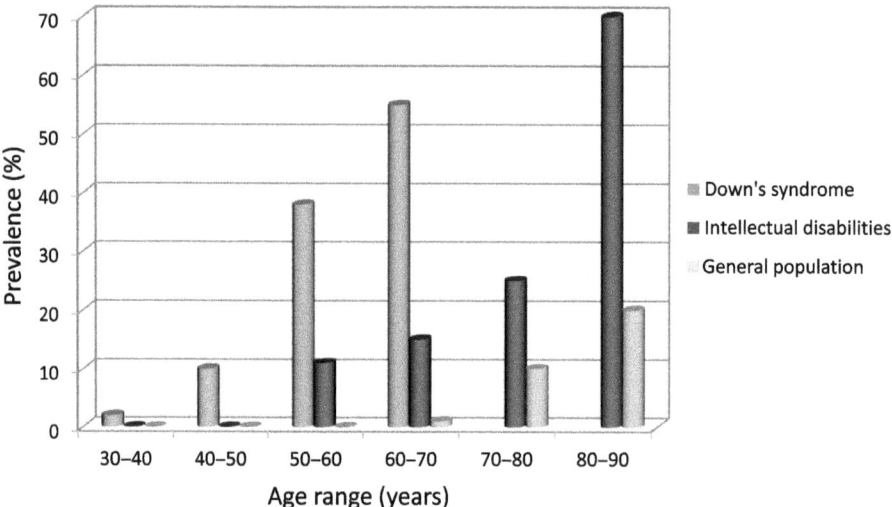

Figure 18.2 Age-related prevalence rates of dementia in Down syndrome, intellectual disability excluding Down syndrome, and general population.

Table 18.3 A Structure for Dementia Assessment in People with Intellectual Disability

Relevant Assessment	Details
Medical history, psychiatric history, and psychosocial history	Medical history to include cardiovascular history, presence of any neurological conditions, history of head injury, evidence of metabolic disorders such as hypothyroidism (including if it is adequately treated if already diagnosed). Psychiatric history to include any evidence of depression either at present or in the past, presence of bipolar disorders or psychotic conditions.

Table 18.3 (cont.)

Relevant Assessment	Details
	Bereavement, changes in social relationships, presence of any stressful events, etc.
Historical description of baseline functioning	Where possible collected using a structured tool covering all areas of functioning.
Picture of current functioning	An informant questionnaire should be used to gather the information systematically. Please see the list of instruments available for this purpose (see Table 18.4).
Review of medications	A thorough of review of medications with a particular focus on newly added medications or changes in the dose. The following medications have a higher risk of causing cognitive impairments: psychoactive, antiepileptic, or anticholinergic, and those with sedating properties.
Family history	Family history of early onset dementia, cardiovascular conditions, stroke, diabetes, rheumatoid arthritis, systemic lupus erythematosus, etc.
Environment	Quality of physical environment, mix of people with intellectual disability in the residential setting, quality, and quantity of day activities. Staffing levels, staff characteristics, including attitudes, competence, etc.
Physical examination	A thorough physical examination where possible, physical health screening where a physical examination is not possible (e.g., OK Physical health check).
Investigations	Full blood count, urea, and electrolytes Blood sugar, thyroid function, Liver function, B12, and folate level Lipid profile, sensory screening Electrocardiograph (ECG), MRI brain scan or CT head if practical Consider additional investigations if they help diagnose dementia subtype, and if this would change management. An issue relevant to people with intellectual disability is their ability to tolerate procedures. With the cautionary note above, additional investigation that could be considered are FDG-PET (fluorodeoxyglucose-positron emission tomography-CT), or perfusion SPECT (single-photon emission CT) if FDG-PET is unavailable. Alternatively, examining cerebrospinal fluid for total or phosphorylate tau protein (elevated) and either amyloid beta 1–42 or amyloid beta 1–42 and amyloid beta 1–40 (depleted). If dementia with Lewy bodies is suspected, use ^{123}I-FP-CIT SPECT. If the latter unavailable, consider ^{123}I-MIBG cardiac scintigraphy.

Table 18.3 (cont.)

Relevant Assessment	Details
	Do not rule out distinct dementia subtypes based solely on the results of structural, perfusion or metabolic imaging tests. It is important to acknowledge here that there are significant challenges while planning for these investigations in people with intellectual disability. Increased anxiety about procedures, and behaviours that challenge may present additional difficulties with timely access to these investigations. After weighing the clinical presentation and available physical examination, investigations, and consulting the patient where possible and where patient lacks capacity, clinicians need to consult all people involved to make a best interest decision.
Mental state examination and cognitive assessment	Several structured tools are available to aid the cognitive assessment in people with intellectual disability (Table 18.4).
Synthesis of information and formulation	Assessments are often undertaken by a number of different professionals (e.g., psychiatry, occupational therapy, speech and language therapy), and therefore information collected by all should be discussed to synthesise all the information to formulate and make a clear diagnosis.

Table 18.4 Instruments used in the assessment of people with intellectual disability and dementia

Questionnaire	Useful Information
Dementia questionnaire for people with learning disabilities (DLD) (Evenhuis, 2018)	Contains 50 items and 8 sub-scales. Carers can complete this questionnaire by themselves. It takes approximately 15–20 minutes to complete and can be repeated every 6 months. Cognitive and non-cognitive scores can be summed up separately. A diagnosis of dementia is considered if the sum of cognitive scores increases by 9 points or the total score increases by 13.
Down syndrome dementia scale (DSDS) (Jozsvai et al., 2009)	60 questions divided up between early, middle, and late stages of dementia. This is the only instrument which attempts to identify the stage of dementia. It requires a trained person (i.e., a psychologist) to administer, and ideally two informants should be interviewed.
Multi-dimensional observation scale for elderly subjects (MOSES) (Sturmey et al., 2003)	A 40-item questionnaire covering 5 areas: self-help skills, disorientation, depression, irritability, and social withdrawal. An informant makes the rating based on one week of direct observation and it can be completed in 10–15 minutes.

Table 18.4 (cont.)

Questionnaire	Useful Information
Daily living skills questionnaire (DLSQ) (National Institute of Aging (NIA), 1989)	A 28-item test assessing the competency in areas of daily living skills. It covers dressing (5 items), manual dexterity (2 items), eating (6 items), personal hygiene (5 items), housekeeping (5 items), and orientation (5 items).
Down syndrome mental state examination (DSMSE) (Haxby, 1989)	This consists of a battery of neuropsychological tests assessing a broad range of skills including recall of personal information, orientation to seasons, day of the week, memory, language, visuo-spatial function, and praxis. A verbal response is required for most of the tests.
Tests for severe impairment (TSI) (Albert & Cohen, 1992)	This was originally developed to measure cognitive impairment in people with severe dementia. The six domains included in this scale are: motor performance, language production, language comprehension, memory, conceptualisation, and general knowledge. The scale has been shown to have validity and reliability for use in intellectual disability.
CAMDEX- DS adapted from CAMDEX-R (Ball et al., 2004)	Includes both direct assessments of the person as well as a structured informant interview. Particular emphasis has been placed on establishing change from the person's best level of functioning.

Case Study 18.1

Peter is a 50-year-old man with mild intellectual disability of unknown aetiology who lives with his parents. He has been reasonably independent until recently. He had been able to look after his personal care with occasional reminders and minimal supervision from his parents. Peter had always helped his parents around the home and helped his father with gardening. He also did voluntary work in the day centre that he attended. He was previously able to go to the nearby town on his own and do some basic shopping as well. He can communicate well, although he can at times struggle to understand the meaning of some words. He has limited reading and writing skills.

Peter presented with forgetfulness and occasional confusion (not knowing where he is, not been able to remember the task he is supposed to do, etc.). In this case, the presentation is somewhat like that in those without intellectual disability. An informant-based Dementia Questionnaire for people with Learning Disability (DLD) was used along with a face-to-face examination with a psychiatrist, which involved a comprehensive mental state examination including Mini Mental State Examination and a physical examination. Peter was able to cooperate with this, and investigations including a brain MRI scan lead to the diagnosis of dementia of the Alzheimer's type.

Case Study 18.2

Mary is fifty two years old and has Down syndrome and moderate intellectual disability. She lives in supported living and attends a day centre. She needs support from carers for her personal care and cannot travel independently. Mary had a vocabulary of 50 words and can use some limited Makaton signs but cannot read or write. She presented with a change in behaviour which included being noisy and disruptive in group sessions, not sleeping well at night, and refusing to accept support for personal care. Once or twice, she hit out at the carers who were trying to provide personal care. A careful history-taking by the psychiatrist showed that there have been subtle changes in her skills (putting on her clothes the wrong way round, difficulty following instructions in the group sessions, reduced ability to engage in a task for a period of time, etc.). There had been several changes in her care staff over the last few months. Unfortunately, there was no clear record of her premorbid skills: she moved into the supported living after her mother died about two years earlier and had not previously had input from health services. Assessment found no evidence of depression or other mental health problems.

Mary would not co-operate with a full physical examination and therefore an 'OK Physical health check' was undertaken by the community nurse. It showed that Mary was having some difficulty in hearing as well as constantly pinching her ears. Apart from the ear problem, the health screening did not show any evidence of physical health problems. Mary would not cooperate with having MRI or CT brain scans.

After desensitisation work by the community nurse, the general practitioner was able to examine Mary's ears and take blood samples. Ear examination showed wax impaction, which was successfully treated using warmed olive oil. This improved her behaviour to some extent (she stopped pinching her ears and was able to follow instructions better than before), but she continued to have the other changes as noted. Blood testing did not reveal any abnormal findings.

Using the Dementia Scale for Learning Disability, a community nurse gathered Mary's level of adaptive skills at the point of original assessment and repeated this after six months. Analysis of the two DLD scores revealed that Mary's cognitive and social scores increased over a six-month period, indicating an increase in impairment over this period. Over the six-month period Mary also started becoming incontinent, slightly unsteady while walking, and unable to feed herself neatly as she used to do.

An occupational therapist also completed an assessment of Mary's motor and processing skills.

A diagnosis of dementia was made by the psychiatrist after analysing the information gathered over a period of nearly a year.

Table 18.5 Evidence base for medication treatment in dementia

Drugs for cognitive symptoms of dementia	Overview of evidence from specific medicine trials of benefits in dementia
Acetyl cholinesterase inhibitors Donepezil Galantamine Rivastigmine	The three-acetyl cholinesterase (AChE) inhibitors donepezil, galantamine, and rivastigmine are recommended as options for managing mild to moderate Alzheimer's disease (National Institute for Health and Care Excellence, 2018). Evidence in people with intellectual disability and dementia is limited. A Cochrane review on pharmacological interventions for

Table 18.5 (cont.)

Drugs for cognitive symptoms of dementia	Overview of evidence from specific medicine trials of benefits in dementia
	cognitive decline in people with Down syndrome in 2015 found only 9 studies that met the selection criteria of a randomised controlled trial. Out of the 9 studies, 4 assessed the effectiveness of donepezil, 2 assessed memantine, one each assessed simvastatin, acetyl L-carnitine and antioxidants. Due to the low quality of evidence, the review was unable to draw any conclusions (Livingstone et al., 2015).
	Double-blind placebo-controlled trial of donepezil showed that the improvement at 24 weeks was statistically non-significant. The sample size of the study was too small to explore the efficacy in the subgroups of mild to moderate disease (Prasher et al., 2002).
	Open-label study on donepezil. Treatment resulted in significant improvement in scores on the Down Syndrome Dementia Scale. However, there were methodological drawbacks (Lott et al., 2002)
	Open-label study on donepezil treatment for people with Down syndrome. Treatment with this antidementia drug was associated with initial improvement in global functioning and adaptive behaviours. Follow-up at 104 weeks found that, while there was deterioration in both treatment and control groups, it was significantly less in the treatment group (Prasher et al., 2003).
	People who were treated with rivastigmine had less decline over 24 weeks in global functioning and adaptive behaviours (Prasher et al., 2005).
	Randomised placebo control trial on 21 Down syndrome patients (45 years of age), treated with 3mg donepezil over 24 weeks concluded that donepezil can help improve general functioning and severe cognitive impairment effectively and safely in people with Down syndrome (Kondoh et al., 2011).
	There were no statistically significant differences between different classes of antidementia medication, although prescription of cholinesterase inhibitors (either alone or in combination with memantine) was consistently associated with a lower hazard ratio of death than prescription of memantine alone (Eady et al., 2018).
NMDA antagonist Memantine	Memantine is recommended as an option for managing Alzheimer's disease for people with moderate Alzheimer's disease who have non-cognitive symptoms and/or behaviour that challenges and are intolerant of or have a contraindication to acetyl cholinesterase inhibitors, as well as people with severe Alzheimer's disease.
	A prospective randomised double-blind control trial comparing memantine with placebo in people with Down syndrome did not find any significant difference (Hanney et al., 2012). However, this study used patients with Down syndrome with and without a clinical diagnosis of dementia and therefore limits the scope of clinical implication.

The Evidence Base for Treatments

The Frith Treatment Guidelines for People with Intellectual Disability

Medications only have a limited role in the management of dementia. Table 18.5 summarises the evidence base in this area. Detailed guidance on the management of dementia in people with intellectual disability is available in the Faculty of Intellectual Disability of the Royal College of Psychiatrists document (see Resource Box). The key principles in the use of medications for dementia in people with intellectual disability are summarised in the following sections.

Medications for the Cognitive Symptoms of Dementia

Several medications are used in delaying the progress of dementia, as in the general population. The evidence base for the use of medication in people with intellectual disability is currently limited and with low evidence. Studies failed to address the impact of these pharmacological interventions on carer stress and institutional/home care.

Algorithm: Medications for the Cognitive Symptoms of Dementia

Figure 18.3 presents an algorithm for guidance in the use of antidementia medication in people with intellectual disability.

Medications for the Behavioural and Psychological Symptoms of Dementia in Intellectual Disability

Behavioural and Psychiatric Symptoms of Dementia (BPSD) are a core part of the syndrome of dementia. These include agitation, aggression, wandering, hoarding, sexual disinhibition, shouting, repeated questioning, sleep disturbance, depression, anxiety, and psychosis. They can cause significant distress and harm to patients and their carers and reduce overall quality of life. The number, type, and severity of BPSD symptoms varies between patients and multiple symptoms often occur at the same time, making it difficult to specifically target each one therapeutically. Management of BPSD is widely debated due to both lack of data and severe adverse drug reactions linked to majority of therapeutic agents, with non-medication interventions being tried before the medication treatment.

Non-Medication Management of Behavioural and Psychiatric Symptoms of Dementia in Intellectual Disability

The National Institute for Health and Care Excellence (2018) recommends non-medication interventions (i.e., aromatherapy, multisensory stimulation, massage, animal therapy and music therapy; Table 18.6) as first-line treatments for BPSD with the use of antipsychotic medications as a last resort. These non-pharmacological interventions not only target specific BPSD behaviour but also improve the quality of live in people with dementia. Given the lack of studies and recommendations around non-pharmacological interventions for BPSD in people with intellectual disability, the recommendations for the general population should be considered.

Diagnosis of probable Alzheimer's disease in adults with Intellectual disability:
- Assessment as outlined in Table 18.3
- Rule out other causes of cognitive decline. Treat other causes if found.
- Bear in mind dementia can co-exist with other conditions.
- Diagnosis of dementia is made by carefully evaluating all information from history, mental state, cognitive assessments, investigations.
- Ideally this should be undertaken through a multidisciplinary discussion to pull together information from all professionals.

Dementia of Alzheimer's type, **consider using anti-dementia drugs** following the NICE guidelines:
- Consider the risks and benefits of treatment with anti-dementia drugs.
- Discuss the risks and benefits with users/carers.
- Gain user consent or best interest for treatment.
- Carry out electrocardiogram (ECG) if necessary.
- Agree the follow up plan and how the effect of medication would be monitored.

Begin treatment with donepezil, galantamine, rivastigmine or memantine at the minimum possible dose.
Monitor closely for any adverse drug reactions – establish telephone link with carers. Additional support from nurses or other professionals for closer monitoring where this is necessary.

Reassess the patient in clinic after 4 weeks:
- Efficacy of treatment, especially in key problem areas
- Any serious adverse drug reactions; stop the drug.
- Consider increasing the dose if needed.

Continue to monitor closely for:
- Clinical improvement
- Any adverse drug reactions

Reassess clinically at end of 3 and 6 months:
- Re-assess key problem areas ideally using a structured instrument like DLD.
- Be prepared to stop drug treatment in those who show no benefit after 24 weeks or earlier if there are severe side effects

Continue treatment in those who show benefit and reassess at the end of 10–12 months:

If treatment is continued beyond 12 months:
- Continue to monitor patient at 6-month intervals as a minimum.
- Prepare carers for possible discontinuation of treatment in the future, e.g., progression to late stage of the disease

Figure 18.3 Algorithm demonstrating the diagnosis and treatment of dementia in adults with intellectual disability

Table 18.6 Non-medication management for Behavioural and Psychiatric Symptoms of Dementia (BPSD). Modified after Cerejeira et al. (2012) and Abraha et al. (2017)

Non-medication treatment	Effect on BPSD symptoms
Cognitive/emotion-oriented interventions (reminiscence therapy, simulated presence therapy, validation therapy)	Improves quality of life, general behaviour, communication, and interaction, albeit with limited evidence in more advanced stages of dementia
Sensory stimulation interventions (acupuncture, shiatsu and acupressure, aromatherapy, light therapy, massage/touch, sensory garden and horticultural activities, music and dance therapy, art and craft therapy, Snoezelen multisensory stimulation, transcutaneous electrical nerve stimulation)	Improves sleep and daytime behaviour, depression and wondering, and may decrease agitation
Behaviour management techniques	Reduction in problematic behaviour (i.e., agitation, wondering, anxiety, aggression)
Other psychosocial interventions such as animal-assisted therapy, doll therapy, environmental modification (i.e., dining room environment), and exercise	Decreases depression, anxiety, and agitation and improves boredom, motor activity, and brings positive emotions

An individually tailored, person-centred approach to meet the needs of the person with intellectual disability and dementia should be the first response to BPSD. This should include both responsive approach and planned activities (Backhouse et al., 2016). The responsive strategies would be beneficial in preventing BPSD or de-escalating behaviours in people who already have Behavioural and Psychiatric Symptoms of Dementia. Strategies could include social relevant activities, such as offering a cup of tea, playing favourite music or a film, playing football, or going out for a walk. These activities all help to de-escalate problem behaviour, such as agitation, wandering, and even aggression. However, people with intellectual disability and dementia experiencing BPSD are usually those with greater physical or mental impairments and may face greater barriers to accessing these interventions than those with higher capacity and functioning. It is thus not surprising that they may be enrolled in prearranged rather than responsive approaches to a non-pharmacological intervention(s) in order to prevent or to de-escalate their BPSD symptoms (Backhouse et al., 2016). One such group activity that has shown good outcomes is mindfulness-based intervention; this has not only beneficial effects (i.e., relaxation, awareness, acceptance, and resilience) in early stages of dementia (Berk et al., 2019) but also reduces anxiety in people with intellectual disability, with this benefit maintained over six weeks of follow-up (Idusohan-Moizer et al., 2015). This suggests that a structured mindfulness-based cognitive therapy group programme adapted for adults with intellectual disability may be a novel non-medication approach in the management of BPSD.

Algorithm for the Treatment of Behavioural and Psychological Symptoms of Dementia

The algorithm in Figure 18.4 is as applied to the general population with dementia and BPSD, but the principle is translational to people with intellectual disability and dementia. Please note that the flow chart does not cover rapid tranquilisation of the acutely disturbed patients.

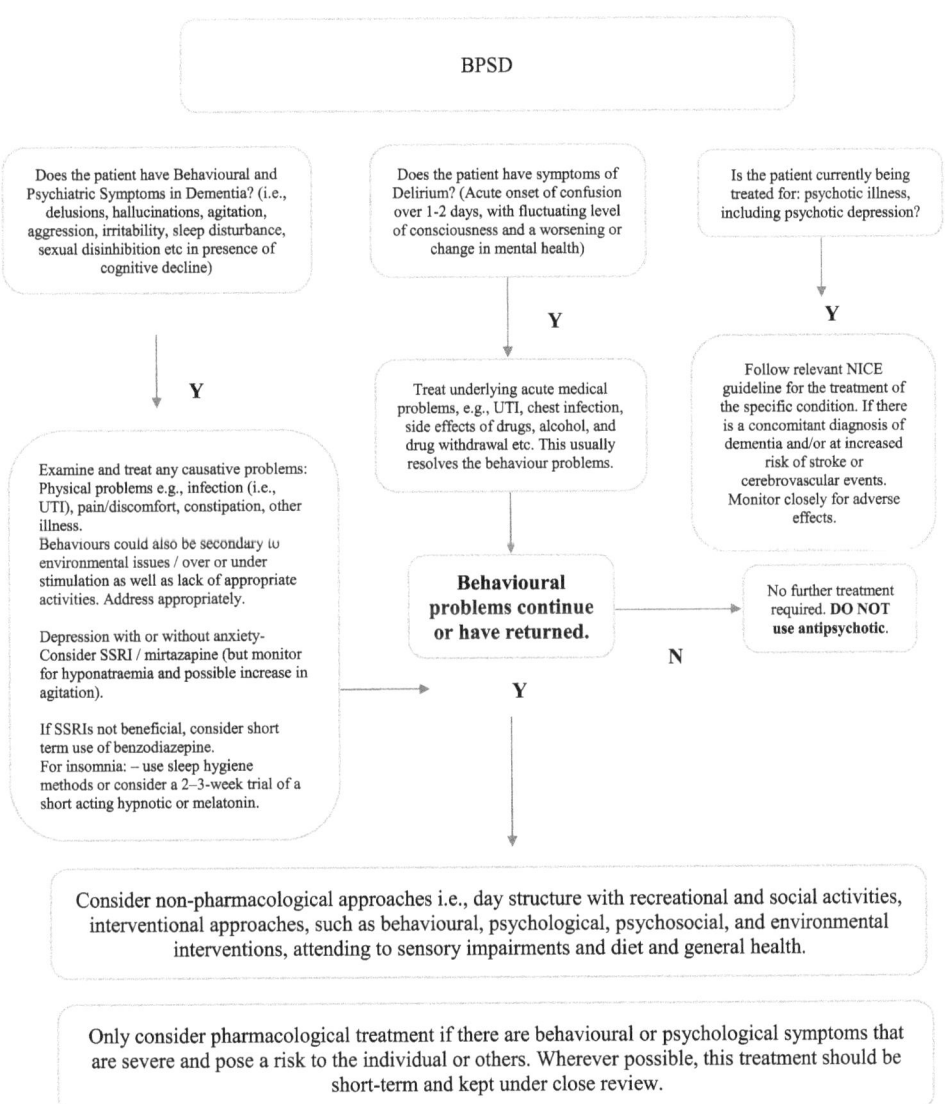

Figure 18.4 Algorithm for the treatment of Behavioural and Psychological Symptoms of Dementia

Medications for Behavioural and Psychiatric Symptoms of Dementia

Medication treatments have only a limited role in the management of BPSD symptoms in people with intellectual disability and dementia. Medication should only be considered if:

- Other environmental/psychosocial approaches have produced limited or no benefits, and
- BPSD pose a significant safety risk or cause a great distress.

Use of medications should only be considered after a careful evaluation of the risks and benefits in each individual circumstance.

The following principles should be utilised:

➢ The risks and benefits should be shared with the individual (if the individual is able to understand the information) and carers. Cerebrovascular risk factors should be discussed highlighting the possible increased risk of stroke/transient ischaemic attack. Possible adverse effects on cognition should be discussed.
➢ Target symptoms are identified and monitored regularly.
➢ Changes in cognition should be assessed and recorded at regular intervals.
➢ Medication should be started at the lowest possible dose and titrated slowly. The effective dose of the medication should be continued.
➢ Treatment should be time limited and regularly reviewed (every 3 months or according to clinical need).

Table 18.7 gives an overview of medications prescribed for the behavioural and psychological symptoms of dementia.

Table 18.7 Medications for behavioural and psychological symptoms of dementia: There is currently no evidence for the use of these medications in people with intellectual disability and dementia. The table therefore summarises the evidence from non-intellectual disability population (National Institute for Health and Care Excellence, 2018; Bessey & Walaszek, 2019).

Drugs for BPSD	Overview of evidence base
Antipsychotics	Second-generation antipsychotics were once widely recommended in dementia-related behavioural disturbances, but their use now is highly controversial. Three reasons for this are: 1. small effect size, 2. poor tolerability and 3. tentative association with increased mortality.
Evidence from non-intellectual disability population: minor effectiveness advantages for olanzapine and risperidone over placebo but all medications were poorly tolerated due to sedation, confusion, and extrapyramidal side effects.
In the United Kingdom and the USA, warnings have been issued regarding increased mortality with olanzapine, risperidone, quetiapine, and aripiprazole when used in dementia due to an association with stroke.
The first-line antipsychotic is risperidone (0.25–2mg/day), and it is the only licenced antipsychotic for short-term treatment of

Table 18.7 (cont.)

Drugs for BPSD	Overview of evidence base
	BPSD. Where risperidone is ineffective or contraindicated consider olanzapine 2.5–10mg/day. In patients with Parkinson's disease or dementia with Lewy bodies, if both the above medications are ineffective or contraindicated, consider quetiapine 12.5–300mg/day; aripiprazole 5–15mg/day. Where all other antipsychotics have been ineffective/contraindicated, consider amisulpiride 25–50mg/day. Clozapine may be used in complex cases or patients with Parkinson's disease/dementia with Lewy bodies where other options have been ineffective.
	Traditional antipsychotic medications like sulpiride have also been used, although sedation and anticholinergic effects can cause deterioration of cognitive impairment.
Acetylcholinesterase inhibitors and memantine	People with mild to moderate Alzheimer's disease who have non-cognitive symptoms (BPSD) may be offered an acetylcholinesterase inhibitor if a non-medication approach is inappropriate or has been ineffective, and antipsychotic drugs are inappropriate or have been ineffective.
	People with moderate to severe Alzheimer's disease who are intolerant of or have a contraindication to acetylcholinesterase inhibitors may be offered memantine.
Antidepressants	To treat symptoms of depression, selective serotonin reuptake inhibitors (SSRIs) and mirtazapine (15–30 mg daily) are preferred but attention is needed to the risk of developing low sodium levels. Sertraline has some evidence for its effectiveness in the treatment of depression in dementia.
	There is emerging evidence that SSRIs may be used for treatment of agitation in dementia. Many clinicians prefer trazodone (50–150mg daily as a single or divided dose), for which also there is some evidence available. However, caution and regular monitoring is recommended in the light of its numerous side effects, including confusion and cardiotoxicity.
Mood stabilisers	Medications such as carbamazepine or sodium valproate may be considered if there is evidence of rapid cycling mood disorder or significant mood fluctuations, and if other options proved to be ineffective or contraindicated.
Analgesics	Paracetamol, 500–1000mg up to four times/day, may be beneficial even in patients without overt pain symptoms. Please note that acetylcholinesterase inhibitors, esp. donepezil, are also known to be efficient analgesics.
Benzodiazepines	Lorazepam, 0.5–2mg daily in divided doses, may be cautiously considered for short periods in severe acute distress.

Case Study 18.1 (cont.)

Peter's psychiatrist discussed the role of antidementia medications with Peter and his parents. They were given accessible information on the medications, which they discussed at home. As Peter lacked capacity to consent, a best interest meeting was held to agree prescribing an antidementia medication. After undertaking an ECG, Peter was prescribed donepezil 5mg. An assessment was agreed after two weeks of prescription to check if Peter is tolerating the medication well, with further assessments at two months and four months to check the response and consider increasing the dose of medication. Peter and his parents were informed that the medication will not cure or stop the progression of dementia but only delay the progress. There were informed of the need for withdrawing this medication once Peter's dementia has progressed to later stages.

Peter benefitted from the use of 10mg of donepezil, and the improvement that it brought enabled the nurse and psychiatrist to work with carers and consider additional strategies to support Peter, which included a communication plan, adaptation of the environment, and a life story book, along with training of family and care staff on dementia and how to support Peter through the various stages of his dementia.

End-of-Life Care in Dementia

Person-centred care with proactive approaches, early identification of the end-of-life status, and effective communication between professionals, carers, and family are essential to providing a good quality support at this stage.

Key focus in end-of-life care includes a clear nutrition and feeding plan, management of pain, management of seizures and recurrent infections, and prevention of inappropriate hospital admissions. Tools to aid assessment of physical symptoms include the DisDAT (Distress Assessment Tool), developed for people with severe communication problems including those with intellectual disability. The REPOS (Rotterdam Elderly Pain Observation Scale) and the Abbey Pain Scale are other options; however, DisDAT is more frequently used in people with intellectual disability Where possible, due consideration should be given to where the person would like to spend their last days of life and any advanced decisions should be respected.

The National Institute for Health and Care Excellence (2015) guideline on 'Care of dying adults in the last days of life' provides guidance on recognising when a person may be in the last days of life and the importance of communication, shared decision making, maintaining hydration, principles of pharmacological interventions, and anticipatory prescribing.

End-of-life care medications (anticipatory medicines) that can be used to manage symptoms are as follows (National Institute for Health and Care Excellence, 2015):

1. Pain can be managed in palliative care with use of morphine, diamorphine, oxycodone, or alfentanil.
2. Breathlessness can be managed with midazolam or an opioid.
3. Anxiety can be managed by midazolam.
4. Delirium and agitation can be managed by haloperidol, levomepromazine, midazolam, or phenobarbital.

5. Nausea and vomiting can be managed by cyclizine, metoclopramide, haloperidol, or levomepromazine.
6. Noisy chest secretions can be managed by hyoscine hydrobromide or glycopyrronium.

Ultimately, it is equally important to get dying right as much as living.

Conclusion

People with intellectual disability in general, and those with Down syndrome in particular, have a higher prevalence of dementia. The timely diagnosis of dementia helps with appropriate management of the cognitive impairment and associated psychological and behavioural symptoms. There are significant challenges to both assessment and making a diagnosis. This chapter provides the principles of assessment and signposts to more detailed guidance. There is generally a lack of evidence for both antidementia medications and treatment of BPSD for people with intellectual disability. This chapter provides evidence relevant to people with intellectual disability where this is available and, where this is lacking, guidance is drawn from evidence that exist for the population without intellectual disability. One needs to consider the use of these approaches in a person-centred manner after carefully evaluating the risk and benefits as well as making every effort to involve the person with intellectual disability and/or their carers.

Finally, apart from assessment and management of dementia, it is equally important to support the patient, family, and carers in a compassionate and therapeutic manner.

The Frith Prescribing Guidelines Editors' Expert Group Consensus Statements

Statements of High Confidence

- There is a high prevalence of dementia in people with intellectual disability, especially those with Down syndrome
- Onset of dementia in people with Down syndrome is significantly earlier than in the general population.

Statements of Medium Confidence

- There is some evidence of the usefulness of current antidementia medications: cholinesterase inhibitors such as donepezil and rivastigmine for treatment of dementia in people with Down syndrome.
- People with Down syndrome experience higher levels of adverse events when treated with the above antidementia medications.

Statements of Low Confidence

- Use of antidementia medications other than donepezil and rivastigmine in the treatment of dementia in people with intellectual disability has no or very limited evidence
- Simvastatin may have a slight improvement in cognitive measures in people with Down syndrome.

For the treatment of BPSD, the use of psychotropic medications and/or memantine has no evidence from intellectual disability population. Therefore, data from general population is extrapolated to give recommendations in this guidance.

> **Resource Box**
>
> The British Psychological Society and the Royal College of Psychiatrists (2009, updated April 2015). Dementia and People with Learning Disabilities; Guidance on the assessment, diagnosis, treatment and support of people with learning disabilities who develop dementia. www.bps.org.uk/guideline/dementia-and-people-intellectual-disabilities
>
> National Institute for Health and Care Excellence. (2015, December 16). Care of dying adults in the last days of life. NICE Guideline [NG31]. www.nice.org.uk/guidance/ng31.
>
> National Institute for Health and Care Excellence. (2018, June 20). Dementia: assessment, management and support for people living with dementia and their carers. NICE Guideline [NG97]. www.nice.org.uk/guidance/ng97.
>
> National Institute of Health and Care Excellence (2011; last updated June 2018), donepezil, galantamine, rivastigmine and memantine for the treatment of Alzheimer's disease, Technology appraisal guidance (TA 217). www.nice.org.uk/guidance/ta217.

References

Abraha, I., Rimland, J. M., Trotta, F. M., et al. (2017). Systematic review of systematic reviews of non-pharmacological interventions to treat behavioural disturbances in older patients with dementia. The SENATOR-OnTop series. *BMJ Open*, 7(3), e012759. https://doi.org/10.1136/bmjo pen-2016-012759.

Albert, M., & Cohen, C. (1992). The Test for Severe Impairment: An Instrument for the Assessment of Patients with Severe Cognitive Dysfunction. *Journal of the American Geriatrics Society*, 40(5), 449–453. https://doi.org/10.1111/j.1532-5415.1992.tb02009.x.

American Psychiatric Association. (2013). *DSM 5 Intellectual Disability*. American Psychiatric Association. www.psychiatry.org/File%20Lib rary/Psychiatrists/Practice/DSM/APA_DS M-5-Intellectual-Disability.pdf.

Backhouse, T., Killett, A., Penhale, B., & Gray, R. (2016). The use of non-pharmacological interventions for dementia behaviours in care homes: findings from four in-depth, ethnographic case studies. *Age and Ageing*, 45(6), 856–63. https://doi.org/10.1093/age ing/afw136.

Ball, S. L., Holland, A. J., Huppert, F. A., et al. (2004). The modified CAMDEX informant interview is a valid and reliable tool for use in the diagnosis of dementia in adults with Down's syndrome. *Journal of Intellectual Disability Research*, 48(6), 611–20. https://doi.org/10.1111/j.1365-2788.2004.00630.x.

Ball, S. L., Holland, A. J., Treppner, P., Watson, P. C., & Huppert, F. A. (2008). Executive dysfunction and its association with personality and behaviour changes in the development of Alzheimer's disease in adults with Down syndrome and mild to moderate learning disabilities. *British Journal of Clinical Psychology*, 47(1), 1–29. https://doi.org/10.1348/014466507X230967.

Berk, L., Warmenhoven, F., Stiekema, A. P. M., et al. (2019). Mindfulness-Based Intervention for People With Dementia and Their Partners: Results of a Mixed-Methods Study. *Frontiers in Aging Neuroscience*, 11. https://doi.org/10.3389/fnagi.2019.00092.

Bessey, L. J., & Walaszek, A. (2019). Management of Behavioral and Psychological Symptoms of Dementia. *Current Psychiatry Reports*, 21(8), 66. https://doi.org/10.1007/s11920-019-1049-5.

Carulla, L. S., Reed, G. M., Vaez-Azizi, L. M., et al. (2011). Intellectual developmental disorders: towards a new name, definition and framework for 'mental retardation/ intellectual disability' in ICD-11. *World Psychiatry*, **10**(3), 175–80. https://doi.org/10.1002/j.2051-5545.2011.tb00045.x.

Cerejeira, J., Lagarto, L., & Mukaetova-Ladinska, E. B. (2012). Behavioral and psychological symptoms of dementia. *Frontiers in Neurology*, **3**. https://doi.org/10.3389/fneur.2012.00073.

Cosgrave, M. P., Tyrrell, J., McCarron, M., Gill, M., & Lawlor, B. A. (2000). A five year follow-up study of dementia in persons with Down's syndrome: early symptoms and patterns of deterioration. *Irish Journal of Psychological Medicine*, **17**(1), 5–11. https://doi.org/10.1017/S0790966700003943.

Deb, S., Hare, M., & Prior, L. (2007). Symptoms of dementia among adults with Down's syndrome: A qualitative study. *Journal of Intellectual Disability Research*, **51**(9), 726–39. https://doi.org/10.1111/j.1365-2788.2007.00956.x.

Eady, N., Sheehan, R., Rantell, K., et al. (2018). Impact of cholinesterase inhibitors or memantine on survival in adults with Down syndrome and dementia: Clinical cohort study. *The British Journal of Psychiatry*, **212**(3), 155–60. https://doi.org/10.1192/bjp.2017.21.

Evenhuis, H. M. (2018). The Dementia Questionnaire for People with Learning Disabilities. In *Neuropsychological Assessments of Dementia in Down Syndrome and Intellectual Disabilities* (pp. 43–56). Springer International Publishing. https://doi.org/10.1007/978-3-319-61720-6_3.

Hanney, M., Prasher, V., Williams, N., et al. (2012). Memantine for dementia in adults older than 40 years with Down's syndrome (MEADOWS): A randomised, double-blind, placebo-controlled trial. *The Lancet*, **379**(9815), 528–36. https://doi.org/10.1016/S0140-6736(11)61676-0.

Berk, L., Warmenhoven, F., Stiekema, A. P. M., et al. (2019). Mindfulness-Based intervention for people with dementia and their partners: Results of a mixed-methods study. *Frontiers in Aging Neuroscience*, **11**. https://doi.org/10.3389/fnagi.2019.00092.

Haxby, J. V. (1989). Neuropsychological evaluation of adults with Down's syndrome: Patterns of selective impairment in non-demented old adults. *Journal of Mental Deficiency Research*, **33** (Pt 3), 193–210. https://doi.org/10.1111/j.1365-2788.1989.tb01467.x.

Livingstone, N., Hanratty, J., McShane, R., & Macdonald, G. (2015). Pharmacological interventions for cognitive decline in people with Down syndrome. *Cochrane Database of Systematic Reviews*, **2015**(10). https://doi.org/10.1002/14651858.CD011546.pub2.

Idusohan-Moizer, H., Sawicka, A., Dendle, J., & Albany, M. (2015). Mindfulness-based cognitive therapy for adults with intellectual disabilities: An evaluation of the effectiveness of mindfulness in reducing symptoms of depression and anxiety. *Journal of Intellectual Disability Research*, **59**(2), 93–104. https://doi.org/10.1111/jir.12082.

Joint Standing Committee of the British Psychological Society and the Royal College of Psychiatrists. (2015). Dementia and People with Intellectual Disabilities: Cover. British Psychological Society. https://doi.org/10.53841/bpsrep.2015.rep77.

Jozsvai, E., Kartakis, P., & Gedye, A. (2009). Dementia Scale for Down Syndrome. In V. Prasher (ed.), *Neuropsychological Assessments of Dementia in Down Syndrome and Intellectual Disabilities* (pp. 53–66). Springer. https://doi.org/10.1007/978-1-84800-249-4_4.

Kondoh, T., Kanno, A., Itoh, H., et al. (2011). Donepezil significantly improves abilities in daily lives of female Down syndrome patients with severe cognitive impairment: A 24-week randomized, double-blind, placebo-controlled trial. *The International Journal of Psychiatry in Medicine*, **41**(1), 71–89. https://doi.org/10.2190/PM.41.1.g.

Livingstone, N., Hanratty, J., McShane, R., & Macdonald, G. (2015). Pharmacological interventions for cognitive decline in people with Down syndrome. *Cochrane Database of Systematic Reviews*, **2015**(10). https://doi.org/10.1002/14651858.CD011546.pub2.

Lott, I. T., Osann, K., Doran, E., & Nelson, L. (2002). Down syndrome and Alzheimer disease. *Archives of Neurology*, 59(7), 1133. https://doi.org/10.1001/archneur.59.7.1133.

Montero-Odasso, M., Ismail, Z., & Livingston, G. (2020). One-third of dementia cases can be prevented within the next 25 years by tackling risk factors. The case 'for' and 'against.' *Alzheimer's Research & Therapy*, 12(1), 81. https://doi.org/10.1186/s13195-020-00646-x.

Moran, J. A., Rafii, M. S., Keller, S. M., Singh, B. K., & Janicki, M. P. (2013). The national task group on intellectual disabilities and dementia practices consensus recommendations for the evaluation and management of dementia in adults with intellectual disabilities. *Mayo Clinic Proceedings*, 88(8), 831–40. https://doi.org/10.1016/j.mayocp.2013.04.024.

National Institute of Aging (NIA). (1989). The Daily Living Skills Questionnaire (DLSQ). www.nia.nih.gov/.

Prasher, V. P., Adams, C., & Holder, R. (2003). Long-term safety and efficacy of donepezil in the treatment of dementia in Alzheimer's disease in adults with Down syndrome: Open label study. *International Journal of Geriatric Psychiatry*, 18(6), 549–51. https://doi.org/10.1002/gps.859.

Prasher, V. P., Fung, N., & Adams, C. (2005). Rivastigmine in the treatment of dementia in Alzheimer's disease in adults with Down syndrome. *International Journal of Geriatric Psychiatry*, 20(5), 496–7. https://doi.org/10.1002/gps.1306.

Prasher, Vee. P., Huxley, A., & Haque, M. S. (2002). A 24-week, double-blind, placebo-controlled trial of donepezil in patients with Down syndrome and Alzheimer's disease – pilot study. *International Journal of Geriatric Psychiatry*, 17(3), 270–8. https://doi.org/10.1002/gps.587.

Prince, M., Knapp, M., Maelenn, G., et al. (2014). Dementia UK: Update (Doctoral dissertation, King's College London).

Robertson, J., Hatton, C., Emerson, E., & Baines, S. (2015). Prevalence of epilepsy among people with intellectual disabilities: A systematic review. *Seizure*, 29, 46–62. https://doi.org/10.1016/j.seizure.2015.03.016.

Strydom, A., Chan, T., King, M., Hassiotis, A., & Livingston, G. (2013). Incidence of dementia in older adults with intellectual disabilities. *Research in Developmental Disabilities*, 34(6), 1881–5. https://doi.org/10.1016/j.ridd.2013.02.021.

Strydom, A., Livingston, G., King, M., & Hassiotis, A. (2007). Prevalence of dementia in intellectual disability using different diagnostic criteria. *British Journal of Psychiatry*, 191(2), 150–7. https://doi.org/10.1192/bjp.bp.106.028845.

Sturmey, P., Tsiouris, J. A., & Patti, P. (2003). The psychometric properties of the Multi-Dimensional Observation Scale for Elderly Subjects (MOSES) in middle aged and older populations of people with mental retardation. *International Journal of Geriatric Psychiatry*, 18(2), 131–4. https://doi.org/10.1002/gps.730.

Visser, F. E., Aldenkamp, A. P., van Huffelen, A. C., et al. (1997). Prospective study of the prevalence of Alzheimer-type dementia in institutionalized individuals with Down syndrome. *American Journal of Mental Retardation*, 101(4), 400–12.

Chapter 19

Eating and Drinking Difficulties

Jennifer Worsfold, Jennifer Roberts, Nicky Calow, and David M. L. Branford

Introduction

The information in this chapter is intended as a guide to (a) help the physician to make a differential diagnosis when someone is presenting with an eating and drinking difficulty, (b) help the physician to decide when to refer to the specialist team for areas which need further investigation, and (c) understanding comorbidity with other conditions.

It is not the intention of this chapter to deal with all aspects of eating and drinking difficulties, just those aspects that impact on the choice or formulation of a medication. These include:

- administration of medications to people with intellectual disability and swallowing difficulties
- administration of medications via tubes (i.e., percutaneous endoscopic gastrostomy (PEG))
- medications that increase or reduce saliva production.

Eating and Drinking Difficulties and Dysphagia

What Are the Eating and Drinking Difficulties in People with Intellectual Disability?

Eating and drinking difficulties are highly prevalent in the intellectual disability population and include all aspects of the eating and drinking process. This can include achieving stable positioning, pacing the meal, and safe swallowing. Dysphagia is a subset of wider eating and drinking difficulties, often seen in the intellectual disability population (Chadwick and Joliffe 2009). Dysphagia presents as a difficulty with chewing and swallowing. It is often the underlying cause of malnutrition, dehydration, weight loss, choking, and aspiration pneumonia, with risks to mental health, social isolation, dignity, and enjoyment.

A deterioration in eating and drinking skills is often a symptom of a broader physical and/or mental health diagnosis. People with eating and drinking difficulties can also experience a cyclical decline in health and an increased risk of malnutrition and dehydration.

Dysphagia can be a contributing factor in recurrent aspiration pneumonia or chest infections (Langmore et al., 1998). 'Aspiration pneumonia is a three-phase process in which the patient (1) colonises pathogenic bacteria in the oropharynx, (2) aspirates the bacteria into the airway, and (3) is unable to clear the material and subsequently develops a bacterial infection in the respiratory system' (Langore, 2002).

Given this, it is clear that aspiration pneumonia can be directly caused by aspiration of any of ingested foods, fluids, infected secretions, vomit, and reflux, if ability to clear these from the lungs is compromised (Gupte, et al. 2022).

How Common Are Eating and Drinking Difficulties in People with Intellectual Disability?

In adults with intellectual disability, choking is often under-recognised and under-reported and represents a major cause of death (Trollor et al., 2017). Adults with intellectual disability are at greater risk of choking episodes compared to the general population (Samuels & Chadwick, 2006; Thacker et al., 2007; Finlayson et al., 2010). Hampshire's multi-agency review in 2010 suggested that choking could be related to five factors: dysphagia, poor oral hygiene, behaviours such as cramming food, pica, and effects of medication. The Belfast Health and Social Care Trust have created a specific set of resources to increase awareness of choking, causal factors and appropriate responses (see toolkit).

Robertson et al. (2017) reported a prevalence of dysphagia in 8.1–11.5% of adults known to formal intellectual disability services. The Learning Disability Mortality Review programme (LeDeR) found that of the people whose death was reported in 2019, 29% had a diagnosis of dysphagia, and dysphagia was included in each of the top three common combinations of long-term health conditions at death (Heslop et al., 2019). Evidence from the NHS digital website (https://digital.nhs.uk/data-and-information/publications/statistical/health-and-care-of-people-with-learning-disabilities/experimental-statistics-2021-to-2022) suggests that prevalence of dysphagia increases in the intellectual disability population as a person ages. The incidence of dysphagia stood at 9.2% of the intellectual disability population in 2021–2. It also suggests that the percentage of patients diagnosed with dysphagia has increased by 4% since 2017/18.

How Are Eating and Drinking Difficulties Different in People with Intellectual Disability?

Around 80% people with intellectual disability have communication difficulties (Royal College of Speech and Language Therapists (RCSLT: www.rcslt.org/wp-content/uploads/media/Project/RCSLT/rcslt-learning-disabilities-factsheet.pdf) and this means that many may not be able to communicate their needs, pain, or eating and drinking difficulties clearly. The clinician needs to consider changes in physical health and behaviour (see the Disability Distress Awareness Tool, DisDAT) as well as what is communicated verbally and carer reports in order to ensure a holistic overview of the presenting issue. For example, a common cause of chest infections can be gastro-oesophageal disease (Hibberd et al., 2009) so it is helpful to rule this out early on by assessment and trial of antireflux medication if there is an indication that reflux is occurring (National institute for Health and Care Excellence (NICE) CG184)).

A deterioration in chewing and swallowing skills is expected in the general ageing population (Feinberg et al., 1990), and in the intellectual disability population dysphagia often presents at an earlier age than in the general population (NHS digital dashboards: Health and Care of People with learning disabilities Jan 2023).

Intellectual Disability Conditions and Syndromes Associated with Eating and Drinking Difficulties

Table 19.1 lists some of the intellectual disability conditions and syndromes associated with eating and drinking difficulties and is adapted with kind permission from Chadwick and Jolliffe (2009).

Table 19.1 Some of the intellectual disability conditions and syndromes associated with eating and drinking difficulties

1: Syndromes and conditions associated with intellectual disability	Potential causes of eating and drinking difficulties
Down syndrome, William's syndrome, Fragile X syndrome, Rubinstein–Taybi syndrome	Associated oro-pharyngeal structural problems involving the palate, teeth and tongue and oral cavity.
Cerebral palsy, epilepsy, Down syndrome, Fragile X, Rett syndrome, and Noonan`s syndrome	Motor processing difficulties giving rise to muscle spasm, changes in muscle tone or muscle coordination, including abnormal tongue movements. Swallowing skills may deteriorate with age.
Intellectual disability and frequently associated impact of care situation	Higher levels of poor oral health are recorded among people with intellectual disability. Respiratory pathogens present in the dental plaque of individuals with very poor dental hygiene may be aspirated and predispose the individual to the development of lung infections. Dependence on others for food and drink; intellectual disability and/or history of institutionalisation making the person more susceptible to choking incidents (e.g., eating too quickly and cramming food).
1a : General medical conditions that can add to eating and drinking difficulties	**Potential causes of eating and drinking difficulties**
Asthma and COPD	Increase in oral transit time (Scarpel and Nóbrega 2021; Sugiya et al., 2022) Reduced tongue strength Increase risk of fatigue (Sugiya et al., 2022) Increased risk of choking. Variable cough strength.
Cardiovascular problems	Increased fatigue during eating and drinking (Ramachandran et al. 2022).

Symptoms Associated with Eating and Drinking Difficulties and Causes to Consider

Table 19.2 lists the symptoms associated with eating and drinking difficulties and the causes to consider.

Table 19.2 Symptoms associated with eating and drinking difficulties and the causes to consider

Symptom domain	Causes to consider
Weight loss	Poor dietary intake Poor positioning for eating and drinking. Infection Weight loss as part of another diagnosis (e.g., carcinoma) Gastrointestinal <ul><li>Malabsorption</li><li>Dietary intolerance</li></ul>Poor dentition Neuromuscular <ul><li>Loss of motor coordination to feed self.</li><li>Dysphagia/swallowing difficulties</li></ul>Iatrogenic <ul><li>Medication side effects</li></ul>Mental health factors <ul><li>Depression, bereavement</li><li>Psychosis</li><li>Eating Disorders including ARFID (Avoidant Restrictive Food Intake Disorder)</li></ul>A means for the patient to control something in their life. Dementia Behavioural issues Distraction due to environment
Dehydration	Poor fluid intake Self-restricting fluid intake to avoid frequent urination or incontinence Poor positioning leading to loss of fluid Kidney disorders Gastrointestinal <ul><li>Malabsorption</li></ul>Dental sensitivity Mental health factors <ul><li>Mood disorder</li><li>Psychosis</li></ul>

Table 19.2 (cont.)

Symptom domain	Causes to consider
	• Eating disorder including ARFID • Dementia, varying levels of alertness Forgetting to drink Embarrassment relating to poor oral control or coughing Neuromuscular • Loss of motor coordination to give oneself a drink • Reduced control of fluid in the mouth leading to anterior loss. Loss of saliva, mouth breathing Fluid loss through body temperature fluctuation
Pain on/after eating	Poor dentition Oral Thrush Gastro-oesophageal stricture Crico-pharyngeal spasm (Feeling of a 'lump in the throat' due to muscle spasm) Gastro-oesophageal disease/reflux Helicobacter pylori infection Muscle tension relating to anxiety
Coughing at meals	Postural and positioning needs Changes to motor skills or muscle tone Overfilling mouth/cramming Rushing – either from self or carer Reduced chewing ability Dysphagia/swallowing disorder Gastro-oesophageal reflux Crico-pharyngeal spasm Pharyngeal pouch Medication-induced dysphagia Changes to cognition, attention, memory or mental health. Structural changes to anatomy Respiratory compromise (e.g., chronic obstructive pulmonary disease (COPD), Chronic asthma) Reduced oral sensitivity
Recurrent chest infections	Asthma COPD and other respiratory conditions Chronic smoking Poor oral hygiene Dysphagia leading to aspiration of food or drink Aspirated reflux Aspirated vomit Regurgitation Aspiration of infected saliva

Table 19.2 (cont.)

Symptom domain	Causes to consider
Choking	Respiratory compromise (e.g., chronic asthma, COPD) Inappropriate food texture Reduced oral sensitivity Overfilling mouth Rushing Dysphagia/swallowing problems Cognition, attention and environment
Food loss from mouth, food on clothes	Poor positioning Loss of motor skills/coordination of motor skills Abnormal muscle tone (Increased or decreased) Tremor, including medication-induced Reduced oral sensitivity

Medications Commonly Used in Intellectual Disability That May Affect Swallowing

Table 19.3 shows the possible side effects of medications commonly prescribed in the intellectual disability population, which may contribute to dysphagia.

> **Case Study 19.1**
>
> Meena, a 45-year-old woman with mild intellectual disability, quadriplegic cerebral palsy with contractures in arms and legs and behaviour that challenges, visits her general practitioner for an annual health check. It comes to light that Meena has suffered three chest infections in the last six months, has reduced appetite, and over that time her weight has dropped from 45 kg (body mass index 18) to 40 kg (body mass index 16)
>
> Following the annual health check, Meena's GP advised her carers to visit the dentist to rule out dentition as a cause for her reduced appetite. The GP examines her mouth and notes she does not have oral thrush, carries out a urine dip test reviews medication, and prescribes interim oral supplements. The GP refers Meena to the dietetic service for nutritional review because the weight loss is above 10% and because of her low body mass index. The GP also refers to the specialist intellectual disability multidisciplinary team for further assessment relating to her chest infections.

Referral to the Multidisciplinary Team

An annual health check is a good place to identify eating and drinking difficulties. It is helpful if the physician can identify if there is:
- a more general deterioration in health occurring and, in which case, begin investigation/treatment

Table 19.3 Possible side effects of medications commonly prescribed in the intellectual disability population which may contribute to dysphagia

Medications	Effect on swallowing mechanism
Muscle relaxants (e.g., benzodiazepines, baclofen)	Reduced tone of swallowing muscles, difficulty in beginning/coordinating muscle movements that allow passage of food bolus from mouth to stomach
Tricyclic antidepressants, some antipsychotics, anticholinergics	Decreased salivation causes dry mouth that can make food bolus 'sticky' and increase risk of choking. May also reduce taste and smell sensations. Drug-induced Parkinsonism (mainly associated with dopamine) Tardive dyskinesia Tardive dyskinesia (from chronic use of antipsychotics) Long-term lithium use can impact on how food tastes and impact sensory feedback leading to cramming behaviours.
Psychotropic medication	Altered levels of alertness
Some antipsychotics, especially clozapine	Increased salivation causing drooling and dribbling, potential to cause choking episodes particularly where swallowing is already compromised (e.g., in cerebral palsy/head injury)

- an underlying gastro-oesophageal reflux issue which can be proactively managed (National Institute for Health and Care Excellence (NICE) CG 184)
- recent behaviour changes, which may indicate the patient is experiencing pain or discomfort.

Triggers for referral to the MDT include:
- Recurrent chest infections
- Diagnosis of aspiration pneumonia
- Weight loss
- Refusal to eat
- Distress at meals
- Coughing at mealtimes
- Changes to eating and drinking support needs.

The Frith Treatment Guideline for People with Intellectual Disability

Management of Eating and Drinking Difficulties

The multidisciplinary team (MDT) should include the person, their family, their carers, and other professionals involved in the assessment. Integrating each member of the team's clinical priorities and risk considerations can be difficult but the clinician must follow the principles of the Mental Capacity Act (2005) and Mental Health Act (2017). A speech therapist can help with ensuring the patient understands, to the best of their ability the risks and the choices available to them, and is able to participate as far as possible in decisions regarding intervention and being able to express their wishes. See toolkit for easy-read health information.

Management of eating and drinking difficulties should be holistic; the care plan should be written by the MDT and strategies embedded in all the areas where the person may eat and drink. The least restrictive interventions need to be always considered first, in line with the Mental Capacity Act and Deprivation of Liberty Safeguards (UK). Examples of management plans and how to make reasonable adjustments can be found in the tool kit (www.gov.uk/government/publications/dysphagia-and-people-with-learning-disabilities/dysphagia-in-people-with-learning-difficulties-reasonable-adjustments-guidance).

The specialist intellectual disability multidisciplinary team can support with dysphagia in the following ways:

Equipment for Independence

Equipment may be recommended by a speech and language therapist (SLT) or occupational therapist (OT) to promote independence and support pacing. Cups, spoons, and specialist plates can be effective tools to support a patient's safe eating and drinking.

Positive Behavioural Support Strategies

Patients may engage in behaviours that increase their risk of choking, aspiration pneumonia, malnutrition, and dehydration. This presentation typically includes food refusal and rushing. Mealtime management should encourage independence and ensure mealtimes are as positive and enjoyable as possible. Strategies can be implemented directly with the patient or with families and carers, considering the patient's skill level and communication skills. For example, supporting a patient to eat and drink at an appropriate speed can sometimes prevent the patient being placed on a more restrictive diet, and restricting the flow of food onto the person's plate can enable a patient to continue to feed themselves but at a safe pace.

Posture and Positioning

Stable posture and positioning are vital to ensure good oral control, swallowing, support with breathing, and aid with digestion. Physiotherapists assess positioning to facilitate and optimise independent eating and drinking in order to:

- Support safe swallowing and reduce risk of aspiration
- Facilitate better chewing and control of the food and drink in the mouth

Positioning can be used after a meal to aid saliva and residue clearance through anterior loss.

Texture Modification

Texture modification and altering the consistency of fluids can be an important compensatory strategy but should be based on person's swallowing skill and other co-occurring conditions and should be assessed by the SLT.

The aim of texture modification is to pre-prepare the bolus based on the patient's chewing ability and swallowing competence. The SLT assesses and recommends according to textures described in the International Dysphagia Diet Standardisation Initiative (IDDSI 2019) to reduce risk of choking and aspiration but maintain the patient's skills. The IDDSI Framework provides a common terminology to describe food textures and drink thickness, it consists of 8 levels (0–7). The IDDSI is recognised globally and ensures consistency of approach.

Thickeners

Thickeners may be used to make management of fluids easier and safer at the oral and pharyngeal stages of the swallow; however, this should only be used when other strategies have been trialled unsuccessfully. A referral should be made to speech and language therapy for consideration of thickener due to the risk of possible contraindications, which include:

- Dehydration
- Constipation
- Refusal of fluids/reduced fluid intake
- Increased effort leading to fatigue
- Possible interactions with prescribed medication uptake
- Possible weight increase. (calories from the thickener)
- Effects on sodium levels (varies according to thickener)

(Beetz, 2003; Robbins et al., 2002; Chichero, 2013; Lazenby-Paterson, 2020).

There are gum and starch-based thickeners and pre-thickened products available to prescribe (see Table 19.4). Patient preference should always be taken into account.

Drinks can be thickened to a range of consistencies, and this will be recommended by the SLT following a detailed assessment according to IDDSI.

Some people with eating and drinking difficulties find swallowing medications in tablet form difficult. Consult with a pharmacist for alternative formulations if this is the case. Dispersible versions, liquid preparations, and syrups should be considered, adhering to guidelines about medication that should not be crushed (see Table 19.6).

Table 19.4 Types of thickeners and examples

Type	Examples
Starch-based	Fresenius Kabi Thick & Easy™ Nestle RESOURCE® THICKENUP®
Xanthan gum-based	NUTRICIA Nutilis Clear Resource®ThickenUp Clear®
Pre-thickened drinks	Slō drinks® Nutilis drinks

Supporting Nutrition and Hydration

Safe and effective management of dysphagia should also consider supporting a patient's nutrition and hydration. Implementing strategies to make mealtimes safer, easier, and more enjoyable will aid in supporting a patient's nutrition and hydration. There are a number of ways to support a patient's nutrition and hydration (see Figure 19.1):

- making a referral to dietetics
- implementing food and fluid monitoring forms
- introducing food fortification for extra calories (see Food fortification/food enrichment and Spotting and Treating Malnutrition in Resource Box)
- ensuring a healthy diet (Eat well Guide, see Resource Box)
- providing advice on fluid-rich foods (jellies, ices cream, sauces, yoghurts, soups, etc.). The SLT will need to assess the suitability of these if the patient has a dysphagia.

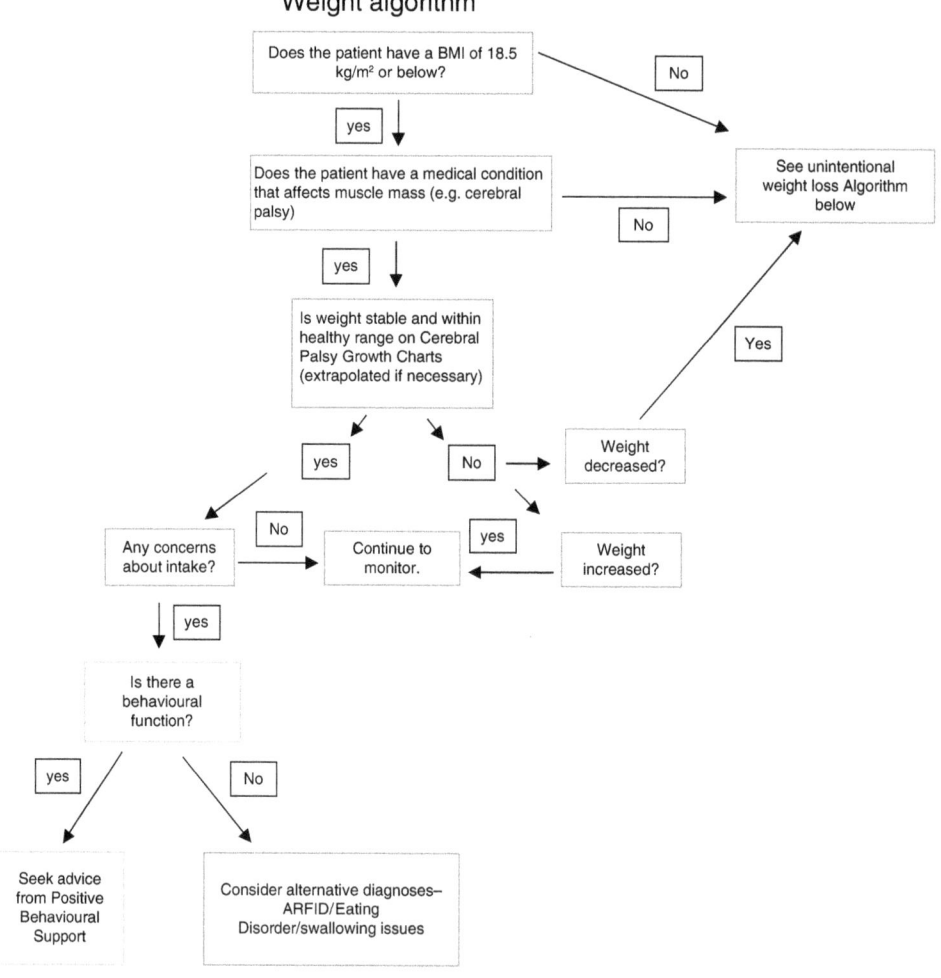

Figure 19.1 (a) Weight algorithm; (b) Unintentional weight loss

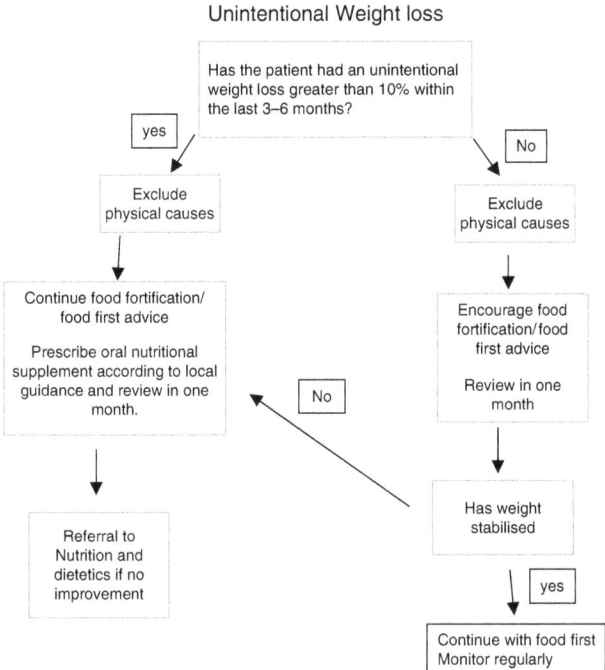

Figure 19.1 (cont.)

Case Study 19.1 (cont.)

A speech therapist from the intellectual disability team assesses Meena and determines there is a risk of aspiration pneumonia and choking due to reduced oral skills and uncoordinated swallow. Using her communication passport and other accessible communication tools, Meena is involved in choosing food and drinks which she can swallow safely. The speech therapist writes a care plan detailing the agreed food texture modifications, pacing needs, and guidance on how best to support Meena at mealtimes.

Meena is taking psychotropic medication that can cause dry mouth. The intellectual disability psychiatrist changes her antipsychotic medication from chlorpromazine to aripiprazole; once Meena is settled on this her procyclidine can also be stopped as it is no longer needed. Both these changes help reduce her mouth dryness.

The dietitian implements oral nutrition supplements.

Eating and Drinking with Acknowledged Risk

Eating and drinking with acknowledged risk (EDAR) refers to the decision to continue eating and drinking despite the associated risks from having dysphagia such as aspiration, malnutrition, dehydration, and choking. Using the EDAR documentation can support a patient who is at the ceiling of care for SLT, on end-of-life care, or who has the capacity to decide they do not want to follow the SLT swallowing advice.

If a patient is deemed to be EDAR, the MDT would work with the patient to create an advanced care plan where appropriate. A document to support decision making is in the Resource Box.

Salivation and Managing Saliva Control (Also Called Drooling or Dribbling)

What Is Salivation and Saliva Control?

Spillage of saliva anteriorly from the mouth onto lips, chin, neck, and clothing can be due to:
- **inability to manage secretions** due to factors such as decreased facial tone, difficulty coordinating facial muscles, facial anatomy, reduced cognitive awareness, altered sensation, difficulties swallowing and moving the saliva to the back of the mouth to swallow
- **increased salivary flow** (sialorrhoea/hypersalivation) as a side effect of medication (e.g., clozapine).

Posterior spillage of secretions relates to when saliva remains in the mouth and spills towards the pharynx causing congestion of breathing, coughing, gagging, vomiting, and, at times, aspiration contributing to recurrent chest infections.

How Common Are Problems With Salivation and Saliva Control in People with Intellectual Disability?

Saliva management issues are found more frequently in those with cerebral palsy (an estimated 10–38% of individuals) and other low-muscle-tone conditions (Erasmus et al., 2009). Research into children with cerebral palsy shows that the flow of saliva is not increased compared to healthy children of the same age, but that spillage related to poor control of salivation (Erasmus 2009).

A third of people with intellectual disability with clinically significant salivation management issues demonstrate evidence of gastro-oesophageal reflux. Boyce (2005) suggests that '[i]ncreased salivary flow occurs as a typically subtle manifestation of gastroesophageal reflux disease'.

Increased flow of saliva is reported as experienced by 31% of patients in the general population using clozapine (Meyler 2016), and flow is reportedly more excessive at night (Safferman et al., 1991). The consequences of saliva management difficulty for people with intellectual disability are summarised in Table 19.5.

The Role of Saliva

Saliva functions as a lubricant and to moisten food ready for swallowing. It also initiates the breakdown of food before entering the stomach. Saliva is important for cleansing the mouth and maintaining good oral health, and plays a defensive role against the gastric acid-induced oesophageal mucosal injury in gastro-oesophageal reflux disorder.

The majority of secretory control of the salivary glands is parasympathetic. This provides a possible avenue for medication treatment, but as many medications used in intellectual disability have side effects involving the parasympathetic system they also have a potential to increase salivary flow.

Table 19.5 Consequences of saliva management difficulty for people with intellectual disability

Irritation and secondary infection may lead to macerated sores around the oral cavity, chin, and neck

Risk of aspiration and choking at night, gurgly/wet voice

Constant wetting of clothes and bed linen can be a significant issue for the person, their families, and their carers

Dehydration; need for extra fluid intake especially in hot weather

Unsightly and unpleasant odour causing social isolation which can have a devastating effect on self-esteem and quality of life

Increased risk of transfer of infection via saliva to others in the environment

Saliva management issues may make swallowing liquid medication unreliable

Due to the complex nature of this condition and often associated polypharmacy, the person with intellectual disability and saliva management problems should be assessed by a MDT. Management should be person-centred, involving an otolaryngologist, an SLT, and a dentist, and for patients with gastro-oesophageal reflux problems medical management should be sought (National institute for Health and Care Excellence (NICE CG 184)).

Management of Saliva

A person needs to have the sensation and cognition to recognise pooling, and to be able to swallow the saliva while maintaining lip closure or having upright posture to prevent the saliva falling forwards. It has been found that people who have difficulty managing saliva have increased difficulty forming a bolus, reduced lip closure, slightly less intra-oral suction, and more oral residue of the swallow. Refer to the MDT for specialist support with the following possible interventions:

- Assessment of and awareness of escaping saliva and sensitisation to help the person recognise when they need to swallow pooled secretions.
- Improving posture to prevent saliva falling forwards out of the mouth.
- Considering posture at night to prevent posterior pooling of secretions (turning to one side, slight elevation of head end of bed).
- Using a functional approach (e.g., use of bandana bibs, sweat bands, or wipes; covering pillows at night with towels). The person may not remember to wipe or swallow, but verbal prompts from a carer may be sufficient.
- If the above strategies are not effective, consider medication treatments.

Medication Treatments for the Management of Saliva

A trial of medication treatment should be attempted for those who have shown an inadequate response with behavioural and postural approaches. The National Centre for Biotechnology (NCBI) bookshelf recommends the following:

- Assess factors that may affect drooling in children and young people with cerebral palsy, such as positioning, medication history, reflux, and dental issues, before starting drug therapy.

- To reduce the severity and frequency of drooling in children and young people with cerebral palsy, consider the use of anticholinergic medication:
    - glycopyrronium bromide (oral or by enteral tube); or
    - transdermal hyoscine hydrobromide; or
    - trihexyphenidyl hydrochloride for children with dyskinetic cerebral palsy, but only with input from specialist services.
- When choosing which medication to use, take into account the preferences of the child or young person and their parents or carers, and the age range and indication covered by the marketing authorisations.
- Regularly review the effectiveness, tolerability, and side effects of all medication treatments used for saliva control.
- Refer the child or young person to a specialist service if the anticholinergic is contraindicated, not tolerated, or not effective, to consider other treatments for saliva control.
- Consider specialist assessment and use of botulinum toxin A injections to the salivary glands with ultrasound guidance to reduce the severity and frequency of drooling in children and young people with cerebral palsy if anticholinergic drugs provide insufficient benefit or are not tolerated.

Evidence for Medication Treatments

- **Anticholinergics** (also called antimuscarinics). An independent systematic review of medical literature (Jongerius et al., 2003) investigating the efficacy of anticholinergic medications to treat salivation management issues found no general conclusion could be reached and that a meta-analysis could not be performed (Jongerius et al., 2003). The authors concluded that there is some evidence that at least two anticholinergics medications (benzatropine, and trihexyphenidyl) are effective in the treatment of salivation management issues. However, other studies (Harvey et al., 2018) have suggested that the high incidence of side effects limit their value. For people with cerebral palsy the use of trihexyphenidyl may have additional benefits for those with rigid or dystonic muscle tone by reduction in muscle tone (Harvey et al., 2018)
- **Hyoscine patches/tablets** can be effective but may have side effects which need to be considered, for example:
    - Reducing salivation reduces the ability to moisten and masticate food, increasing the risk choking and negative health consequences. It is important to make sure that food is moistened with gravies and sauces, or table sauces are offered.
    - Reducing the amount of saliva produced can increase the concentration of bacteria in the saliva, making it more potent if aspirated and decreasing its cleansing affect.
    - It can also make saliva sticky and difficult to swallow and the mouth can feel dry and uncomfortable, making swallowing effortful.
    - Parr et al. (2018) compared the use of hyoscine and glycopyrronium in management of saliva in children and found hyoscine to have more problematic side effects. They recommend use of glycopyrronium as the first-choice medication.

- **Surgical relocation or rerouting of the salivary duct.** Bilateral tympanic neurectomy with sectioning of the chorda tympani destroys parasympathetic innovation of the gland, but this may cause loss of taste sensation in the anterior two-thirds of the tongue.
- **Intra-glandular botulinum toxin.** Small studies involving the use of botulinum toxin injections have been found to be effective. Botulinum toxin A can be injected into the parotid glands, reducing saliva production for 3–6 months after each injection (Lakraj et al., 2013).

Case Study 19.2

Simon is a 34-year-old man with cerebral palsy and epilepsy who uses a moulded wheelchair and has a sleep system in place from physiotherapy. He was referred to speech and language therapy due to coughing during and after meals and at night. The skin around his chin was red and his GP prescribed a topical cream for this.

A swallow assessment suggested that the current SLT recommendations were continuing to manage the risk of negative health consequences, but as well as coughing post-meal and in between meals, carers noted that they were changing Simon's neckerchief several times a day which was not usual for him.

The SLT asked the GP to consider a trial of proton pump inhibitor to treat any gastro-oesophageal reflux and referred to physiotherapy for a review of Simon's positioning at night. Cough charts were also implemented to monitor coughing.

Coughing charts showed a reduction in coughing after meals and carers reported that Simon's neckerchiefs were dryer, and they were only needing to change them twice a day.

Feeding Tubes

Individuals with severe swallowing difficulties may require to completely bypass oral intake of food, fluids, and medications and have either a nasogastric tube or insertion of a gastrostomy or jejunostomy tube.

The use of enteral feeding tubes has increased both for short- and long-term feeding, due to increasing awareness of the importance of ensuring adequate nutritional intake for promotion and maintenance of good health. Gastrostomy tubes provide a means of improving nutritional intake when oral intake is very poor or when there is restricted access to the gastrointestinal tract either due to swallowing difficulties or an obstruction. Dietitians are essential members of the MDT to ensure people with gastrostomy tubes receive adequate fluid and nutrition, and will prescribe a diet based on individual requirements and relevant disease states. The gastrostomy tube itself needs to be looked after to maintain good hygiene and prevent infection, as well as to reduce the risk of the tube blocking or coming out.

The feeding regime needs to be considered when prescribing medication; ideally, there should be a gap around medication administration, and medications such as phenytoin require two hours either side of administration as they will bind to proteins in feeds. Some medications will react with feeds to cause insoluble precipitates that could potentially block the tube. Some of the most common problems are:

- Osmotic diarrhoea from liquid medicines that contain sorbitol. The dose is cumulative, so the risk increases with the more medicines there are. The patient can experience painful cramping with the diarrhoea.
- Poor absorption, especially with percutaneous endoscopic gastro-jejunostomy feeds, as the medication may enter the gastrointestinal tract too low down to be adequately absorbed.
- Altered bioavailability when converting from some tablets to liquids.
- Changing from a modified-release preparation to a liquid will mean reduced doses but more frequent intervals.
- Risk of tube blocking from viscous liquids.
- Risk of the medication binding to the plastic tube: these medications will require dilution prior to administration.

A person with intellectual disability on a modified or enteral diet will often require careful thought around choice of formulation. It might be that there is an alternative route of administration available (e.g., changing tablets to patches). Many liquid formulations are relatively thick and will be safe for administration to an individual requiring a modified diet; however, it may be necessary to thicken liquid medication. If there is no liquid formulation available, tablets may need to be crushed or capsules opened and then mixed with water for administration. Altering the manufacturer's formulation of a medication by thickening, crushing, or opening capsules can render it an unlicenced product, and some medications must never be crushed or opened.

For people with intellectual disability with enteral tubes who receive all fluids, nutrition and medications via a gastrostomy, it is important to ensure that the feeding regimen does not adversely affect the medication (e.g., phenytoin binding to proteins in feeds). It is important that carers of individuals with swallowing difficulties/gastrostomy tubes have clear guidance on how to safely administer medication; this will require multidisciplinary input from speech and language therapy, dietetics, and pharmacy as well as the relevant prescribers, and it might be useful to provide written information. Many pharmaceutical companies will have information on administering their medication to individuals with swallowing difficulties/gastrostomy tubes, but will emphasise that they will not have stability information and that it is an unlicenced use. There are a number of useful reference sources that have information on prescribing and administration of medications for people with swallowing difficulties/gastrostomy tubes as well as very useful monographs for individual medication, including antiepileptic and psychotropic medications.

Table 19.6 Some medication that should never be crushed or opened

Formulations with any kind of enteric coating: these medications could be an irritant or be affected by environmental conditions

Modified or sustained release formulations: the pharmacokinetics of these formulations will be altered

Hormones or cytotoxic medications: due to the risk of harm to the person administering the medication

Nitrates: due to the theoretical risk of explosion

Guidance on the Administration of Medication via Percutaneous Endoscopic Gastrostomy Tubes

There are many guidelines and resources available to guide the administration of particular medications. For that reason we have not provided a table of such guidance here. Regularly updated sources include:

- White, R., and Bradnam, V. *Handbook of medication administration via enteral feeding tubes.* London: RPS Publishing; 2007 (www.rlandrews.org/pdf_files/handbk_of_enteralfeeding.pdf).
- Smyth, J. *The NEWT Guidelines for administration of medication to patients with enteral feeding tubes or swallowing difficulties.* Wrexham: North East Wales NHS Trust; 2006 (www.newtguidelines.com/splash.html).
- SHPA, *Don't rush to crush handbook: Therapeutic options for people unable to swallow solid oral medicines.* The Society of Hospital Pharmacists of Australia (shpa.immij.com/dont-rush-to-crush).

If medication is to be administered via a PEG tube, the following is recommended:

- Make the prescriber aware that:
  - The person has a PEG tube
  - The formulations of the medications prescribed are appropriate to go into the PEG tube.
- Not all liquids are suitable for administration via a PEG tube because they may be too thick.
- Medication that must not be crushed/opened to be administered via a PEG tube include:
  - Enteric-coated tablets: these tablets have a coating on them to either protect the medication or to prevent gastric irritation.
  - Controlled/modified/sustained release, long-acting, retard, or chrono formulations: these formulations allow decreased dosing frequency and encourage more consistent blood levels of a medication.
  - Hormones and cytotoxics, because of possible harm to the person administering the medication.

The following points should be remembered when administering medications via a PEG tube:

- They should not be added to a feed
- Only one should be administered at a time. They should not be mixed
- A 50-millilitre syringe should be used to reduce the likelihood of strong pressure rupturing the tube
- Cooled boiled water should be used when dispersing tablets and flushing the tube:
  - flush tube with a minimum of 15 ml of water between medication
  - flush tube with 50 ml of water after administration of the last medication.

Always flush the PEG tube pre/post and between medicines.

It is often easier to prepare all of the medications for administration in an area away from the person with intellectual disability so that they can then be administered consecutively with the minimum amount of disruption.

Directions for Administration of Tablets

Crushing tablets:
1. Crush the tablets in a tablet crusher.
2. Add 15–30 mls of cooled boiled water to the crusher and mix with the powder.
3. Draw up the solution in an oral or bladder syringe or suitable administration container.
4. Rinse out the crusher with cooled boiled water using the same syringe and dispense into the suitable administration container.

Dispersible/Disintegrating Tablets

Tablets may disintegrate in water without crushing. If this is the case the tablet should be prepared as follows:
1. Place intact tablet into the barrel of an oral/bladder syringe.
2. Replace the plunger and draw up 10–15 mls of cooled boiled water.
3. Replace cap, allow tablet to dissolve.
4. Shake well and administer dose down the enteral feeding tube.
5. Flush the tube post-dose with 15–30 mls of water.

Effervescent Tablets

Tablets will effervesce and disperse when placed in water. The resulting gases need to be allowed to escape.
1. Pour 50 mls cooled boiled water into a glass/beaker
2. Add the tablet to the water
3. Wait for the effervescent reaction to finish
4. Swirl the solution and draw it all up into a 50 ml oral/bladder syringe
5. Administer the dose down the enteral feeding tube

What Not to Do with tablets

- Do not crush the tablet in a plastic container other than the tablet crusher supplied as the medication may adhere to the plastic
- Do not use boiling water to dissolve tablets as it may affect bioavailability
- Do not leave oral medications unattended in syringes
- Do not administer any medication that you have not prepared yourself

The Frith Prescribing Guidelines Editors' Expert Group Consensus Statements

Statements of High Confidence

- Dysphagia causes negative health consequences such as malnutrition and dehydration.

- Respiratory compromise (e.g., COPD, smoking) is an influencing factor in whether a patient with dysphagia develops aspiration pneumonia.
- In addition to dysphagia, other causative factors associated with aspiration pneumonia include dependence on others for feeding, multiple medical conditions, smoking, tube feeding, dependence for oral care, polypharmacy, and presence of reflux.
- Individuals with severe swallowing difficulties may require to completely bypass oral intake of food, fluids, and medications and have either a nasogastric tube or insertion of a gastrostomy or jejunostomy tube.

Statements of Medium Confidence
- Thickeners should be used with caution. Thickeners increase the risk of dehydration due to factors such as a negative response to texture and increased feelings of fullness which result in little motivation and reduced drive to consume thickened liquids.
- Some medications such as antipsychotics can cause extra-pyramidal symptoms which can lead to a dysphagia.
- Dysphagia was reported in 23% of deaths from initial review, making it the fifth most common long-term health condition in people who died in 2021 (White et al., 2022).

Statements of Low Confidence
- Anticholinergic (antimuscarinic) medications may have value in saliva management. An independent systematic review of medical literature investigating the efficacy of anticholinergic medications to treat salivation management issues found no general conclusion.

Resource Box
- NICE nutrition and hydration guideline Full guideline | Nutrition support for adults: oral nutrition support, enteral tube feeding and parenteral nutrition. www.nice.org.uk/guidance/cg32
- The Disability Distress Assessment Tool: DisDAT
- Royal College of Speech and Language Therapists (RCSLT) Eating and drinking with acknowledged risk. www.rcslt.org/wp-content/uploads/2021/09/EDAR-multidisciplinary-guidance-2021.pdf
- Reducing the risk of choking for people with learning disability. A multi-agency review in Hampshire (2018). https://documents.hants.gov.uk/adultservices/safeguarding/Reducingtheriskofchokingforpeoplewithalearningdisability.pdf
- British Dietetic Association (BDA). www.bda.uk.com/
- Spotting malnutrition: Spotting and treating malnutrition | British Dietetic Association (BDA). www.bda.uk.com/resource/malnutrition.html
- Belfast Health and Social Care Trust Help stop Choking resources. http://helpstopchoking.hscni.net/pages/resources
- In England, the National Patient Safety Agency (NPSA) produced a wide range of documents to assist with the assessment and management of dysphagia. These include a risk assessment guide and form; a dysphagia report form; an eating, drinking, and swallowing care plan; mealtime information forms; a protocol for general practitioners; and a consent form. The NPSA no longer exists, but the documents are still available via http://psychology-resources.wlvpsych.co.uk/?projects=intellectual-disability-dysphagia-research%2F and https://choiceforum.org/docs/dysphnpasp.pdf

- The Eatwell Guide – NHS. www.nhs.uk/live-well/eat-well/food-guidelines-and-food-labels/the-eatwell-guide/
- Food first/Food enrichment. www.bapen.org.uk/nutrition-support/nutrition-by-mouth/food-first-food-enrichment
- Easy Health. www.easyhealth.org.uk/
- International Dysphagia Diet Standardisation Initiative (IDDSI) 2019. https://iddsi.org/framework/
- Dysphagia in people with learning difficulties: reasonable adjustments guidance. www.gov.uk/government/publications/dysphagia-and-people-with-learning-disabilities/dysphagia-in-people-with-learning-difficulties-reasonable-adjustments-guidance
- NICE guideline CG184 Gastro-oesophageal reflux disease and dyspepsia in adults: investigation and management (2019). www.nice.org.uk/guidance/cg184
- NICE guideline CG32 Nutrition support for adults: oral nutrition support, enteral tube feeding and parenteral nutrition (2017). www.nice.org.uk/guidance/cg32
- NICE guideline NG48 Oral health for adults in care homes (2016). NICE NG62 Cerebral Palsy in under 25s: assessment and management London 2017 https://www.ncbi.nlm.nih.gov/books/NBK533231
- Eating and Drinking with acknowledged risk Learning Disability Guidance RCSLT. www.rcslt.org/members/clinical-guidance/eating-and-drinking-with-acknowledged-risks-risk-feeding/
- International Dysphagia Diet Standardisation Initiative (IDDSI) 2019. https://iddsi.org/framework/

References

Aaronson, J. K. (ed.) (2016) *Meyler's side effects of drugs: The international Encyclopaedia of adverse drug reactions and Interactions*, 16th ed. www.sciencedirect.com/referencework/9780444537164/meylers-side-effects-of-drugs.

Beetz, R. (2003) Mild dehydration: a risk factor of urinary tract infection? *European Journal of Clinical Nutrition*; 57 Suppl 2, S52–S58.

Belfast Health and Social Care Trust Help stop Choking resources. Resources | Help Stop Choking (hscni.net).

Boyce, H. W., & Bakheet, M. R. (2005) Sialorrhea: A review of a vexing, often unrecognized sign of oropharyngeal and oesophageal disease. *J Clin Gastroenterol*. Feb; 39(2), 89–97.

Chadwick, D. D., Jolliffe, J. A. (2009) Descriptive investigation of dysphagia in adults with intellectual disabilities. *JIDR*; 53(1), 29–43.

Cichero, JA. (2013) Thickening agents used for dysphagia management: effect on bioavailability of water, medication and feelings of satiety. *Nutr J. May*; 1(12), 54.

Erasmus, C. E. et al. (2009) Drooling in cerebral Palsy: hypersalivation or dysfunctional oral motor control? *Developmental Medicine and Child Neurology*, 51(6).

Feinberg, M. J., Knebl, J., Tully, J., & Segall, L. (1990) Aspiration and the elderly. *Dysphagia*; 5, 61–71.

Finlayson, J., Morrison, J., Jackson, A., Mantry, D., Cooper, S. A. (2010) Injuries, falls and accidents among adults with intellectual disabilities. Prospective cohort study.*J Intellect Disabil ResNov*; 54(11), 966–80.

Gupte, T., Knack, A. & Cramer, J. D. (2022) Mortality from aspiration pneumonia: Incidence, trends, and risk factors. *Dysphagia*; 37, 1493–500.

Hampshire County Council (2018). Reducing the risk of choking for people with learning disability. A multi-agency review in

Hampshire. https://documents.hants.gov.uk/adultservices/safeguarding/Reducingtheriskofchokingforpeoplewithalearningdisability.pdf.

Harvey, A. R., Baker, L. B., Reddihough, D., Scheinberg, A., & Williams, K. (2018) Trihexyphenidyl for dystonia in cerebral palsy. *Cochrane Database of Systematic Reviews*, Issue 5. Art. No.: CD012430. https://doi.org/10.1002/14651858.CD012430.pub2

Health and Care of People with learning disabilities (n.d.) General practice data dashboards – NHS Digital. https://digital.nhs.uk/data-and-information/data-tools-and-services/data-services/general-practice-data-hub.

Heslop, P., Calkin, R., Byrne, V., Huxor, A., & Gielnik, K. (2019) The learning disabilities mortality review (LeDeR) programme, Annual Report Bristol University.

Hibberd, J., Fraser, J., Chapman, C., et al. (2013) Can we use influencing factors to predict aspiration pneumonia in the United Kingdom?. *Multidiscip Respir Med*; **8**, 39.

International Dysphagia Diet Standardisation Initiative (IDDSI) (2019) IDDSI – IDDSI Framework. https://iddsi.org/Framework.

Jongerius, P. H., van Tiel, P., van Limbeek, J., Gabreëls, F. J., & Rotteveel, J. J. (2003) A systematic review for evidence of efficacy of anticholinergic drugs to treat drooling. *Arch Dis Child*. Oct; **88**(10), 911–14. https://doi.org/10.1136/adc.88.10.911. PMID: 14500313; PMCID: PMC1719306.

King, l., Maya, A. & Lazenby-Paterson, T. (2023) Position statement on the use of thickened fluids in the management of people with swallowing difficulties. www.rcslt.org/wp-content/uploads/2023/03/Position-statement-thickened-fluids-1.pdf.

Lakraj, A. A., Moghimi, N., & Jabbari, B. (2013) Sialorrhea: Anatomy, pathophysiology and treatment with emphasis on the role of botulinum toxins. *Toxins (Basel)*. May 21; **5**(5), 1010–31.

Langmore, S. E., Skarupski, K. A., Park, P. S., Fries, B. E. (2002) Predictors of aspiration pneumonia in nursing home residents. *Dysphagia*. Fall; **17**(4), 298–307.

Langmore, S., Terpenning, M., Schork, A., et al. (1998) Predictors of aspiration pneumonia: How important is dysphagia? *Dysphagia*; **13**, 69–81.

Lazenby-Paterson, T. (2020). Thickened liquids: Do they still have a place in the dysphagia toolkit?. *Current Opinion in Otolaryngology & Head and Neck Surgery*; **28**, 145–54.

Marik, P. E. (2001) Aspiration pneumonitis and aspiration pneumonia. *N Engl J Med*. Mar 1; **344**(9), 665–71.

NBCI (n.d.). Managing saliva control – Cerebral palsy in under 25s: assessment and management. https://www.ncbi.nlm.nih.gov/books/NBK533231/.

Parr, J. R., Todhunter, E., Pennington, L., et al. (2018) Reduction Intervention randomised trial (DRI): comparing the efficacy and acceptability of hyoscine patches and glycopyrronium liquid on drooling in children with neurodisability. *Arch Dis Child*; **103**, 371–6. https://doi.org/10.1136/archdischild-2017-313763.

Ramachandran, G, Prasad, C. H. R. K., Garre, S., & Sundar, A. S. (2022) Oxygen management in heart failure patients. *Indian Journal of Clinical Cardiology*; **3**(3), 150–6.

Robbins, J., Langmore, S., Hind, J. A., & Erlichman, M. (2002) Dysphagia research in the 21st century and beyond: Proceedings from Dysphagia Experts Meeting, August 21, 2001. *J Rehabil Res Dev*. Jul–Aug; **39**(4), 543–8.

Robertson, J., Chadwick, D., Baines, S., Emerson, E., & Hatton, C. (2017) Prevalence of dysphagia in people with intellectual disability: A systematic review. *Intellect Dev Disabil*. Dec; **55**(6):377–91.

Safferman, A., Lieberman, J. A., Kane, J. M., et al. (1991) Update on the clinical efficacy and side effects of clozapine. *Schizophr Bull*; **17**(2), 247–61.

Samuels, R. & Chadwick, D. (2006) Predictors of asphyxiation risk in adults with intellectual disabilities and dysphagia. *Journal of Intellectual Disability Research*, **50**(5), 362–70.

Scarpel, R. D., Nóbrega, A. C., Pinho, P., et al. (2021) Oropharyngeal swallowing dynamic findings in people with asthma. *Dysphagia*; 36, 541–50.

Sokoloff, L., & Pavlakovic, R. (1997) Neuroleptic-induced dysphagia. *Dysphagia*; 12, 177–9.

Sugiya, R., Higashimoto, Y., Shiraishi, M., et al. (2022). Decreased tongue strength is related to skeletal muscle mass in COPD patients. *Dysphagia*; 37, 636–43.

Thacker, A. Abdelnoor, A. Anderson, C. White, S. & Hollins, S. (2007) Indicators of choking risk in adults with learning disabilities: A questionnaire survey and interview study. *Disability and Rehabilitation*; 30(15), 1131–8.

Trollor, J., Srasuebkul, P., Xu, H., & Howlett, S. (2017) Cause of death and potentially avoidable deaths in Australian adults with intellectual disability using retrospective linked data. *BMJ Open*. Feb 7; 7(2).

White, A., Sheehan, R., Ding, J., et al. (2022) LeDeR Learning from lives and deaths – People with a learning disability and autistic people Annual report for 2021 Kings College London. www.kcl.ac.uk/ioppn/assets/fans-dept/leder-main-report-hyperlinked.pdf.

Chapter 20

Children and Adolescents

Mark Lovell, Ashley Liew, and Keir Jones

Introduction

Almost all the clinical presentations detailed throughout this book can present in children and adolescents with intellectual disability. Of note, many comorbid neurodevelopmental disorders (e.g., attention deficit hyperactivity disorder and autism) are first identified and diagnosed in childhood. Mental illnesses such as psychosis often have onset in late adolescence and may present with attenuated or prodromal symptoms in childhood. As such, the treatments discussed in this chapter require a careful approach to assessment, formulation, and diagnosis in the first instance. This chapter will focus on selected mental disorders presenting in children with intellectual disability to help illustrate relevant treatment principles.

How Common Are Mental Health Problems in Children and Young People with Intellectual Disability?

Reviews of epidemiological studies consistently note rates of mental health problems in up to 50% in children with intellectual disability (Buckley et al., 2020). These rates are always much higher compared to children without intellectual disability (Einfeld et al., 2011) and are distributed across many of the same disorders seen through childhood (see Figure 20.1).

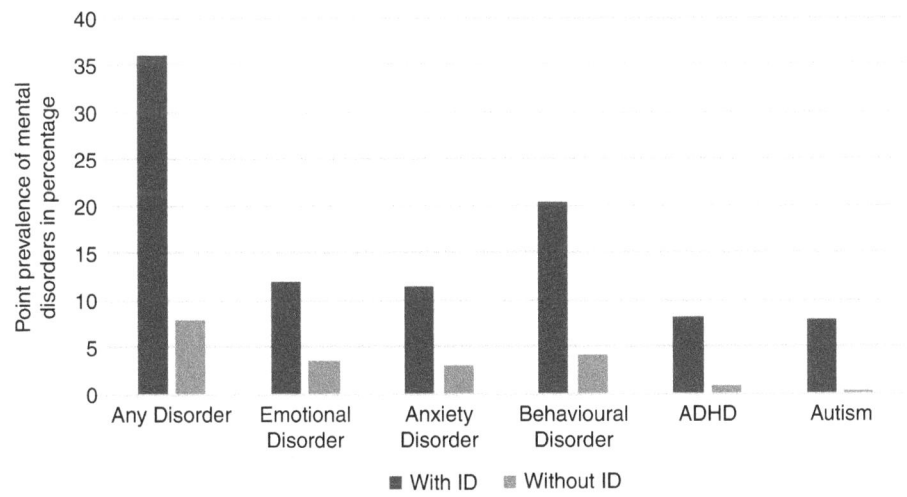

Figure 20.1 Prevalence of mental disorders in children with and without intellectual disability. Graph adapted from data in Emerson and Hatton, 2007

Clinical Presentation

Many of the same mental health, behavioural, and neurodevelopmental disorders can occur in children and adolescents with intellectual disability that are seen in the adult population with intellectual disability, except for those disorders that present specifically later in life, such as Huntington's disease or dementia. Like in adults with intellectual disability, these disorders are more common in children and young people with intellectual disability compared to typically developing peers. However, as seen in children without intellectual disability, the prevalence of mental health and behaviour disorders vary by age.

Much like in adults with intellectual disability, children with intellectual disability can present with more biological/somatic symptoms and behavioural manifestations rather than psychological symptomatology. Presentation is also affected by developmental stage as well as chronological age. In children without intellectual disability, presentations of mental disorders typically become more complex and focused on psychological symptoms with advancing age, rather than biological or behavioural changes dominating the picture; intellectual disability can clearly impact this development, however, and must be borne in mind when assessing presentations and making diagnoses in this group of young people.

Most mental health, neurodevelopmental and behavioural disorders also present for their first time in childhood or adolescence, often not starting as fully diagnosable conditions, but rather as prodromes or at the milder end of presentation, worsening in severity over time.

Neurodevelopmental disorders are life-long and start from birth; however, their presence may not be detected until certain developmental phases have occurred and a difference from neurotypical development is seen, or symptoms are distinguishable from the presence of the child's intellectual disability. Of course, not all of these can be treated with medication, but some can.

These early presentations may pose diagnostic conundrums to clinicians, with overlaps in presentations, diffuse symptomatology, and below diagnostic threshold for the frequency or severity of symptoms.

Neurodevelopmental Disorder Example: Attention Deficit Hyperactivity Disorder

Attention Deficit Hyperactivity Disorder (ADHD) is a neurodevelopmental condition that has evidence-based pharmacological treatment options. In a child with intellectual disability, ADHD presents as increased inattention, hyperactivity, and impulsivity compared to other children of the same age with the same level of intellectual disability. This symptom cluster is the same as for other children. The complicating factor is establishing the developmental equivalence of the child. Younger children are more impulsive, less attentive, and more active than older children, so developmental delays can present like ADHD if the degree of developmental delay is not known or underestimated. In children without intellectual disability, ADHD isn't generally diagnosed until at least age 5 or 6, since distinguishing pathological or significant difference is difficult until the child is developmentally more able. Those with intellectual disability may remain below the developmental equivalent of a 5- or 6-year-old for much longer, and if the intellectual disability is not appropriately recognised ADHD may be incorrectly diagnosed. Conversely, recognising the intellectual disability may diagnostically overshadow the ADHD if the child is not compared with other children of the same ability. It is important to recognise both diagnoses if they are present, as the ADHD has potential treatments.

Behaviour Disorder Example: Behaviour That Challenges Others

Behaviour that challenges others is an extreme presentation of behaviour that limits an individual's access to the community. It is generally associated with more severe intellectual disability. Examples of behaviours that challenge others include self-injury, aggression, damage to property, and running away. These usually occur for identifiable reasons (e.g., communication difficulties, sensory sensitivities, pain or discomfort, confusion, irritation, ending a preferred activity, or simply being told no). Some of these behaviours are seen in typically developing children at younger developmental phases (e.g., toddler 'temper tantrums'), but may be considered challenging in a child with intellectual disability by virtue of the child's age or the chronicity of the difficulties or the extreme level of distress shown by the child. This child, however, is not a toddler and has more years of experience of triggers and learning from the consequences to their behavioural presentation, so behaviours that would ordinarily be a phase in toddlers, may persist for many years. Though the mainstay of management of behaviour that challenges others is non-pharmacological, in more extreme cases where non-pharmacological approaches have had a sub-optimal effect, pharmacological approaches may be used to manage hyperarousal levels. Medications may also be considered to support the child or young person at earlier points in the escalation chain to address intermediate phases between the trigger and end response (e.g., where they are experiencing significant anxiety). Where there is an identifiable cause for the behaviours that challenge, then this needs to be the focus of treatment. Some of the contributory factors for behaviour that challenges may be mental disorders or neurodevelopmental disorders that have pharmacological treatments in their own right, or physical health issues such as pain or discomfort that need addressing. Using psychotropics to sedate someone in pain (e.g., due to ear infection or tooth pain) is unethical and should be avoided.

Diagnosis

Diagnosis following an assessment of presenting symptomatology and signs (often behaviours) in children and adolescents with intellectual disability is very similar to the processes used for adults with intellectual disability. The Diagnostic Criteria for people with Intellectual Disability (DC-LD), which is a modified version of International Classification of Diseases (ICD-10), was originally written only for adults. The principles still generally stand, but they haven't been validated for children and adolescents. The next version that will accompany the International Classification of Diseases (ICD-11) is planned to include children and adolescents with intellectual disability too, but at the time of writing this has not been developed.

When undertaking assessments, reasonable adjustments will often be required, alongside an additional focus on observation and history, rather than rating scales. For more able and/or older children, a history from the young person and a description of symptoms may be elicited. For those who are younger or less able, a collateral history will be required. Usually in children this will be from parents and school, but may involve carers or a wide range of involved professionals. Often a change of behaviours will be presented and the nature of these will require interpretation as to whether they represent a mental illness, neurodevelopmental disorder, a reaction to a trigger, or, indeed, developmentally appropriate behaviours.

Observation is often key to the understanding of a presentation. It may help to establish antecedents, the nature and severity of a presentation, and whether there were consequences that may prove reinforcing. The purpose or meaning of a behaviour may also become evident. Observation may be required across multiple settings or multiple occasions. This will direct diagnosis and formulation and, thus, evidence-based treatment/management options.

Understanding the broader context is key. This takes the diagnostician beyond diagnosis and into the territory of formulation, considering not only the presenting factors, but also considering predisposing, precipitating, perpetuating, and preventative factors in the three domains: biological, psychological, and social/environmental. This approach is often more important for understanding the wider context of a child's presentation and to direct potential advice, management, or treatments than a series of diagnoses. Of course, diagnosis can still be very helpful, as evidence-based treatment is usually diagnosis or symptom specific, but wider formulation can set these diagnoses into context and ensure more person-centred and holistic care.

The developing child not only has a changing neurological and physical biology, but also many areas of function are still developing (e.g., receptive and expressive language and communication, ability to rationalise, albeit sometimes at a slower rate in children and adolescents with intellectual disability).

Some disorders commonly start in the developmental phase (e.g., ADHD, autism, sibling rivalry and conduct disorders), although not all of these have pharmacological treatments. Occasionally they may be limited to childhood, or progress into adulthood but take on a different diagnostic term in adulthood (e.g., conduct disorder that persists into adulthood may be reframed as an antisocial personality disorder if accompanied by wider personality features).

Mental or neurodevelopmental disorders in childhood may resemble each other, with the same biological or behavioural presentations potentially seen in a variety of conditions. Some features of intellectual disability or autism may resemble ADHD, for example, and features commonly seen in autism may resemble depression or anxiety. Care must be taken to avoid diagnostic overshadowing, where one established diagnosis masks the presence of another either due to overlapping symptomatology or by blinkering the diagnosing clinician. Provisional diagnoses can be helpful, as well as working hypotheses and narrative formulations while there is uncertainty, using the adage that the more common a diagnosis, the more likely it is to be the cause. Pragmatic trials of different therapeutic approaches may be required, and an openness to change the diagnosis or formulation. In addition, many disorders co-occur, so any presentation may be an amalgamation of multiple co-occurring conditions (e.g., intellectual disability, autism, ADHD, anxiety).

In childhood, decision making regarding engagement with an assessment and/or treatment may be guided by different legislation compared to adults. For example, in England and Wales, The Children Act will be the starting point for under 18s, which enshrines in law the role of parents in consenting for children and adolescents. At a developmental equivalent of about age 13, Gillick or Fraser competency, originally set out by case law, allows children to opt into health care if mature enough to do so without parental consent/involvement; however, many children with intellectual disability won't reach this developmental stage. It also generally doesn't allow refusal of care. From age 16, the Mental Capacity Act applies regarding capacity to consent, with an adolescent's understanding, ability to retain pertinent information, ability to weigh up the pros and cons of a decision, and to communicate that decision being the core parts of the competency framework. Capacity is assumed unless there is a reason to doubt it. Having intellectual disability is grounds to consider a Mental Capacity Act assessment. If someone over 16 years of age lacks capacity, then decisions to assess or treat need to be made in their best interests, involving the Court of Protection if needed. Mental Health Act legislation may be used at any age if assessment or treatment of a mental disorder is required in an inpatient setting or for the safety of the person or others.

> **Case Study 20.1**
>
> Feroz, a 12-year-old boy with tuberous sclerosis, moderate intellectual disability, autism, and epilepsy, was referred by his special school paediatrician to the child and adolescent mental health services (CAMHS) intellectual disability (CAMHS-ID) service as he had been displaying increasing behaviours of running out of the classroom, biting his hands, and delayed sleep onset since the start of the new school year.
>
> He was assessed by a psychiatrist and a speech and language therapist in clinic who also noted that he was eating more, had gained weight, was not engaging in favourite activities like water play, and was communicating less. The psychiatrist noted that a paediatric neurologist had recently increased Feroz's antiepileptic medication, which is an agent which can have adverse effects on mood.
>
> A psychologist from the CAMHS-ID observed Feroz in class and noticed that he tended to bite his hands whenever his teacher held up the visual timetable board to indicate breaktimes, and that he attempted to leave the classroom when the teacher started distributing musical instruments for an activity. She hypothesised that Feroz would get anxious in anticipation of unstructured and noisy situations and was not able to communicate his anxiety effectively. Feroz's teacher explained that he had transitioned from a primary school which had much smaller classes.
>
> A diagnosis of anxiety was made. The psychologist and the speech and language therapist started to develop a behaviour support and communication plan in cooperation with Feroz's family and teachers. The psychiatrist contacted the neurologist to alert her about Feroz's change in mental state.

Management

Guidance for any treatments may come from a variety of sources. In England and Wales, there is National Institute for Health and Care Excellence (NICE) guidance, and in Scotland there are the Scottish Intercollegiate Guidelines Network guidelines. Many other countries have their own guidelines. Most of these are either for adults, adults with intellectual disability or children and adolescents in general, but rarely children and adolescents with intellectual disability. This means that often guidance and its associated evidence base has to be extrapolated for children and adolescents with intellectual disability. This is far from an ideal situation, but warranted nevertheless to meet their needs. Some specific NICE guidelines reference children with intellectual disability, such as the guidance documents for ADHD and challenging behaviour. However, even these guidance documents direct those that work with children with intellectual disability to use their expert judgement and explain that the guidance don't necessarily apply in their full form (e.g., National Institute for Health and Care Excellence guideline for Attention Deficit Hyperactivity Disorder: www.nice.org.uk/guidance/ng87).

Given this lack of formal guidance, many clinicians working in the field rely on the Bolam test – that is, to ensure they are operating within the practice parameters of a reasonable body of peers. This approach uses collective clinical expertise and established practice. Though not ideal, this should be considered preferable to experimental and potentially unsafe therapeutic approaches. Groups like the Child and Adolescent Intellectual Disability Psychiatry Network (CAIDPN), a special interest group of the Association for Child and Adolescent Mental Health, is such a group of worldwide psychiatrists and paediatricians with appropriate knowledge and expertise to reference one's practice against.

With regards to medications, the British National Formulary for Children (BNF-C) has a list of medications that are appropriate for use in children, including those licenced and where prescribing is off label or off-licence (e.g., for a different indication or where the doses used are sometimes higher or lower than those included in the original licence). Doses, ranges, and differences between diagnoses are included and sometimes titration timescales and licenced duration of prescription (e.g., for short term only). There may also be dose differences by age or weight.

Reasonable adjustments may be required for children with intellectual disability, for example to allow for their complex physical health or sensory needs. These may include using micro dosing; using liquid, oro-dispersible, or melting preparations; sprinkling capsule contents; patches; or covert medication. These options may be considered if a young person cannot or will not take a tablet/capsule or where they are refusing to take any form of medication due to the required routine change, or the taste, for example. Appropriate legislation should be considered when medications are being hidden (e.g., in food or drink). This can cause some issues where a younger child had medication covertly administered, but at the age where legal consent is possible if capacious, confessing to hiding their medication when they didn't want it may erode trust in service or a change in treatment compliance. Therefore, it is always preferable to be as honest as possible with a child about them having medication, even if they don't fully understand its purpose.

Implications of legislation for assessment were discussed earlier. These have the same implications for the management/treatment of mental health disorders and consent to access these. There are occasions where treatments in children and adolescents require additional legislation. In England and Wales for example, a Second Opinion Approved Doctor is required to continue treatment for a prolonged period under the Mental Health Act where the young person is refusing or unable to consent or in special circumstances (e.g., electroconvulsive therapy). Some treatments may be banned altogether for under 18s. For example, at the time of writing, many gender reassignment treatments are restricted to adults only, irrespective of the capacity of the young person.

For children and young people with intellectual disability, using lower doses, slower dose changes, and careful monitoring of positive effects and side effects is potentially even more important than in typically developing children, due to some having complex physical health comorbidities and difficulties in communicating any benefits or concerns by conventional means. Most structured tools available rely on self-report, and this may not be possible so collateral information (e.g., from a parent) is often required. Some medications have age limits for prescribing and may have different maximum doses by age too.

Modified medication information and assessment and monitoring tools may be required with adjustments made for language and communication level (e.g., using simplified information and symbols or pictures). Ideally monotherapy would be used, rather than polypharmacy, to reduce interactions and likelihood of cumulative side effects. If using polypharmacy, only one medication should be changed at a time so that effect and side-effect monitoring of that particular medication change can occur and be responded to accordingly. There are some medications that can alter the level of others and care needs to be taken to combine medications appropriately, particularly when prescribing for two presentations like anxiety as well as psychosis or hyperarousal: for example, aripiprazole and sertraline or risperidone and fluoxetine are appropriate combinations but aripiprazole and fluoxetine or risperidone and sertraline should be avoided unless the selective serotonin reuptake inhibitor is started first as it has the potential to increase the level of the antipsychotic medication.

Medication treatment may not be directed towards a specified diagnosis but rather to modify a child's presenting behaviours or a specific symptom. Medication may be chosen to manage the symptom either through known effects (e.g., in reducing anxiety in specified anxiety disorders) or using the side-effect profile of a medication (e.g., sedation to reduce hyperarousal or aggression levels). Pragmatic trials of medications may also be used when a cause of a presentation is not known. These are usually based upon the use of the evidence available, and likelihood of the medication chosen to improve the child's presentation.

The STOMP–STAMP (Stopping Over Medication of People with a learning disability, autism, or both- Supporting Treatment and Appropriate Medication in Paediatrics) campaign has a pledge for services to sign up to. Owing to psychoactive medications often having long durations of being prescribed with poor monitoring or review in people with intellectual disability, the campaign encourages the stopping of the over prescribing of medications in people with intellectual disability, as well as the starting of more appropriate ones. Both approaches can improve prescribing practices and help reduce inappropriate overprescribing.

The Evidence Base for Medication Treatments

The two mental disorder areas with the most evidence for prescribing pharmacological treatments in children and adolescents with intellectual disability are in ADHD and in behavioural disorders (typically irritability and agitation associated with the intellectual disability and/or autism). We present key evidence in these areas in Boxes 20.1 and 20.2.

Box 20.1 Evidence for ADHD Medication Treatment in Children and Adolescents with Intellectual Disability

- A 1993 double-blind crossover trial of Methylphenidate in 84 children with intellectual disability and with mean age 8.8 demonstrated improvements in ADHD symptoms (Aman et al., 1993)
- A 1999 double-blind crossover trial of Methylphenidate in 33 children with intellectual disability (including severe intellectual disability), with mean age 4.9, demonstrated improvement in ADHD symptoms (Handen et al., 1999)
- A 2010 16-week prospective study of atomoxetine in 48 children with intellectual disability with mean age 8.8 demonstrated improvement in ADHD symptoms (Fernández-Jaén et al., 2010)
- A 2013 16-week randomised controlled trial of methylphenidate in 122 children with intellectual disability (IQ between 30 and 68), and with mean age 10.83, demonstrated improvements in ADHD symptoms (Simonoff et al., 2013)

> **Box 20.2** Evidence for Medication Treatment for Behaviour Disorders (Particularly Involving Irritability and Agitation) in Children and Adolescents with Intellectual Disability
>
> - A 2002 double-blind randomised controlled trial of risperidone in 118 children with intellectual disability demonstrated reductions in severely disruptive behaviours, including irritability and hyperactivity (Aman et al., 2002)
> - A 2004 48-week open-label extension study of 107 children from the above 2002 study demonstrated long-term benefits for managing irritability (Findling et al., 2004)
> - A 2017 double-blind randomised controlled trial of aripiprazole in 92 children (of which 58 had intellectual disability) demonstrated significant reductions in irritability (Ichikawa et al., 2017)
>
> Research findings are often extrapolated from adult intellectual disability or child and adolescent (without intellectual disability) research. Medication research in children with intellectual disability has historically been challenging to conduct due to research ethical issues such as consent, but it is notable that many of the studies listed herein were not extensions from existing adult intellectual disability or child (without intellectual disability) literature. There have also been determined efforts by medicine regulators and the research community to advance high-quality empirical evidence to guide clinical treatments in this group of underserved children.

Non-Medication Treatments

Most of the support, care, and treatments offered for children and young people with intellectual disability is non-psychopharmacological. Though this chapter focuses on pharmacological management, it should be noted that in children and young people with intellectual disability, rather than a bio-psycho-socio approach, the order is often reversed with environmental approaches to management occurring first (socio-), then psychological (psycho-) and biological treatments (bio-) (e.g., medications being third line or in addition to the other approaches, but rarely in isolation). Even if the evidence-based approach is medication first line, the wider system often still requires education and support to manage the child and their presentation owing to the presence of the intellectual disability and or co-occurring diagnoses (e.g., autism).

The emphasis of behaviour management is towards positive behavioural support, which includes understanding the function of presenting behaviours and the use of positive approaches to management. Social interventions may include family interventions, adjusting to sensory issues, appropriate education, and home support. Psychological interventions may include anger management or anxiety management, speech and language interventions, and so forth. Biological interventions may include sedating agents (e.g., antipsychotics, sedating antihistamines or benzodiazepines), anxiolytics (e.g., selective serotonin reuptake inhibitors) or the treatment of physical causes for the behaviour (e.g., analgesia, anti-constipation, sleep).

Many have co-occurring physical ailments are managed through general practitioners, paediatricians, nurses, and a range of allied health professionals (e.g., speech and language therapists, physiotherapists, dietitians, occupational therapists, and health visitors). These include pharmacological treatments for underlying conditions that may also have an impact on mental state or behaviour (e.g., epilepsy, sleep, iron deficiency in pica or ADHD). Some genetic disorders with known behavioural phenotypes including aggression or self-injury may have physical health treatments to reduce behaviours (e.g., Cornelia de Lange syndrome and the use of proton pump inhibitors for reflux; and the use of betablockers, light boxes, and melatonin to alter the sleep-wake cycle in Smith–Magenis syndrome). Research in these areas point towards correlations but not specifically causality.

> **Case Study 20.2**
>
> Ann is a 9-year-old girl who was diagnosed with Smith–Magenis syndrome (SMS) last year. She has moderate intellectual disability, autism, and ADHD. Ann was referred to her local CAMHS-ID service as she was displaying poor sleep and increased behaviours that challenge, including self-injury, agitation, and aggression directed at others, which was having a significant impact on her accessing education and causing her to look increasingly unhappy, as well as increasing her parents' stress.
>
> After a comprehensive multidisciplinary assessment including a function-based assessment of behaviours, clinicians delivered the following interventions:
>
> (a) Nurse liaison with school professionals to implement communication strategies like visual timetables, and behavioural strategies like regular movement breaks and small achievable targets with incentives.
> (b) Psychology sessions with Ann's parents to implement equivalent behavioural and communication strategies at home, as well as to consider the impact of Ann's behaviour on family wellbeing and responding by scheduling parental inputs with some respite support.
> (c) Psychiatry commencing ADHD medication and liaising with a tertiary sleep service to prescribe melatonin and a beta blocker to help shift the characteristic inverted melatonin secretion pattern seen in Smith–Magenis syndrome.
>
> Positive outcomes following this multi-modal and multidisciplinary intervention plan included a reduction in Ann's behaviours that challenge, improved sleep, progression in her educational learning, and improved parental wellbeing and resilience.

How Long Should Treatment Continue?

Treatment should continue for as long it is needed. The STOMP–STAMP campaign guides prescribers to reduce over prescribing and to support appropriate prescribing. This includes the consideration of whether a medication should be reduced or stopped. Once a prescription is stable, generally it should continue for a period of time; often this is at least a year in children and young people with an intellectual disability. At each review, continuing effects and side effects should be considered. This should be backed up by multiagency information and observation. At the same time, a discussion should occur regarding whether the time is right to consider a trial reduction in medication. The ideal circumstances are when the young person's wider social and educational circumstances are in a period of stability and when no major changes are expected. A meeting with those involved in decision making for the child should be held and ideally a consensus should be reached about trialling a reduction. In the same way that starting and increasing medications may be done slowly with lots of monitoring, reductions should follow the same principles to minimise the likelihood of causing harm by reducing a medication. If there is a return of previous symptomatology, reinstatement of the previous dose may help. There are a variety of guidelines that recommend minimum timescales for consideration of need for a medication (e.g., the Prescribing Observatory for Mental Health audit).

Sometimes stopping a medication for a short period can be helpful for certain medications such as melatonin. This can allow a re-evaluation of whether it is still required and may actually improve the response (particularly when a medication has become habituated to). However, timing this is important – often during the longer school holidays is best, when the impact of possible reduced sleep on education will be limited.

There may be occasions where responsibility for prescribing and monitoring of medication is transferred to either primary care (general practitioner), another specialist care prescriber (e.g., non-medical prescriber), or when a young person graduates to adult services. It is important to summarise the original indication, what legislation is being used for decision making or consent, what effects and side effects have been seen, any results from physical parameter monitoring, how stable the prescription is, and what you would do next had you continued prescribing (e.g., frequency of prescribing, any planned dose changes and/or specialist monitoring required).

Case Study 20.3

Nguyen presented to services aged 6 with high levels of impulsivity, hyperactivity, and inattention compared to her school peers and some immaturity in her behaviours. She was in a mainstream educational setting with no additional support. A diagnosis of ADHD was made. She was prescribed a variety of ADHD medications, with some effect on her concentration, impulsivity, and hyperactivity, and no side effects. Over a number of years her level of learning was getting further and further behind her peers and ADHD medications were being increased gradually with limited improvements with each dose increase. She was delayed by about 5 years when she was aged 10. Cognitive assessments and assessments of her adaptive functioning were conducted. The results showed that she had an IQ of 49 and she was diagnosed with a moderate intellectual disability.

Owing to the limited effect of the ADHD medications, trial reductions were made, with observations put in place to compare her over time. Eventually, her medication was stopped by the time she was 13. There was no discernible difference in her presentation before and after stopping the medication. Nguyen's diagnoses were reviewed, and ADHD removed. It was estimated that at age 6, she would have been functioning at the developmental equivalent of a 3-year-old.

The Frith Prescribing Guidelines Editors' Expert Group Consensus Statements

Statements of High Confidence

- Methylphenidate is an effective treatment for ADHD in children with intellectual disability.
- The following principles of management from the general children population apply to children with intellectual disability as well:
    - An evidence-based framework like Positive Behaviour Support is crucial in devising a clinical formulation.
    - Antipsychotic medications can be helpful adjunctive medications to a comprehensive behaviour support plan in reducing irritability and behaviours that challenge.

Statements of Medium Confidence

- Risperidone and aripiprazole can be helpful adjunctive medications in reducing irritability and behaviours that challenge.

Statements of Low Confidence

- Atomoxetine is an effective treatment for ADHD in children with intellectual disability.

Resource Box

Key References and Guidelines

- NICE Guideline (2015) – Challenging Behaviour and Learning Disabilities: Prevention and interventions for people with learning disabilities whose behaviour challenges. www.nice.org.uk/guidance/ng11.
- NICE Guideline (2016) – Mental health problems in people with learning disabilities: prevention, assessment and management. www.nice.org.uk/guidance/ng54.
- Totsika, V., Liew, A., Absoud, M., Adnams, C. & Emerson, E. (2022) Mental health problems in children with intellectual disability. *The Lancet Child & Adolescent Health* 6, 432–44. https://doi.org/10.1016/S2352-4642(22)00067-0.
- Siegel, M., McGuire, K., Veenstra-VanderWeele, J., et al. (2020) Practice parameter for the assessment and treatment of psychiatric disorders in children and adolescents with intellectual disability (intellectual developmental disorder). *Journal of the American Academy of Child & Adolescent Psychiatry* 59, 468–96. https://doi.org/10.1016/j.jaac.2019.11.018.
- Allington-Smith, P. (2006) Mental health of children with learning disabilities. *Advances in Psychiatric Treatment* 12, 130–8. https://doi.org/10.1192/apt.12.2.130.

References

Aman, M. G., De Smedt, G., Derivan, A., et al. 2002. Double-blind, placebo-controlled study of risperidone for the treatment of disruptive behaviors in children with subaverage intelligence. *AJP* **159**, 1337–46. https://doi.org/10.1176/appi.ajp.159.8.1337.

Aman, M. G., Kern, R. A., McGhee, D. E., & Arnold, L. E., 1993. Fenfluramine and methylphenidate in children with mental retardation and ADHD: Clinical and side effects. *Journal of the American Academy of Child & Adolescent Psychiatry* **32**, 851–9. https://doi.org/10.1097/00004583-199307000-00022.

Buckley, N., Glasson, E. J., Chen, W., et al. 2020. Prevalence estimates of mental health problems in children and adolescents with intellectual disability: A systematic review and meta-analysis. *Aust N Z J Psychiatry* **54**, 970–84. https://doi.org/10.1177/0004867420924101.

Einfeld, S. L., Ellis, L. A., & Emerson, E., 2011. Comorbidity of intellectual disability and mental disorder in children and adolescents: A systematic review. *Journal of Intellectual & Developmental Disability* **36**, 137–43. https://doi.org/10.1080/13668250.2011.572548.

Emerson, E., & Hatton, C., 2007. Mental health of children and adolescents with intellectual disabilities in Britain. *British Journal of Psychiatry* **191**, 493–9. https://doi.org/10.1192/bjp.bp.107.038729.

Fernández-Jaén, A., Fernández-Mayoralas, D. M., Calleja Pérez, B., Muñoz Jareño, N., & del

Rosario Campos Díaz, M., 2010. Atomoxetine for attention deficit hyperactivity disorder in mental retardation. *Pediatric Neurology* **43**, 341–7. https://doi.org/10.1016/j.pediatrneurol.2010.06.003.

Findling, R. L., Aman, M. G., Eerdekens, M., et al. 2004. Long-term, open-label study of risperidone in children with severe disruptive behaviors and below-average IQ. *AJP* **161**, 677–84. https://doi.org/10.1176/appi.ajp.161.4.677.

Handen, B. L., Feldman, H. M., Lurier, A., & Murray, P. J. H., 1999. Efficacy of methylphenidate among preschool children with developmental disabilities and ADHD. *Journal of the American Academy of Child and Adolescent Psychiatry* **38**, 805–12.

Ichikawa, H., Mikami, K., Okada, T., et al. 2017. Aripiprazole in the treatment of irritability in children and adolescents with autism spectrum disorder in Japan: A randomized, double-blind, placebo-controlled study. *Child Psychiatry Hum Dev* **48**, 796–806. https://doi.org/10.1007/s10578-016-0704-x.

Simonoff, E., Taylor, E., Baird, G., et al. 2013. Randomized controlled double-blind trial of optimal dose methylphenidate in children and adolescents with severe attention deficit hyperactivity disorder and intellectual disability: Methylphenidate for hyperkinetic disorder in children with intellectual disability. *Journal of Child Psychology and Psychiatry* **54**, 527–35. https://doi.org/10.1111/j.1469-7610.2012.02569.x.

Chapter 21: Prescribing for Health Issues in Women with Intellectual Disability

Sowmy Murickal, Nnenna Kalu-Nsi, and Amala Jesu

Introduction

For women with intellectual disability, the expression and recognition of their mental distress may be complicated not only by their gender and intellectual disability but also by their communication needs and dependency on others and society at large. (O'Hara, 2004)

It is well known that individuals with intellectual disability have more physical and mental health ailments, higher morbidity, earlier mortality, lower access to primary care services, and, hence, require more attention (Hanlon et al., 2018; Perera et al., 2019). The requirements of women with intellectual disability are not hugely dissimilar to those of other women; however, services are often not responsive to the needs of women with intellectual disability. This consequently leads to a plethora of issues related to parenting, sexual relationships, caring for others, bereavement, and loss (Brown, 1996). Women are often excluded from vital interventions by virtue of their intellectual disability – for example, use of services for breast and cervical screening for cancer were noted to be poor among women with intellectual disability (Plourde et al., 2018; Maltais et al., 2020).

In this chapter, the following conditions will be discussed in more detail:

- Premenstrual disorders, including menstrual period-linked psychosis and premenstrual dysphoric disorder (PMDD)
- Problems related to childbearing years, contraception, and education
- Polycystic ovary syndrome (PCOS)
- Catamenial epilepsy
- Perimenopausal problems

Premenstrual Disorders

Premenstrual symptoms have been recognised since the time of Hippocrates when menstruation was thought as a process of 'purging melancholic humours' (Stolberg 2000); it wasn't until the latter part of twentieth century that they gained widespread recognition among the scientific community (Paul & Pal, 2022).

Premenstrual syndrome (PMS) can be broadly defined as the constellation of psychological and physical symptoms that recur regularly in the luteal phase of the menstrual cycle, remit for at least one week in the follicular phase, and cause distress and functional impairment. The symptoms should be of at least moderate intensity and cause functional impairment. When these symptoms become severe, they are referred to as premenstrual dysphoric disorder (PMDD).

The International Classification of Diseases (ICD-11) defines PMDD as 'a pattern of mood symptoms (depressed mood, irritability), somatic symptoms (lethargy, joint pain, overeating), or cognitive symptoms (concentration difficulties, forgetfulness) that begin several days before the onset of menses, start to improve within a few days after the onset of menses, and then become minimal or absent within approximately 1 week following the onset of menses'.

The prevalence of premenstrual disorders is estimated to be between 20% and 50%, and PMDD significantly lower at around 2–8%, across several studies around the globe. (Gao et al., 2021). It is difficult to know the prevalence rates in women with intellectual disability due to limited research in this population group. Arguably, recognition of menstrual period-related problems in women with intellectual disability may be poor due to associated comorbidities (e.g., epilepsy treatment, communication difficulties).

There have been case reports of episodic psychosis linked to the menstrual period, which have the following characteristics: acute onset, short in duration with full recovery in between episodes, and psychotic features (delusions, hallucinations, and mood changes) which tend to recur in rhythm with the menstrual cycle.

The cause of premenstrual disorders is poorly understood. The brain cells of patients with PMDD show abnormal expression of hormone-processing genes and there is altered functioning of the brain's serotonin and GABA systems across the menstrual cycle. Studies have shown that it is likely that several neurotransmitters may be involved, but there is no conclusive evidence (Dilbaz & Aksan, 2021).

Problems Related to Childbearing Years

These are similar to the general population; however, additional issues for women with intellectual disability include ethical, legal (capacity to consent), and social issues, which may have a major impact on their mental well-being, as well as behaviours seen as challenging. Key issues to consider are capacity to consent, use of sterilisation, therapeutic amenorrhoea, and developing parenting skills, plus the mental health impact consequent to a child being removed for fostering/adoption.

It has been found that women with intellectual disability use a limited range of contraceptive methods, have reduced knowledge about options regarding contraceptives, commence contraception earlier, and often utilise it before becoming sexually active compared to women without disabilities. Women with intellectual disability are frequently on contraceptives for menstrual suppression. Evidence confirms that people with intellectual disability are likely to have fewer and delayed sexual experiences than people without intellectual disability.

Family planning counselling, though vital, is often not offered to women with intellectual disability based on the notion that they might not be sexually active. Additionally, there is the obstacle of health professionals not trained in intellectual disability having limited knowledge, confidence, and experience in offering advice and information around contraception, as well as limited numbers of women with intellectual disability requesting this. Women with intellectual disability having accessible and equitable sexual and reproductive health education around menstruation, contraceptive decision making, and menopause is fundamental to achieving health equality (Wiseman & Ferrie, 2020).

Polycystic Ovary Syndrome

Polycystic ovary syndrome (PCOS) is a common endocrine disorder affecting women at reproductive age, with an estimated prevalence of 6–10% (Gurkan 2016). It is a complex disorder characterised by androgen excess (hirsutism and acne) and ovarian dysfunction leading to oligomenorrhoea or amenorrhoea and infertility. Follicular cysts in ovaries do not necessarily have to be present to make the diagnosis. Women with polycystic ovary syndrome are at greater risk of developing long-term health problems due to insulin resistance, obesity, metabolic disorders, and cardiovascular risk factors. There are high rates of psychological morbidity and associated medical problems like asthma and migraine. Despite being a common condition with a high morbidity risk, the syndrome often remains underdiagnosed and is therefore underrepresented in the general population let alone women with intellectual disability. There are also reports of an association of developing polycystic ovary syndrome in women taking sodium valproate for epilepsy during their young adulthood.

Catamenial Epilepsy

Catamenial epilepsy is defined as a 'pattern of seizures that changes in severity during particular phases of the menstrual cycle, wherein oestrogens are proconvulsant, increasing the neuronal excitability; and progesterone is anticonvulsant, enhancing GABA-mediated inhibition' (Verrotti et al., 2012). The prevalence ranges widely between 10% and 70% of women with epilepsy who are of reproductive age (Duncan 1993). The rates are likely to be higher if there is the comorbidity of intellectual disability. Three patterns of catamenial seizures have been noted: perimenstrual, peri-ovulatory, and luteal phase in anovulatory cycles (Cooper et al., 2019). Knowledge of the effects of sex hormones on epilepsy is key to understanding novel therapeutic approaches, in addition to antiepileptic drugs, for women with catamenial seizures.

Perimenopausal Issues

Perimenopause is the period when there is an initial change to the menstrual pattern: the menstrual cycle length may shorten to 2–3 weeks or lengthen to many months. The amount of menstrual blood loss may change, and commonly increases slightly. Menopause is diagnosed after 12 months of amenorrhoea resulting from the permanent cessation of ovarian function.

The phase of irregular menstrual activity which directly precedes menopause is characterised by widely fluctuating hormone levels amidst a significant decline in circulating oestrogen. This phase is typically accompanied by physical discomfort, including vasomotor symptoms, such as headaches, insomnia, and hot flushes, as well as genital atrophy. Additionally, studies also suggest a significant increase in mood lability for women during this period.

This phase may be difficult to recognise in women with intellectual disability especially when they have associated behaviour seen as challenging, anxiety problems, or communication difficulties. Menopause is usually earlier in women with intellectual disability, with higher rates of premature menopause for those with Down syndrome. Discussions about hormone replacement therapy often exclude the needs of women with intellectual disability and their views are not considered in decision making. More research is needed in this area for better recognition and management of menopause-related health issues (Martin 2003).

Key Issues Related to Menstrual Period during Adolescence/Puberty

The onset of adolescence and puberty can be a particularly challenging time for young women with intellectual disability and their family/carers. Understanding and dealing with hormonal and bodily changes can prove difficult. The key issues on this topic are shown in Figure 21.1.

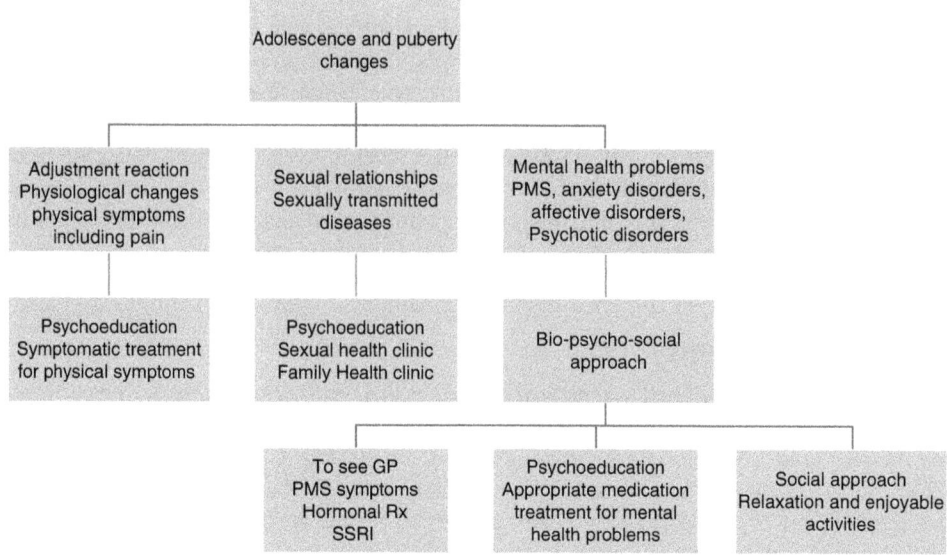

Figure 21.1 Key issues related to menstrual period during adolescence/puberty and their management

Menstrual Cycle-Related Issues Specific to Intellectual Disability

- Most frequently reported symptoms are pain, mood changes, generally feeling unwell or tired, and heavy blood loss.
- Women with severe/profound intellectual disability are more likely to have more period-related problems at some stage as compared to women with mild/moderate intellectual disability.
- Women with a coexisting physical impairment are more likely to experience marked or severe problems with their periods.
- In women with communication difficulties, symptoms may present as behavioural challenges around the menstrual period.
- Younger women are more likely to experience menstrual problems compared to women over the age of 35.
- Women with intellectual disability may experience menopause earlier than women in the general population.
- The prevalence of epilepsy in people with intellectual disability is higher than in the general population; in women with intellectual disability this can be associated with catamenial epilepsy.
- There is a higher risk of developing polycystic ovary syndrome in younger women with epilepsy who are prescribed sodium valproate. New MHRA Regulations on the prescribing of sodium valproate in females came into force in the UK in 2024.

The Frith Treatment Guideline for People with Intellectual Disability

The common menstrual cycle problems in different life stages are summarised in Table 21.1.

Table 21.1 The common menstrual cycle problems encountered at different life stages and a general treatment approach to follow

Timeline	Key issues related to menstrual cycle at different stages of life	What to do/who to consult
Adolescence/ puberty changes	• Adjustment reaction to pubertal changes (hormonal and physiological bodily changes) • Mental and physical health problems related to onset of menarche and menstrual period (e.g., premenstrual disorders, dysmenorrhoea, acne, mastalgia, etc.) • Sexual relationship and risk of sexually transmitted disease • Contraception	• Psychoeducation • For physical symptoms, see general practitioner • For mental health problems, psychoeducation/sexual health clinic • To consult general practitioner/family planning clinic
Childbearing Age	• Sexual relationship and risk of sexually transmitted disease • Premenstrual syndrome, dysmenorrhoea, acne, mastalgia, catamenial epilepsy • Pregnancy and childbirth, contraception, sterilisation, problems with medications crossing the placenta barrier and breast milk. • Mental health problems: associated with puerperium, postnatal depression, puerperal psychosis • Postnatal 'blues', stress, and adjustment reaction related to parental responsibility and sleepless nights • Affective disorder, psychotic disorder, and anxiety disorders.	• Psychoeducation/sexual health clinic • For physical symptoms, see general practitioner • Epilepsy: general practitioner/neurologist/psychiatrist • See general practitioner/family clinic • See psychiatrist • Psychoeducation/general practitioner • Referral to psychiatrist; see relevant chapters of this *Guideline*
Older age group (menopausal changes)	• Age-related physical health: mobility problems, higher risk of osteoporosis after menopause • Mental health problems related to menopause	• See general practitioner for physical symptoms and menopausal symptoms • Psychiatrist referral; see relevant chapters of this *Guideline*

Medication Management

Table 21.2, which provides information on the role of medications used in general in the management of menstrual period-related problems, is for information and guidance only. Hormonal treatment and treatment for metabolic disorders are included in the table for information only as these areas of treatment are normally recommended by general practitioners and gynaecologists.

Table 21.2 Guidance on the role of medications used in general in the management of menstrual period-related problems

Problem	Medications used in management	Evidence
Premenstrual syndrome/ premenstrual dysphoric disorder	**Mild premenstrual disorders symptoms:** Pain relief (i.e., paracetamol, non-steroidal anti-inflammatory drugs (NSAID)) if predominant symptom is pain **Moderate premenstrual disorders symptoms:** New-generation combined oral contraceptive, especially if the woman requires contraception (off-label use if used solely to treat premenstrual disorders symptoms) **Severe premenstrual disorders symptoms:** Selective serotonin reuptake inhibitors (SSRI) (off-label use) to be taken continuously or just during the luteal phase (e.g., on days 15–28 of the menstrual cycle, depending on its length) Other psychotropics, serotonin and norepinephrine reuptake inhibitors (SNRI), and buspirone Hormone treatment: Combined oral contraceptive Danazol Spironolactone Oestradiol patches and GnRH agonists GABAergic system and therapies: dutasteride	National Institute for Health and Care Excellence guidelines (CKS) The Royal College of Obstetricians and Gynaecologists (RCOG) recommends the use of new-generation combined oral contraceptives because they produce fewer adverse effects and there is some evidence supporting their efficacy in the treatment of premenstrual syndrome (Green et al., 2017) There is increasing evidence that SSRIs and SNRI are helpful in managing premenstrual disorder symptoms in general population (Tiranini & Nappi, 2022) Venlafaxine has shown efficacy for the treatment of premenstrual dysphoric disorder in one open-label trial. However, it is associated with a higher risk of withdrawal effects compared with other antidepressants Buspirone has been shown to be superior to placebo but less effective than SSRIs (Landen et al., 2001) The rationale for combined hormonal contraceptive is the blockade of an ovulatory surge of sex steroids since premenstrual symptoms are not observed during anovulatory cycles

Table 21.2 (cont.)

Problem	Medications used in management	Evidence
		There is evidence that danazol is effective for treating premenstrual syndrome. However, caution is needed as it is an off-label use and there is a risk of irreversible virilising adverse effects (such as weight gain, acne, hirsutism, and voice changes) associated with its use (Green et al., 2017)
		The Royal College of Obstetricians and Gynaecologists recommends spironolactone for treating physical symptoms in women with premenstrual syndrome (BJOG, 2016). Off-label use, specialist prescription only
		Oestrogen patches (given with a progestogen to prevent endometrial hyperplasia) are offered as an option in the Royal College of Obstetricians and Gynaecologists guideline (Green et al., 2017). Specialist prescription only
		At present, dutasteride is a potential off-label option for women experiencing side effects or lacking benefits of SSRIs
Catamenial epilepsy	Titrate up antiepileptic dose. Intermittent clobazam around menstrual period Cessation of menstruation using synthetic hormones (e.g., medroxyprogesterone (Depo-Provera)) or gonadotropin-releasing hormone (GnRH) analogues (triptorelin and goserelin)	In double-blind crossover study, intermittent use of clobazam versus placebo around the time of menstruation appeared to be superior to placebo (Feely et al., 1982) Continuous use of combined oral contraceptives is thought to decrease the frequency of the seizures by achieving amenorrhea, but again there is inadequate data to reach a robust conclusion (Dural et al., 2020; Christian et al., 2020)

Table 21.2 (cont.)

Problem	Medications used in management	Evidence
Polycystic ovary syndrome (PCOS)	The 'new therapeutic tools' Insulin sensitisers: metformin, thiazolidinediones	The new guideline encourages combining metformin with combined oral contraceptives, especially in overweight or obese women with polycystic ovary syndrome 3-component treatment, including diet, exercise, and cognitive behaviour therapy, improved depression and self-esteem in obese women with polycystic ovary syndrome (Hoeger et al., 2020) Therapeutic management should be individualised and not targeted on specific symptoms. Currently available treatments for polycystic ovary syndrome are not fully able to treat all the metabolic consequences (Bargiota et al., 2012)
Perimenopausal symptoms	Non-hormonal treatment • SSRIs • SNRI Hormone replacement therapy (HRT)	SSRIs or SNRI compared to placebo, were found to be effective in reducing severe menopausal hot flushes among postmenopausal women (Nelson, 2006; Goodman, 2011) Serotonergic antidepressants are generally the first-line treatment for depression in the perimenopause Hormone replacement therapy is currently the most effective treatment for vasomotor symptoms in postmenopausal women. There is a clear beneficial effect with oestrogen replacement compared to placebo (Hickey, 2012; Panay et al., 2013) Oestrogen treatment is widely believed to improve depressive symptoms in menopausal women, but study results are inconclusive

Case Study 21.1

Penny is a 35-year-old woman with moderate intellectual disability presenting with complex epilepsy and significant behaviour seen as challenging (aggression towards others) who is living in a residential care home. Her seizures have been well controlled for many years, but over the last six months she has been having clusters of partial seizures happening around the time of her menstrual period. She has been on a regime of antiseizure medication including lamotrigine and carbamazepine that has not changed in the past five years. The antiseizure medications have also had a mood stabilising effect which is helpful in managing the behaviours.

Penny has regular input from the local intellectual disability team and during psychiatry review the increase in seizure frequency was reported by carers. On further questioning, it transpired that her periods have been heavy and irregular as well during the last six months. Alongside this there was a clear increase in behavioural challenges around the time of periods. Physical examination was normal and further blood tests were completed which picked up anaemia. The general practitioner also completed a gynae referral in view of the heavy periods and resultant anaemia.

The psychiatrist suggested the use of adequate pain relief during periods and use of PRN clobazam to manage the clusters of seizures. Further scans revealed uterine fibroids which explained the heavy periods, and this was successfully treated using medications. Following this the seizures stabilised and clobazam was cautiously withdrawn.

The Frith Prescribing Guidelines Editors' Expert Group Consensus Statements

Statements of High Confidence

- The prevalence of menstrual cycle-related disorders in women with intellectual disability is at least as high as that of women without an intellectual disability.
- Women with Down syndrome are likely to develop early menopause.
- The following guidance for the general population applies to women with intellectual disability as well:
  - Treatment for premenstrual syndrome (PMS)/premenstrual dysphoric disorder (PMDD) include:
    - Offer adequate pain relief where indicated
    - In women with severe premenstrual syndrome, consider prescribing a selective serotonin reuptake inhibitor (SSRI, off-label use) to be taken continuously or just during the luteal phase
    - Management of premenstrual syndrome should be tailored to the severity and type of symptoms, the woman's treatment preferences, and any desire to become pregnant
  - There is good evidence to combine metformin with combined oral contraceptives, especially in overweight or obese women with polycystic ovary syndrome (PCOS).
  - Hormone replacement therapy is currently the most effective treatment for vasomotor symptoms in postmenopausal women.

Statements of Medium Confidence
- There is some benefit to use of venlafaxine and buspirone in premenstrual syndrome/PMDD, though caution is needed in women with intellectual disability due to withdrawal effects.
- Intermittent use of clobazam has its benefits in catamenial epilepsy.

Statements of Low Confidence
- The role of cognitive behavioural therapy/psychological intervention for moderate or severe symptoms of premenstrual syndrome alongside medical management in women with intellectual disability is poorly understood.
- The following guidance for the general population applies to women with intellectual disability as well:
  - In catamenial epilepsy, use of continuous combined oral contraceptives is thought to decrease the frequency of the seizures by achieving amenorrhea
  - There is limited evidence to support the use of complementary treatments for some women with premenstrual syndrome, especially those in whom hormonal therapy is contraindicated, may benefit from a holistic approach.

Resource Box

Important Guidelines
1. NICE Clinical Knowledge Summaries (CKS): Management of Polycystic ovary syndrome in adults (last revised February 2022) and Management of premenstrual syndrome (last revised May 2019)
2. Premenstrual Syndrome, Management (Green-top Guideline No. 48). www.rcog.org.uk/guidance/browse-all-guidance/green-top-guidelines/premenstrual-syndrome-management-green-top-guideline-no-48/

References

Bargiota, A. & Diamanti-Kandarakis, E. (2012) The effects of old, new, and emerging medicines on metabolic aberrations in PCOS. *Therapeutic Advances in Endocrinology and Metabolism*, 3(1), 27–47.

Bozdag, G., Mumusoglu, S., Zengin, D., Karabulut, E., & Yildiz, B.. (2016) The prevalence and phenotypic features of polycystic ovary syndrome: a systematic review and meta-analysis, *Human Reproduction*, 31(12), 2841–55.

Brown, H. (1996). Ordinary women: Issues for women with learning disabilities. *British Journal of Learning Disabilities*, 24(2), 47–51. https://doi.org/10.1111/j.1468-3156.1996.tb00201.x

Christian, C. A., Reddy, D. S., Maguire, J., & Forcelli, P. A. (2020). Sex differences in the epilepsies and associated comorbidities: Implications for use and development of Pharmacotherapies. *Pharmacological Reviews*, 72(4), 767–800. https://doi.org/10.1124/pr.119.017392

Cooper, N. C., Balachandran Nair, D., Egan, S., Barrie, A., & Perera, B. (2019). Current evidence for the identification and management of premenstrual syndrome in women with intellectual disabilities: A systematic review. *Advances in Mental Health and Intellectual Disabilities*, 13(6), 268–83. https://doi.org/10.1108/amhid-05-2019-0015

Dilbaz, B., & Aksan, A. (2021). Premenstrual syndrome, a common but underrated entity: Review of the clinical literature. *Journal of the Turkish-German Gynecological Association*, **22**(2), 139–48. https://doi.org/10.4274/jtgga.galenos.2021.2020.0133

Duncan, S., Read, C. L., & Brodie, M. J. (1993). How common is catamenial epilepsy? *Epilepsia*, **34**(5), 827–31.

Dural, Ö., Taş, İ. S., & Akhan, S. E. (2020). Management of menstrual and gynecologic concerns in girls with special needs. *Journal of Clinical Research in Pediatric Endocrinology*, **12**(1), 41–5. https://doi.org/10.4274/jcrpe.galenos.2019.2019.s0174

Feely, M., Calvert, R., & Gibson J. (1982). Clobazam in catamenial epilepsy. A model for evaluating anticonvulsants. *Lancet*, **10**(2), 71–3. https://doi.org/10.1016/s0140-6736(82)91691-9.

Gao, M., Cheng, X., Zhang, H., et al. (2021). Global and regional prevalence and burden for premenstrual syndrome and premenstrual dysphoric disorder: A study protocol for systematic review and meta-analysis. *Medicine (Baltimore)*, **101**(1), e28528. https://doi.org/10.37766/inplasy2021.12.0065

Goodman, A. (2006). SNRI antidepressant reduces postmenopausal hot flashes. American Congress of Obstetricians and Gynecologists (ACOG) 59th Annual Clinical Meeting.

Goodman, N. F., Cobin, R. H., Ginzburg, S. B., et al. (2011). American Association of Clinical Endocrinologists Medical Guidelines for Clinical Practice for the diagnosis and treatment of menopause. *Endocrine Practice*, **17**, 1–25.

Green, L. J., O'Brien, P. M.S., Panay, N., & Craig, M. on behalf of the Royal College of Obstetricians and Gynaecologists (2017). Management of premenstrual syndrome. *BJOG*, **124**, e73–e105.

Hanlon, P., MacDonald, S., Wood, K., Allan, L., & Cooper, S.-A. (2018). Long-term condition management in adults with intellectual disability in primary care: A systematic review. *BJGP Open*, **2**(1). https://doi.org/10.3399/bjgpopen18x101445

Hoeger, K. M., Dokras, A., & Piltonen, T. (2020). Update on PCOS: Consequences, challenges, and guiding treatment. *The Journal of Clinical Endocrinology & Metabolism*, **106**(3). https://doi.org/10.1210/clinem/dgaa839

Hickey, M., Elliott, J., & Davison, S. L. (2012) Hormone replacement therapy. *BMJ*; **344**, e763.

Landen, M., Eriksson, O., Sundblad, C., et.al. (2001) Compounds with affinity for serotonergic receptors in the treatment of premenstrual dysphoria: A comparison of buspirone, nefazodone and placebo. *Psychopharmacology*; **155**, 292–8.

Maltais, J., Morin, D., & Tassé, M. J. (2020). Healthcare services utilization among people with intellectual disability and comparison with the general population. *Journal of Applied Research in Intellectual Disabilities*, **33**(3), 552–64. https://doi.org/10.1111/jar.12698

Martin, D. M., Kakumani, S., Martin, M. S., & Cassidy, G. (2003). Learning disabilities and the menopause. *The Journal of the British Menopause Society*, **9**(1), 22–6. https://doi.org/10.1258/136218003100322107

Maguire, M. J., & Nevitt, S. J. (2021). Treatments for seizures in catamenial (menstrual-related) epilepsy. *Cochrane Database of Systematic Reviews*, 9. Art. No.: CD013225. https://doi.org/10.1002/14651858.CD013225.pub3.

Nelson, H. D. et al. (2006) Nonhormonal therapies for menopausal hot flashes systematic review and meta-analysis. *Journal of American Medical Association, JAMA*, **295**(17), 2057–71.

O'Hara, J. (2004) Mental Health needs of women with learning disabilities: Services can be organised to meet the challenge; (Commentary) – *Learning Disability Review*: **9**(4), 20–3.

Panay, N., Hamoda, H., Arya, R. & Savvas, M. (2013) The 2013 British Menopause Society Women's Health concern and recommendations on Hormone Replacement Therapy. Published online, **19**(2), 59–68. http://min.sagepub.com/content/19/2/59.full.pdf+html

Paul, S. & Pal, A. (2022). Premenstrual syndrome and premenstrual dysphoric disorder: A review of their history with an eye on future. *Annals of Indian Psychiatry.* https://doi.org/10.4103/aip.aip_16_22.

Perera, B., Audi, S., Solomou, S., Courtenay, K., & Ramsay, H. (2019). Mental and physical health conditions in people with intellectual disabilities: Comparing local and national data. *British Journal of Learning Disabilities,* **48**(1), 19–27. https://doi.org/10.1111/bld.12304

Plourde, N., Brown, H. K., Vigod, S., & Cobigo, V. (2018). The association between continuity of primary care and preventive cancer screening in women with intellectual disability. *American Journal on Intellectual and Developmental Disabilities,* **123**(6), 499–513. https://doi.org/10.1352/1944-7558-123.6.499.

Stolberg, M. (2000). The monthly malady: A history of premenstrual suffering. *Medical History,* **44**(3), 301–22.

Tiranini, L., & Nappi, R. E. (2022). Recent advances in understanding/management of premenstrual dysphoric disorder/premenstrual syndrome. *Faculty Reviews,* **11**. https://doi.org/10.12703/r/11-11

Verrotti, A., D'Egidio, C., Agostinelli, S., Verrotti, C., & Pavone, P. (2012). Diagnosis, and management of catamenial seizures: A review. *International Journal of Women's Health,* **4**, 535–41. https://doi.org/10.2147/IJWH.S28872.

Wiseman, P., & Ferrie, J. (2020). Reproductive (in)justice and inequality in the lives of women with intellectual disabilities in Scotland. *Scandinavian Journal of Disability Research,* **22**(1), 318–29. https://doi.org/10.16993/sjdr.677.

World Health Organization. (2019/2021). *ICD-11: International classification of diseases* (11th revision). https://icd.who.int/.

Chapter 22

Older People

Gemma Lewin, Elizabeta Mukaetova-Ladinska, Rohit Gumber, and Satheesh K. Gangadharan

Introduction

The life expectancy for people with intellectual disability is increasing due to advances in medical treatment and social care (O'Leary et al., 2018). However, significant discrepancies in life expectancy between people with intellectual disability and the general population remain, and there continues to be scope to close the inequality gap (Tyrer et al., 2020). This was confirmed in the recent 2021 Learning Disability Mortality Review (LeDeR) report (White et al., 2022). The standardised mortality ratio for people with intellectual disability ranges from 2 to 5, which draws a comparison against the general population. Those with additional comorbidities such as epilepsy, genetic syndromes, and functional impairments have a lower age of death (O'Leary et al., 2018).

The leading causes of death in older adults (at or over 65 years of age) between 2018 and 2021 were reviewed in the 2021 Learning Disability Mortality Review report. In comparison to the general population, a higher proportion of deaths in older adults with intellectual disability were due to COVID-19 (Coronavirus disease), cancers, and influenza or pneumonia. Unsurprisingly, dementia (in particular Alzheimer's disease), cerebrovascular disease, chronic lower respiratory tract infections and diseases of the urinary system were more common causes of death in older people with intellectual disability compared to that reported in their younger counterparts (White et al., 2022).

Increasing life expectancy among people with intellectual disability poses new clinical challenges concerning the care they require in their middle and late age, as many face age-associated health problems similar to older people without intellectual disability (Lim et al., 2018). The intellectual disability population has a higher prevalence of multiple long-term conditions when compared to the general population, and these are much more common in older age groups (Mann et al., 2022). These include sleep problems, major depressive disorders, dysphagia, obesity, suboptimal nutritional intake, and low physical activity levels (de Leeuw et al., 2022), as well as chronic constipation, severe challenging behaviour, and hearing and visual impairment (Hermans & Evenhuis, 2014).

The social implications of the ageing process among the intellectual disability population should not be underestimated. An older person with intellectual disability who has been looked after in the home environment may also be cared for by an ageing caregiver, who may now not be able to cater to their care needs due to their own ill health or frailty. Death or loss of a carer may consequently lead to a sudden and poorly prepared move to a residential care facility, as well as challenges associated with bereavement for the person with intellectual disability. Financial difficulties may be further exacerbated by retirement of the caregiver or household contributor. Increased life expectancy in turn adds higher demands on residential care facilities, which may mean that people are moved to general elderly care facilities that may not be specific to, or well supported for, the person with intellectual disability.

Key Issues Related to Prescribing in Older People with Intellectual Disability

Frailty and Accelerated Ageing in People with Intellectual Disability

People with intellectual disability age prematurely and become frail at a much younger age compared to the general population. Thus, the frailty of the >50 years intellectual disability population is comparable to that of the >70 years general population (Schoufour et al., 2021). Frailty is an important predictor of adverse health outcomes and should form part of the regular clinical review for people with intellectual disability to identify and intervene where possible at the earliest stage. An intellectual disability frailty index (ID-frailty index) has been created by Schoufour et al. (2013). When the scale was used in the intellectual disability population, the ID-frailty index appears to predict mortality more effectively than general population frailty scales, which were previously used. The ID-frailty index predicts a decline in mobility, increased disability, polypharmacy, and increased care intensity. Access information for the ID-frailty scale is provided in the Resource Box.

A unique example of accelerated ageing in a person with intellectual disability is that seen in Down syndrome. Down syndrome increases the risk of many chronic diseases that are typically associated with older age: premature skin wrinkling, greying of hair, hearing loss, early menopause, declining immune function, and Alzheimer's disease. This accelerated ageing involves some but not all organs and tissues. DNA damage accumulation, telomere shortening, loss of protein homeostasis, oxidative stress and mitochondrial dysfunction, cellular senescence, stem cell ageing, inflammation, and epigenetic changes have all been documented (Gensous et al., 2019).

Pharmacokinetics and Pharmacodynamics Related to Ageing

In an ageing population, there are physiological changes which can impact prescribing in a multifactorial manner. These can be broadly separated into those that affect pharmacokinetics and pharmacodynamics. Pharmacokinetics describes what the body does to the medication, including absorption, distribution, metabolism, and excretion, whereas pharmacodynamics describes the effects of medications on the body and their mechanisms of action which are affected by target receptor availability, binding, post-receptor signal effects, and chemical interactions (Drenth-van Maanen et al., 2019).

This section summarises the pharmacokinetic and pharmacodynamic changes related to ageing in general. Due to their accelerated ageing process, multiple medical comorbidities, and polypharmacy, people with intellectual disability are particularly vulnerable to these changes. Considering the lack of more detailed information relating to these changes in intellectual disability population, the information presented is drawn from the general body of literature (see Table 22.1).

Table 22.1 Summary of pharmacokinetic and pharmacodynamic changes in the ageing general population

Process and general description	Relevant consideration in ageing population
Absorption (the principal route of absorption is gut but could also be skin, muscle, subcutaneous layer or the lungs based on the route of administration of medication)	Drenth-van Maanen et al. (2019); Ruscin and Linnebur (2019) 1. Reduced acid production and increase of pH (a scale used to specify the acidity or basicity of an aqueous solution) in the stomach reduces dissolution of the medication and its bioavailability. 2. Reduced gastric motility, small intestinal surface area, blood flow to the gut and delayed gastric emptying reduces the absorption. 3. The above changes, however, are not likely to be clinically significant for most medications.
Distribution (this describes the movement of a medication from blood to and from various tissues of the body)	Drenth-van Maanen et al. (2019); Jansen and Brouwers (2012) 1. There is an increase in body fat proportion with ageing. Lipophilic medications like benzodiazepines will have an increased volume of distribution, meaning that there is an increased amount of medication remaining in the tissues leading to an increase in half-life elimination and prolonged adverse effects. 2. Reduction in lean body mass and total body water leads to a smaller volume of distribution for hydrophilic medications such as lithium leading to higher serum concentration. The dose should therefore be reduced. 3. Albumin may be reduced and α–1 acid glycoprotein may be increased. Acidic medications like diazepam and phenytoin which bind to albumin will have an increase in unbound (active) volume. When α–1 acid glycoprotein is increased, basic medications like clozapine and propranolol will have a decrease in unbound (active) volume.
Metabolism (the process of breakdown of medications by the body)	Ruscin and Linnebur (2019) 1. Ageing leads to reduced hepatic mass (up to 30%), reduced hepatic blood flow and decreased cytochrome P-450 and other metabolic enzymes. Medications like benzodiazepines and propranolol which have a significant first pass metabolism (extensive metabolism during the medication's first pass through the liver) could have an increase in bioavailability. Reduced hepatic metabolism increases the bioavailability of medications that depend principally on hepatic metabolism, such as chlordiazepoxide, diazepam, imipramine, levodopa, nortriptyline, and trazodone.
Excretion (the process of the removal of medications by the body)	Ruscin and Linnebur (2019) 1. Reduced glomerular filtration rate (GFR) and overall renal function affect the medications which are excreted mainly through kidney un-metabolised. An example is lithium.

Table 22.1 (cont.)

Process and general description	Relevant consideration in ageing population
	The narrow therapeutic range of lithium makes this particularly risky as levels can accumulate. Kidney function (GFR) should therefore be monitored, and the dose/dose intervals of medications should be altered appropriately. 2. Due to reduced muscle mass, serum creatinine could be normal in the elderly despite renal dysfunction. As renal function could be affected by acute illnesses, a constant vigil is essential. 3. Examples of the psychoactive medications affected by impaired renal functions include gabapentin, lurasidone, paliperidone, risperidone and lithium.
Pharmacodynamics (the process that describes effects of medications on the body and their mechanisms of action)	Drenth-van Maanen et al. (2019) 1. Some neuroleptic medications cause increased sedation and higher risk of extrapyramidal side effects in elderly. 2. Benzodiazepines cause sedation, postural sway, and memory impairment. Reduced doses and short-acting preparations are therefore preferred when used in older people (Jansen and Brouwers, 2012). 3. Increased sensitivity to anticholinergic side effects leads to confusion, sedation, blurred vision, constipation, urinary retention, orthostatic hypotension, and a dry mouth. These can be caused by tricyclic antidepressants, neuroleptic medications, and sedating antihistamines. Medications with similar side effects profile could cause a cumulative effect, especially in the context of polypharmacy.

Polypharmacy

Multimorbidity is common in an ageing person with intellectual disability. As comorbidities accumulate and preventative strategies are implemented, it is easy to see how the number of pharmacological treatments that a person receives can increase dramatically. With increased sensitivity to medications and changes to pharmacokinetics and pharmacodynamics as a person ages, caution should be exercised when prescribing in this population. The British National Formulary (2022) reports that adverse reactions are often vague and non-specific in the older general population, with confusion being a frequently presenting symptom caused by most of the commonly used medications. Constipation, postural hypotension, and falls are also noted as common side effects.

Schoufour et al. (2018) determined that polypharmacy is an independent and strong predictor of mortality in the intellectual disability population, independent of multimorbidity. A cross-sectional observational study of adults with intellectual disability between 41 and 90 years of age reports that excessive polypharmacy was observed in 20.1% of participants. Living in a residential institution and having a psychiatric or neurological comorbidity were strongly associated with excessive polypharmacy (O'Dwyer et al., 2016a).

Psychotropic medications are a significant contributor to polypharmacy in the older intellectual disability population. Psychotropic medications are often prescribed in the absence of severe mental illness and are regularly prescribed for challenging behaviour alone. In a large study of more than 33,000 adults with intellectual disability, 49% had a record of psychotropic prescribing despite only 21% of the cohort having documented mental illness. New prescriptions for neuroleptics were significantly more common in the older cohort (Sheehan et al., 2015). A further study observing 405 older adults with intellectual disability and epilepsy noted nearly one-third were prescribed a neuroleptic in addition to an average of two antiseizure medications. Completed epilepsy care plans and reviews were less common in the elderly with intellectual disability (Watkins et al., 2022).

As part of the initiative to reduce psychotropic prescribing in intellectual disability people, NHS England (2019) recommends Stopping the Over-Medication of People with a learning disability, autism, or both (STOMP) and Supporting Treatment and Appropriate Medication in Paediatrics (STAMP) principles. Although these principles were initially developed for younger people with intellectual disability, they are transferrable and relevant to the older age cohort. The guidance comprises a comprehensive set of recommendations when starting, reviewing, and stopping psychotropic medication with the aim of 'the right medication, at the right time, for the right reason.'

Comparisons can be drawn between the STOMP and STAMP criteria, and the BNF-recommended STOPP/START criteria, which have been created to review medication regimens in the general elderly population. STOPP (Screening Tool of Older Persons' potentially inappropriate Prescriptions) provides recommendations to review and stop medications if indicated, with the aim to reduce adverse events. Conversely, START (Screening Tool to Alert to Right Treatment) is used to prevent omissions of clinically indicated medications in older people (O'Mahoney et al., 2014).

Both STOMP and STAMP and STOPP/START guidance are recommended resources when commencing, reviewing, or discontinuing medication in the older intellectual disability population and access information is available in the resources section at the end of the chapter.

The Frith Treatment Guideline for People with Intellectual Disability

Medication Considerations

Older people with intellectual disability require lower doses of medication, similarly to the older general population. Particular attention should be paid to medication–medication interactions as well as to prescribing multiple medications from the same group of medications. Regular review and optimisation of medications is recommended to minimise unwanted effects and medication associated morbidities.

Medications which are commonly prescribed in older people and have a significant adverse effect or risk profile include medications with anticholinergic side effects. Medications with anticholinergic properties encompass a wide range of pharmaceuticals and are often used to treat conditions which are prevalent in older people with intellectual disability. Examples of these medications include those frequently used for pain relief (i.e., co-codamol, morphine), anxiety and sedation (neuroleptic medication, some antidepressants, such as amitriptyline, selective serotonin reuptake inhibitors (SSRI) and serotonin and norepinephrine reuptake inhibitors (SNRI)), and urge incontinence (i.e., solifenacin). Anticholinergic medications have a side-effect profile which includes both central and peripheral effects, such as sedation, confusion, blurred vision, orthostatic hypotension, constipation, and difficulty urinating. With increasing anticholinergic exposure, the risk of adverse outcomes including falls, delirium, and admission to hospital increases (Boustani et al., 2008; Best et al., 2013), as well as cognitive impairment and increased mortality (Ruxton et al., 2015).

The deleterious effects of anticholinergic medications are cumulative, and the effects are described as the 'anticholinergic burden'. The anticholinergic burden score (ACB score) is a tool that was developed to calculate the total burden of anticholinergic medication on an individual, with a score of 3+ indicating significant cholinergic burden, warranting an urgent review of the anticholinergic medication (Boustani et al., 2008). The anticholinergic burden score for some commonly prescribed is shown in Table 22.2, though this list is not

Table 22.2 Anticholinergic burden score (ACB) for commonly prescribed medications in the elderly population with intellectual disability

Examples of medications with anticholinergic properties	Anticholinergic burden score 1	Anticholinergic burden score 2	Anticholinergic burden score 3
Antidepressants	sertraline citalopram fluoxetine venlafaxine duloxetine mirtazapine bupropion		paroxetine amitriptyline clomipramine imipramine nortriptyline
Neuroleptics	haloperidol aripiprazole risperidone		clozapine olanzapine quetiapine chlorpromazine
Antiepileptics	sodium valproate lithium	carbamazepine	
Sedatives	diazepam clonazepam lorazepam		
Painkillers	codeine morphine		
Other			promethazine solifenacin oxybutynin

exhaustive. Access information for the anticholinergic burden score has been provided in the Resource Box at the end of the chapter. O'Dwyer et al. (2016b) determined that in elderly people with intellectual disability, the median anticholinergic burden score was 4, and 29.1% had an anticholinergic burden score of 5+. Neuroleptics contributed to 35.4% of the cumulative anticholinergic burden score, with other anticholinergics medications, including antidepressants, and antiepileptics being the additional most prescribed classes.

The Maudsley Prescribing Guidelines in Psychiatry (Taylor et al., 2021) contain a nine-page guide to medication doses of commonly used psychotropics in older adults, which due to the lack of formal prescribing guidance for the older person with intellectual disability may be utilised when considering commencing psychotropic medication. The guide contains information regarding starting doses, usual maintenance doses, and maximum doses generally accepted in the elderly alongside any specific considerations. Further information is available in the Resource Box at the end of the chapter. These guidelines should be used with additional caution and contemplation when prescribing for people with intellectual disability. Table 22.3 summarises some considerations when prescribing psychotropic medication in both the general and intellectual disability elderly populations.

Table 22.3 A summary of considerations when prescribing in the elderly population

Medication class	Considerations in the elderly
Analgesia	General population: • Paracetamol is considered a safe and well-tolerated medication in the elderly. • Caution should be used when prescribing NSAIDs in the elderly; consider bleeding risk and renal function. Consider short-term use with gastroprotection, or whether a topical preparation may be used. • Opiates can increase the risk of falls, cognitive side effects including sedation, medication–medication interactions, and constipation. Additional considerations for elderly people with intellectual disability: • Pain (particularly headaches, musculoskeletal pain, or pain related to the circulatory and respiratory systems) often goes undetected and undertreated in this group so index of suspicion should be high (Axmon et al., 2018a).
Antidepressants	General population: • May require prolonged medication treatment before desired effect (10–12 weeks) (Nelson et al., 2008). • Increased risk of side effects or complications from commonly prescribed antidepressants such as hyponatraemia, gastrointestinal bleeding, increased blood pressure, increased QTc (in particular citalopram and escitalopram) and sedation (NICE, 2022). • At risk groups for hyponatraemia: female, increasing age, previous or current hyponatraemia, coadministration of diuretics (Mottram et al., 2006).

Table 22.3 (cont.)

Medication class	Considerations in the elderly
	• Consider the anticholinergic burden of commonly prescribed antidepressants, particularly tricyclic antidepressants.
Antiepileptics	General population: (Kaur et al., 2019)
	• Consider medication–medication interactions as antiepileptic medications are inducers and inhibitors of the cytochrome P450 enzyme superfamily, as well as being subject to metabolism by the cytochrome P450 system (therefore levels are affected by other inducers and inhibitors of the system).
	• Hepatic changes in the elderly as described in the pharmacokinetics section of this chapter may influence the metabolism and availability of antiepileptic medications.
	• Lamotrigine and levetiracetam are noted to be virtually free of cognitive side effects that are present in other antiepileptics.
	• Additional caution in the elderly is required when considering properties of antiepileptics: for example, sodium channel blockade, which can exacerbate heart block or other conduction abnormalities. Some antiepileptics may be contraindicated in this instance. Hyponatraemia can be aggravated, particularly with concordant diuretic use.
	• Another relevant complication of antiepileptic use is decreased bone strength and bone mineral density. Serum vitamin D, calcium, phosphate, and alkaline phosphatase should be measured at least annually and supplementation of calcium and vitamin D3 should be prescribed.
	Additional considerations for elderly people with intellectual disability:
	• Unique issues that need to be addressed for intellectual disability elderly patients include higher frequencies of epilepsy that may be refractory to treatment, atypical presentation of symptoms, seizures of multiple types, and the presence of comorbidities (O'Dwyer et al., 2018).
Neuroleptics	General population:
	• Both first- and second-generation neuroleptics have been associated with an increased risk of stroke when used in the longer term, though it is uncertain as to whether this risk is transient (returning to base level after three months) or cumulative (Taylor et al., 2021).
	• The risk of tardive dyskinesia in elderly adults is around 5–6× higher than the general adult population (Jeste, 2000). Age, duration of neuroleptic treatment, high potency, and first-generation preparations are risk factors for developing tardive dyskinesia (Ghosn et al., 2021).
	• When prescribing clozapine in the elderly, there is an increased risk of agranulocytosis and neutropenia. Older people are also vulnerable to the side-effect profile, including hypotension, oversedation, and constipation (Kirrane et al., 2018).

Table 22.3 (cont.)

Medication class	Considerations in the elderly
	• Be wary of the 'prescribing cascade' whereby movement disorders attributed to neuroleptic use are treated with anticholinergic medications, contributing to anticholinergic burden (O'Dwyer et al., 2018). • Consider the broader actions of nonselective neuroleptics, which may cause hypotension, oversedation, and anticholinergic effects. • Consider the impact of extrapyramidal side effects in the elderly person (of which they are at increased risk of developing); these are likely to worsen mobility, increase falls, and decrease capability for activities of daily living. Additional considerations for elderly people with intellectual disability: • Adults with intellectual disability experience an increased risk of adverse effects associated with high anticholinergic burden of neuroleptics (Ward et al., 2022). • There is substantial potential for side effects such as tardive dyskinesia, akathisia, and pseudo-Parkinsonism in the case of first-generation neuroleptics, and increased risk of metabolic side effects and weight gain in the case of second-generation neuroleptics (O'Dwyer et al., 2018).
Sedatives	General population: (O'Mahony et al., 2014) • Risk of prolonged sedation, confusion, impaired balance, and falls. • For use no longer than 4 weeks unless specific indication. • To stop by withdrawing gradually in those who have been treated with benzodiazepines for more than 4 weeks, to reduce risk of withdrawal syndrome. • Consider stopping if a person has had a fall in the past 3 months, or in those with respiratory failure. Additional considerations for elderly people with intellectual disability: • Increased risk of falls, fall-related fractures, and other fall-related injuries than the general adult population (Axmon et al., 2018b).
Lithium	General population: (Mohandas and Rajmohan, 2007) • Aim for plasma levels 0.4–0.7 mmol/L in the elderly. • Lithium levels are higher in the elderly when compared to a similar dose in the general adult population due to a combination of factors, including a smaller volume of distribution (a result of lower total body water), dehydration in the elderly, and reduced GFR (associated with ageing but also the long-term use of lithium). • Medications commonly used in the elderly population such as diuretics, non-steroidal anti-inflammatories, and ACE inhibitors can alter the serum levels of lithium. Additional considerations for elderly people with intellectual disability:

Table 22.3 (cont.)

Medication class	Considerations in the elderly
	• Phlebotomy in intellectual disability patients can be challenging due to anxiety, phobia, hypersensitivity or movement disorders, and reasonable adjustments, desensitisation work, and a modified frequency of blood tests for lithium should be considered.
Z-medications	General population: • The British National Formulary (2022) recommends caution when prescribing in the elderly, particularly those preparations with a longer half-life which may lead to prolonged hangover effects of drowsiness, unsteady gait, slurred speech, and confusion. Additional considerations for elderly people with intellectual disability: • The sleep-wake rhythm in this population is less stable and more fragmented than in older adults in the general population. • Visual impairment, severe hearing impairment, epilepsy, and spasticity are independently associated with a less stable or more fragmented sleep-wake rhythm in older adults with intellectual disability specifically (van de Wouw-Van Dijk, 2013).
Other	General population: • Promethazine is a first-generation antihistamine and is nonselective with significant anticholinergic activity. • Hyoscine hydrobromide is an anticholinergic medication. *The Maudsley Prescribing Guidelines in Psychiatry* (Taylor et al., 2021) recommend pirenzepine and sublingual atropine for the management of hypersalivation in the elderly population with dementia. • Please note that the use of antidementia medications will be covered in Chapter 18 on Dementia.

Other Practical Considerations

Considering health changes that occur both physiologically with ageing and those which are already prevalent in the intellectual disability population, there are practical considerations that may assist in medication prescribing. With age, people with intellectual disability may acquire further deterioration in vision or hearing, cognition, self-care ability, and motor functions such as swallowing and coordination. The following strategies may help with this:

- Large print or easy-read medication information leaflets should be given and discussed with the patient.
- Cognitive deficits or difficulties experienced when taking medication could have implications on medication compliance. Every effort to maintain independence should be given. For this, reminder charts, medication alarms, and (if required) multi-compartment compliance aids (MCAs) may be considered before caregiver involvement to support the administration of medication.

- MCAs should be discussed with and ideally prepared at the pharmacy to minimise risk associated with user error, and to negate the use of unsuited medications in MCAs. (N.B. Some medications should not be removed from their outer packaging and transferred into an MCA as the exposure to light or moisture may make the medication unstable).
- Reduced mobility and frailty may lead to difficulty in accessing medication. Considerations such as a postal pharmacy service or allocating medications to be sent to a local pharmacy may be helpful.
- Impaired vision and hearing, and difficulties with swallowing, coordination, and motor functions may affect the ease of taking certain formulations of medication. This could involve the practicalities of handling medication, opening the packaging, preparing the preparation, and swallowing the medication.
- If tablets are left in the mouth for prolonged periods of time, ulcers may develop. Alternative formulations such as oro-dispersible tablets and liquid preparations may need to be sought.
- Medication administration technique should be observed: for example, if medications require preparation (i.e., adding a medication to liquid) or skill in administration (i.e., inhaler technique and use of aids such as a spacer device).
- Difficulties which can lead to the user altering the preparation of the medication (e.g., crushing a large, modified-release tablet or emptying the content of a capsule into liquid), could lead to unintentional overdose and toxic effects of medications.

Medication initiation, titration, and monitoring should be rigorously discussed with the patient and caregiver at each clinical encounter to reduce occasions whereby poor compliance leads to suboptimal levels, or mismanagement of medication leads to user error and unintentional overdose.

Non-Medication Approaches

This section gives considerations/strategies which are not directly related to prescribing but may reduce the unnecessary reliance on the use of medications in this population.

Diagnostic overshadowing is a well-versed topic in the intellectual disability population, and it is essential to rule out physical conditions which may give rise to disturbed behaviour. An atypical presentation should be considered when older people with intellectual disability present with functional decline. Functional decline may often be attributed to dementia or challenging behaviours; however, it may be a result of treatable conditions such as delirium, depression, and sensory impairments (Lim et al., 2018). Holistic principles should be implemented with elderly people with intellectual disability, similarly to how they are implemented in the general population. Thus:

- Regular screening for both visual and auditory deficits may help to establish a baseline and thus detect any early decline of the senses, in a population where sensory deficits are prevalent.
- Regular assessments for mobility will provide the opportunity for early detection of a decline in mobility, the ability to provide assistive equipment with aims to increase quality of life, mobility, and engagement, and to reduce falls.

A systematic literature review by Schepens et al. (2019) informs on the effects of support strategies on the quality of life of elderly people with intellectual disability. Quality of life was determined by eight established domains (Schalock et al., 2005) as well as existential and spiritual well-being (see Table 22.4).

Table 22.4 Support strategies affecting quality of life of elderly people with intellectual disability (compiled using information from Schepens et al. 2019)

With noted positive effect on quality of life:	With noted negative effect on quality of life:
Ageing in place (remaining in the same residence). If relocation is necessary, then this should be prepared alongside the person and their caregiver network.	High staff turnover, unsuitable accommodation, care networks falling apart.
Provision of aids, equipment, and adaptations for physical and mobility changes. Provision of cognitive devices.	Staff decide how free time is organised and provide a schedule rather than encouraging choices.
Deinstitutionalization leading to a more favourable staff: resident ratio.	Relocation, unplanned moves, or hospital admissions.
Provision of accessible community environment and more community activities, as well as developing networks in the community. Provision of more meaningful social activities.	Being housed in regular services for older people highlights a need for intellectual disability-specific elderly residential housing, specialist training of staff and/or development of community intellectual disability networks for inclusive activities in the community.
More choice around determining routine and activities that the person wishes to engage in. Self-determination work.	Activities focused only on health promotion and not social stimulation or enjoyment.
Retirement planning, active mentoring on the topic.	Transportation or financial constraints.
Physical health promotion. Attendance of physical health monitoring and screening appointments.	Ageist ideas and moving older people into larger residential placements.
Supporting communication.	
Life Story Work. Reminiscence groups.	
Giving spiritual care to the anxious elderly who are dying, advanced care planning, DNA-CPR (Do not attempt cardiopulmonary resuscitation) decisions. End of life care collaboration and adequate treatment of needs.	
Appointing a key person to coordinate care who knows the person well.	
Where hospital admission is required, good interdisciplinary care and communication to patient and caregivers.	

Conclusion

The life span of people with intellectual disability is increasing. People with intellectual disability are also prone to an accelerated ageing process. The impact of ageing, multimorbidity, and polypharmacy imply a strong need to be vigilant to the side effects of medications in this population. There can be distinct changes in the pharmacokinetics of the medications necessitating the need to monitor the effects and side effects as well as body metabolic parameters. Presence of organ dysfunction (such as renal impairment) should necessitate increased vigilance. In addition, there can be significant pharmacodynamic considerations such as increased sensitivity to anticholinergic side effects.

Medication use in elderly persons with intellectual disability is essential and can be life-saving, but it needs to be carefully monitored to reduce the unwanted use of medications (number of medications used and how long medications used) to minimise the risk of unwanted side effects, medication-related morbidities/mortality as well as to improve the quality of life. A guiding consideration should be the quality of life of the individual, and this needs to be considered in discussion with the person and other people in the individual's circle of support.

Case Study 22.1

David is a 60-year-old man with intellectual disability, Down syndrome, autism, and epilepsy. David was prescribed sodium valproate 1600 mg for epilepsy and has done well with this. Five years ago, he had an episode of depression and was started on venlafaxine 150 mg. David also has medications for bronchial asthma which has remained controlled.

David's carer reported that he has been becoming forgetful for the past few months. David used to go to the nearby shops by himself and return home. Over the last four months, he has wandered off a few times and had to be returned home by neighbours who knew him. He has also become very confused a couple of times, throwing objects at other people and appearing to be very fearful.

On assessment David was found to have had a steady loss of skills over the last few months. David's mood was euthymic although he was anxious about not being able to do things like going to the shop on his own anymore. The physical examination and blood tests were normal. David would not cooperate for an MRI (magnetic resonance imaging) or CT (computerised tomography) scan of his head. An initial diagnosis of dementia was considered based on his decline in cognitive performance compared to his usual baseline, and in absence of underlying physical and mental health problems that could have impaired his cognition. His psychiatrist used the Dementia Scale in Learning Disability (DLD) to check the decline in the cognitive and social domains along with the negative results from examination and blood tests to arrive at the diagnosis.

David was started on donepezil 5 mg as antidementia medication. He did not show any side effects (i.e., confusion, change in sleeping patterns, diarrhoea, nausea and vomiting, fatigue, or muscle cramps) and after one month the dose was increased to 10 mg. A review after six months did not show notable change. At this time, after careful consideration and discussion with the carers, a decision was made to withdraw venlafaxine. Withdrawal of venlafaxine had a notable change in David's appearance and behaviour, with him becoming more alert and regaining some of the skills he had lost. A re-evaluation using the DLD four months after stopping venlafaxine showed significant improvement in cognitive and social domains. Further follow-up and discussion with carers took place to consider reducing the dose of sodium valproate and if seizures recurred replacing it with a non-sedating antiepileptic medication. With the optimisation of David's medications, David stopped having periods of confusion as well as regained some of the skills. This provided David with another two years of life with reasonable independence, although he could still not go out on his own. David's memory continued to deteriorate which confirmed that he did also have dementia.

The Frith Prescribing Guidelines Editors' Expert Group Consensus Statements

Statements of High Confidence
- The life expectancy for people with intellectual disability is increasing.
- The intellectual disability population has a higher number of multiple long-term conditions in comparison to the general population, and this increases with age.
- Polypharmacy is common in the intellectual disability population, especially in older people with intellectual disability.
- Psychotropic medications contribute significantly to the anticholinergic burden.
- People with intellectual disability are frailer at an earlier age when compared to the general population.
- As in the general population, age-related changes affect pharmacokinetics and pharmacodynamics in people with intellectual disability as well, which may require an adjustment in prescribing.

Statements of Medium Confidence
- Medications with anticholinergic effects are commonly prescribed in the intellectual disability population.
- Psychotropic medications are commonly prescribed in the intellectual disability population in the absence of severe mental illness, including for challenging behaviour alone.
- STOMP principles are transferrable and relevant to the older age cohort with intellectual disability.

Statements of Low Confidence
- Recommendations are gleaned from the general elderly population, though this guidance should still be used with additional caution and consideration.

Resource Box

Prescribing Principles
STOMP and STAMP principles for prescribing in people with learning disability, autism or both: www.england.nhs.uk/learning-disabilities/improving-health/stomp/
STOPP/START principles for prescribing in older people: https://bnf.nice.org.uk/medicines-guidance/prescribing-in-the-elderly/

Rating Scales and Calculators
ID-frailty index: https://dx.doi.org/10.1016/j.ridd.2013.01.029
Anticholinergic burden calculator: www.acbcalc.com/

Easy-Read Documents
STOMP and STAMP principles: www.england.nhs.uk/wp-content/uploads/2018/02/stomp-easy-read-leaflet.pdf

Treatment Recommendations

The Maudsley Prescribing Guidelines in Psychiatry (2021) provides a guide to prescribing recommendations of commonly used psychotropic medications in older adults: www.maudsley-prescribing-guidelines.co.uk

References

Axmon, A., Ahlström, G. & Westergren, H. (2018a). Pain and pain medication among older people with intellectual disabilities in comparison with the general population. *Healthcare*, **6**(2), 67. https://doi.org/10.3390/healthcare6020067.

Axmon, A., Sandberg, M., Ahlström, G. & Midlöv, P. (2018b). Fall-risk-increasing drugs and falls requiring health care among older people with intellectual disability in comparison with the general population: A register study. *PLOS ONE*, **13**(6), e0199218. https://doi.org/10.1371/journal.pone.0199218.

Best, O., Gnjidic, D., Hilmer, S. N., Naganathan, V. & McLachlan, A. J. (2013). Investigating polypharmacy and drug burden index in hospitalised older people. *Internal Medicine Journal*, **43**(8), 912–918. https://doi.org/10.1111/imj.12203.

Boustani, M., Campbell, N., Munger, S., Maidment, I. & Fox, C. (2008). Impact of anticholinergics on the aging brain: A review and practical application. *Aging Health*, **4**(3), 311–20. https://doi.org/10.2217/1745509x.4.3.311.

British National Formulary (2022). Prescribing in the elderly. NICE. https://bnf.nice.org.uk/medicines-guidance/prescribing-in-the-elderly/.

de Leeuw, M. J., Oppewal, A., Elbers, R. G., et al. (2022). Healthy Ageing and Intellectual Disability study: Summary of findings and the protocol for the 10-year follow-up study. *BMJ Open*, **12**(2), e053499. https://doi.org/10.1136/bmjopen-2021-053499.

Drenth-van Maanen, A. C., Wilting, I. & Jansen, P.A.F. (2019). Prescribing medicines to older people – How to consider the impact of ageing on human organ and body functions. *British Journal of Clinical Pharmacology*, **86**(10), 1921–30. https://doi.org/10.1111/bcp.14094.

Gensous, N., Franceschi, C., Salvioli, S., Garagnani, P. & Bacalini, M. G. (2019). Down Syndrome, ageing and epigenetics. *Sub-Cellular Biochemistry*, [online] **91**, 161–93. https://doi.org/10.1007/978-981-13-3681-2_7.

Ghosn, O., Ye, E. & Huege, S. (2021). Evaluating and managing tardive dyskinesia in the older adult'. *Current Geriatrics Reports*, **10**(3), 108–15. https://doi.org/10.1007/s13670-021-00364-8.

Hermans, H. & Evenhuis, H. M. (2014). Multimorbidity in older adults with intellectual disabilities. *Research in Developmental Disabilities*, **35**(4), 776–83. https://doi.org/10.1016/j.ridd.2014.01.022.

Jansen, P. A. F. & Brouwers, J. R. B. J. (2012). Clinical pharmacology in old persons. *Scientifica*, **2012**, 1–17. https://doi.org/10.6064/2012/723678.

Jeste, D. V. (2000). Tardive dyskinesia in older patients. *The Journal of Clinical Psychiatry*, **61**(4), 27–32. https://pubmed.ncbi.nlm.nih.gov/10739328/.

Kaur, U., Chauhan, I., Gambhir, I. S. & Chakrabarti, S. S. (2019). Antiepileptic drug therapy in the elderly: A clinical pharmacological review. *Acta Neurologica Belgica*, **119**(2), 163–73. https://doi.org/10.1007/s13760-019-01132-4.

Kirrane, A., Majumdar, B. & Richman, A. (2018). Clozapine use in old age psychiatry. *BJPsych Advances*, **24**(3), 204–11. https://doi.org/10.1192/bja.2017.26.

Lim, J. C., Bessey, L. J., Joshi, P. & Boyle, L. L. (2018). Intellectual disability in the elderly. In R. Tampi, D. Tampi, & L. Boyle (eds.), *Psychiatric Disorders Late in Life*. Springer, 253–262. https://doi.org/10.1007/978-3-319-73078-3_23.

Mann, C., Jun, G. T., Tyrer, F., et al. (2022). A scoping review of clusters of multiple long-term conditions in people with intellectual disabilities and factors impacting on outcomes for this patient group. *Journal of Intellectual Disabilities*, 174462952211072. https://doi.org/10.1177/17446295221107275.

Mohandas, E. & Rajmohan, V. (2007). Lithium use in special populations. *Indian Journal of Psychiatry*, **49**(3), 211. https://doi.org/10.4103/0019-5545.37325.

Mottram, P. G., Wilson, K. & Strobl, J. J. (2006). Antidepressants for depressed elderly. *Cochrane Database of Systematic Reviews*. https://doi.org/10.1002/14651858.cd003491.pub2.

National Institute for Health and Care Excellence (2022). BNF. NICE. Available at: https://bnf.nice.org.uk.

Nelson, J. C., Delucchi, K. & Schneider, L. S. (2008). Efficacy of second-generation antidepressants in late-life depression: a meta-analysis of the evidence. *The American Journal of Geriatric Psychiatry: Official Journal of the American Association for Geriatric Psychiatry*, **16**(7), 558–67. https://doi.org/10.1097/JGP.0b013e3181693288.

NHS England (2019). STOMP and STAMP principles. www.england.nhs.uk/wp-content/uploads/2019/02/STOMP-STAMP-principles.pdf.

NICE (2022). Selective serotonin reuptake inhibitors (SSRIs). NICE. https://cks.nice.org.uk/topics/depression/prescribing-information/ssris/.

O'Dwyer, M., Maidment, I. D., Bennett, K., et al. (2016b). Association of anticholinergic burden with adverse effects in older people with intellectual disabilities: An observational cross-sectional study. *British Journal of Psychiatry*, **209**(6), 504–10. https://doi.org/10.1192/bjp.bp.115.173971.

O'Dwyer, M., McCallion, P., McCarron, M. & Henman, M. (2018). Medication use and potentially inappropriate prescribing in older adults with intellectual disabilities: A neglected area of research. *Therapeutic Advances in Drug Safety*, **9**(9), 535–57. https://doi.org/10.1177/2042098618782785.

O'Dwyer, M., Peklar, J., McCallion, P., McCarron, M. & Henman, M.C. (2016a). Factors associated with polypharmacy and excessive polypharmacy in older people with intellectual disability differ from the general population: A cross-sectional observational nationwide study. *BMJ Open*, **6**(4), e010505. https://doi.org/10.1136/bmjopen-2015-010505.

O'Leary, L., Cooper, S.-A. & Hughes-McCormack, L. (2018). Early death and causes of death of people with intellectual disabilities: A systematic review. *Journal of Applied Research in Intellectual Disabilities: JARID*, **31**(3), 325–42. https://doi.org/10.1111/jar.12417.

O'Mahony, D., O'Sullivan, D., Byrne, S., et al. (2014). STOPP/START criteria for potentially inappropriate prescribing in older people: Version 2. *Age and Ageing*, **44**(2), 213–18. https://doi.org/10.1093/ageing/afu145.

Ruscin, J. M. & Linnebur, S.A. (2019). Pharmacokinetics in Older Adults. MSD Manual Professional Edition. www.msdmanuals.com/en-gb/professional/geriatrics/drug-therapy-in-older-adults/pharmacokinetics-in-older-adults.

Ruxton, K., Woodman, R. J. & Mangoni, A. A. (2015). Drugs with anticholinergic effects and cognitive impairment, falls and all-cause mortality in older adults: A systematic review and meta-analysis. *British Journal of Clinical Pharmacology*, **80**(2), 209–20. https://doi.org/10.1111/bcp.12617.

Schalock, R. L., Verdugo, M. A., Jenaro, C., et al. (2005). Cross-cultural study of quality-of-life indicators. *American Journal on Mental Retardation*, **110**(4), 298. https://doi.org/10.1352/0895-8017(2005)110[298:csoqol]2.0.co;2.

Schepens, H. R. M. M., Van Puyenbroeck, J. & Maes, B. (2019). How to improve the quality of life of elderly people with intellectual disability: A systematic literature review of support strategies. *Journal of Applied Research in Intellectual Disabilities*, **32**(3), 483–521. https://doi.org/10.1111/jar.12559.

Schoufour, J. D., Maes-Festen, D., Oppewal, A. & Evenhuis, H. M. (2021). Towards untangling the ageing riddle in people with intellectual disabilities: An overview of research on frailty and its consequences. In M. Putnam & C. Bigby (Eds.), *Handbook on ageing with disability*. Routledge.

Schoufour, J. D., Mitnitski, A., Rockwood, K., Evenhuis, H. M. and Echteld, M. A. (2013). Development of a frailty index for older people with intellectual disabilities: Results from the HA-ID study. *Research in Developmental Disabilities*, **34**(5), 1541–55. https://doi.org/10.1016/j.ridd.2013.01.029.

Schoufour, J. D., Oppewal, A., van der Maarl, H. J. K., et al. (2018). Multimorbidity and polypharmacy are independently associated with mortality in older people with intellectual disabilities: A 5-year follow-up from the HA-ID Study. *American Journal on Intellectual and Developmental Disabilities*, **123**(1), 72–82. https://doi.org/10.1352/1944-7558-123.1.72.

Sheehan, R., Hassiotis, A., Walters, K., et al. (2015). Mental illness, challenging behaviour, and psychotropic drug prescribing in people with intellectual disability: UK population-based cohort study. *BMJ*, **351**(8023), h4326. https://doi.org/10.1136/bmj.h4326.

Taylor, D. M., Barnes, T. R. & Young, A. H. (2021). *Prescribing in older people: In Maudsley Prescribing Guidelines in Psychiatry*. Wiley-Blackwell.

Tyrer, F., Kiani, R. & Rutherford, M. J. (2020). Mortality, predictors and causes among people with intellectual disabilities: A systematic narrative review supplemented by machine learning. *Journal of Intellectual & Developmental Disability*, **46**(2), 1–13. https://doi.org/10.3109/13668250.2020.1834946.

van de Wouw-Van Dijk, E. (2013). Circadian sleep-wake rhythm in older adults with intellectual disabilities. In *Sleep and Sleep-wake rhythm in older adults with intellectual disabilities*. Erasmus University, pp. 103–18. https://repub.eur.nl/pub/40241.

Ward, M. L., Cooper, S.-A., Henderson, A., et al. (2022). A study on prescriptions contributing to the risk of high anticholinergic burden in adults with intellectual disabilities: retrospective record linkage study. *Annals of General Psychiatry*, **21**(1). https://doi.org/10.1186/s12991-022-00418-x.

Watkins, L. V., Henley, W., Sun, J. J., et al. (2022). Tackling increased risks in older adults with intellectual disability and epilepsy: Data from a national multicentre cohort study. *Seizure*, **101**, 15–21. https://doi.org/10.1016/j.seizure.2022.05.022.

White, A., Sheehan, R., Roberts, C., et al. (2022). Learning from Lives and Deaths – People with a learning disability and autistic people (LeDeR) report for 2021. King's College London. www.kcl.ac.uk/ioppn/assets/fans-dept/leder-main-report-hyperlinked.pdf.

Index

Abbey pain scale, 270
Aberrant Behaviour Checklist (ABC), 64, 135
acceptance and commitment therapy, 121
adverse life events
 increased occurrence in intellectual disability, 61
 see also trauma
affective disorders, 15, 87
aggression, 131–52
 bipolar disorder, 103
 case studies, 147–7, 149–50
 definition, 131
 diagnostic criteria, 132
 expert group consensus statements, 150–1
 medication treatment evidence base, 136–8
 withdrawal of, 148–9
 personality disorders, 163
 prevalence, 131–2
 psychological therapies, 135
 resources, 151–2
 risk factors, 132
 symptom of mental illness/disorder, 55
 treatment algorithm, 146
 see also challenging behaviour; self-injurious behaviour
alcohol use disorders
 medication treatments, 192
 NICE guidelines, 185
 prevalence, 183
 Wernicke–Korsakoff syndrome, 185
Alzheimer's disease, 258
American Psychiatric Association (APA), diagnostic criteria for intellectual disability, 2
Angelman syndrome
 risk factor for autism, 210
 sleep disorders, 225
annual health check, 31

anticholinergic burden score (ACB), older people, 326
anticholinergics, 288
 side effect profile, 326
anti-dementia drugs, monitoring recommendations, 35
antidepressants
 anxiety disorders, 78
 duration of treatment, 95
 monitoring recommendations, 32
 obesogenic risk, 42
 overprescribing, 148
 prescribing in intellectual disability, 90
 prescribing rates, 14, 15
 sleep disorders, 232
 withdrawing medication, 6, 97–8
antihistamines, sleep disorders, 232
antipsychotics
 alcohol use disorder, 192
 anxiety disorders, 77
 association with constipation, 45
 autism, 211, 216
 autism, NICE guidelines, 218
 behavioural disturbances, 4
 bipolar disorders, 107, 109, 112
 challenging behaviour, 54–5
 epilepsy, 245
 monitoring recommendations, 33, 35–6
 obesogenic risk, 42
 overprescription of, 248
 paraphilic disorders, 173
 personality disorders, 158
 potential impact on sleep, 225
 prescribing rates, 14, 15
 PTSD, 66
 reduction/discontinuation programmes influencing factors, 19

 reviews, 19
 schizophrenia, 122
 sleep disorders, 233
 withdrawing medication, 6
antiseizure medications (ASM)
 adverse effects, 245
 choice, 247–8
 classification, 246
 evidence base, 245
 mood stabilisers, 103
 newer medications, 246
 off-licence prescribing, 249
 overview, 242
 polypharmacy, 249
 polytherapy, 244
 prescribing principles, 247
 prescribing rates, 14, 15
 specific epilepsy syndromes, 248
 traffic light system, 245–6
 withdrawal, 249
anxiety disorders, 74–84
 overview, 74
 aetiology, 74–5
 assessment, 79
 behavioural disturbances, 74
 case studies, 76, 81
 clinical presentation, 74
 differential diagnosis, 75
 duration of treatment, 81
 expert group consensus statements, 83
 medication treatments, 78–9, 80–1
 NICE recommendations, 77, 79
 non-medication treatments, 77–8, 80
 prevalence in intellectual disability, 76
 resources, 83–4
 treatment algorithm, 82
 treatment guidelines, 79–81
 treatments in the general population, 76–7
anxiety, symptom of mental illness/disorder, 55
anxiolytics
 anxiety disorders, 78

338

monitoring
 recommendations, 35
aripiprazole
 autism, 216
 RCT, 304
aspiration pneumonia, 275,
 276, 282, 285
atomoxetine, 193, 203–4, 205,
 303, 307
attention deficit and
 hyperactivity
 disorder (ADHD), 34,
 199–207
 atomoxetine, 204
 case studies, 149, 202, 205,
 305, 306
 clinical presentation
  in childhood, 298–9
  in intellectual
   disability, 202
 clonidine, 204
 definition, 199
 diagnostic classifications,
  200, 201
 differential diagnosis, 200–2
 duration of treatment, 205
 expert group consensus
  statements, 206
 guanfacine, 204
 iron deficiency, 304
 medication treatments,
  202–4, 303
 methylphenidate, 203–4
 NICE guidelines, 206
 non-medication treatments,
  204–5
 paraphilic disorders,
  171
 prevalence, 199
 resources, 207
 sexual offending, 171
 similarities with other
  disorders, 300
 sleep disorders, 225
 treatment guidelines, 206
autism spectrum disorder
 (ASD), 209–19
 age of onset, 209
 assessment, 215–16
 case study, 218
 causes, 210
 challenging behaviour,
  63, 211
 differential diagnosis, 210
 duration of treatment,
  216–18

employment-related
 interventions, 213
evidence base for treatment,
 212–15
expert group consensus
 statements, 219
genetic syndromes
 associated with
 increased risk of, 210
medication treatments
 evidence base, 213–15
 treatment guidelines, 216
 NICE guidelines, 211–12
non-medication treatments
 evidence base, 212–13
 treatment guidelines, 216
personality disorders, 156
prevalence, 211
prevalence estimates for co-
 occurring mental
 health and
 neurological
 conditions, 210
prevalence of paraphilic
 fantasies and
 behaviours, 171
psychotropic medications, 4,
 211, 217
resources, 219
risk factor for PTSD, 62
risk factors in pregnancy and
 birth, 210
self-injurious behaviour, 133
sensory hypersensitivities
 and trauma, 61
sexual offending, 171
sleep disorders, 224–5
social skills
 interventions, 213
trauma and, 66
treatment algorithm, 217
treatment guidelines, 215–18
treatment in general
 population, 211–12
autonomic nervous system
 (ANS), impact of
 trauma on, 62, 63–4

bariatric surgery, 44
behaviour disorders, 138, 298
 clinical presentation, 299
 medication treatment,
  evidence base, 304
Behaviour Problems
 Inventory, 135
behavioural disturbances

antipsychotics, 4
anxiety disorders, 74
constipation, 44
sleep disorders, 235
Belfast Health and Social Care
 Trust, 276
benzodiazepines
 adjunctive therapy, 125
 alcohol abuse disorders, 185,
  191, 195
 anxiety disorders, 77, 81
 insomnia, 232
 prescribing rates, 15
 PTSD, 66
 withdrawal, 24, 234
bipolar disorders, 102–13
 acute mania, 105–6
 case studies, 104, 107,
  111–12
 combination therapy, 107
 comorbidities, 110
 definition, 102
 depression, 108
 differential diagnosis, 103
 discontinuing
  medication, 110
 duration of treatment, 110
 electroconvulsive
  therapy, 110
 expert group consensus
  statements, 112–13
 long-term treatment
  bipolar I, 109
  bipolar II, 109
 maintenance treatment,
  108–9
 medication treatment, 105
 monotherapy, 106–7
 NICE guidance, 108,
  110, 112
 prevalence, 102
 prophylaxis, 109
 rapid cycling bipolar
  disorder, 103, 108–9
 resources, 113
 screening tools, 103–4
 treatment refractoriness,
  109–10
buprenorphine, 187
bupropion, 186

cancer, under-detection of in
 intellectual
 disability, 31
cannabis use disorder
 focus of treatment, 186

cannabis use disorder (cont.)
  non-medication treatments, 193
  proposed medication treatments, 193
cannabis use, prevalence in intellectual disability, 184
carbamazepine
  alcohol abuse disorders, 185, 191
  bipolar disorder, 109
cardiography, 227
carer support in using medication, 7
case studies
  ADHD, 149, 202, 205, 305, 306
  aggression, 134–5, 147–7, 149–50
  anxiety disorders, 76, 81–2
  autism, 218
  cerebral palsy, 147–7, 280, 289
  childhood mental health problems, 301, 305, 306
  dementia, 261–2, 270, 333
  depression, 89, 97, 98
  Down syndrome, 228–9, 333
  eating and drinking difficulties, 280, 285, 289
  epilepsy, 89, 97, 242, 248, 250, 289, 317, 333
  insomnia, 228–9, 233, 234
  older people, 333
  personality disorders, 156–7, 164
  positive behaviour support, 23, 194
  prescribing of psychotropic medications, 23–4
  PTSD, 66–7
  schizophrenia, 126
  self-injurious behaviour, 134–5, 305
  sleep disorders, 228–9, 233, 234
  Smith-Magenis syndrome, 305
  substance use disorders, 184, 194–5
  women's health issues, 317
catamenial epilepsy, 311
cerebral palsy

as cause of intellectual disability, 2
  case studies, 147–7, 280, 289
  eating and drinking difficulties, 280, 288–9
  epilepsy, 240
  salivation management, 286, 287–8
challenging behaviour
  antipsychotics, 54–5
  autism, 63, 211
  behaviour support plan, 142
  bipolar disorder and, 103
  clinical presentation in childhood, 299
  definition of challenging behaviour, 52
  diagnostic assessment, 53
  effectiveness of pharmaceutical treatments, 13
  emotional regulation and, 63
  formulation and understanding, 53
  interventions, 54
  mental health conditions and, 52
  NICE guidance, 20, 141–7, 148
  offending behaviour, 52
  positive behaviour support, 54
  Prader Willi syndrome, 63
  prescribing, 54–6
    clear mental illness/ disorder, 55
    general points, 56
    no mental illness present, 54–5
    off label, 55–6
    some features of mental illness/disorder, 55–6
  prevalence in selected settings, 52
  psychiatric disorders and, 2–3
  psychotropic medications
    negative consequences, 61
    potential overuse, 6
    prescription rates, 3, 54
    supporting role, 3
  resources, 58
  restraint and, 61
  risk factors, 141
  schizophrenia, 119–20

social effects, 53
trauma, 61, 63–4
see also aggression; self-injurious behaviour
'chemical straitjacketing', 4
chest infections, 276
dysphagia as contributing factor, 275
Child and Adolescent intellectual disability Psychiatry Network (CAIDPN), 302
childhood
  abuse, 61, 157, 170
  aggression, 132
  Gillick competency, 300
childhood mental health problems, 297–307
  ADHD, 298–9
  capacity assessment, 300
  case studies, 301, 305, 306
  challenging behaviour, 299
  clinical presentation, 298
  diagnosis, 299, 301
  duration of treatment, 305–6
  examples of, 297
  expert group consensus statements, 306
  management, 301–3
  medication treatments
    appropriate, 302–3
    evidence base, 303–4
  Mental Health Act, 302
  NICE guidance, 301
  non-medication treatments, 304–5
  prevalence, 297
  resources, 307
  STOMP-STAMP campaign, 303, 305
Children Act (1989), 300
choking, 276, 282–3
chromosomal disorders, 2, 204
Clinical Global Impression (CGI) scale, 56
clomethiazole, 185
cocaine use
  prevalence in intellectual disability, 184
  self-help groups, 187
cognitive behaviour therapy (CBT)
  obesity, 41
  schizophrenia, 121
  sexual offenders, 171
  trauma, 65

cognitive disorders compared with developmental disorders, 1
communication aids, 7
communication difficulties
  prescribing medication, 6–7
  prevalence, 276, 281
constipation, 44–6
contraception, 310
Cornelia de Lange syndrome, 133, 305
COVID-19 (Coronavirus disease), 321

dementia, 254
  anti-dementia medications, 35
  assessment, 258–61
    instruments, 261
    structure, 258
  behavioural and psychiatric symptoms
    algorithm, 267
    medication treatments, 264, 268–9
    non-medication management, 264–6
  case studies, 261–2, 270, 333
  cause of death in intellectual disability, 321
  clinical presentation, 254
  clinical stages, 255
  cognitive symptoms, medication treatments, 264
  definition, 254
  differential diagnosis, 255–6
  end-of-life care, 270–1
  expert group consensus statements, 271–2
  medication treatments, 262–3
  mimicked in Down syndrome, 255
  most common causes in intellectual disability, 257
  prevalence, 87, 256–8
  resources, 272
  treatment guidelines, 264–9
depression, 87–99
  antidepressants
    comorbid illnesses, 95
    discontinuation, 97
    case study, 98
    prescribing, 90
    withdrawal symptoms, 98
  case studies
    discontinuation of antidepressants, 98
    presentation, 89
    treatment, 97
  characteristic, 87
  differential diagnosis, 87–9
  expert group consensus statements, 98–9
  key guidelines, 99
  medication treatments
    evidence base, 91
    first line, 92–3
    resistance to, 94
    second line, 93
  NICE guidelines, 92
  non-medication treatments, 91–2
  prevalence, 87–8
  rating scales, 89
  resources, 99
  symptoms in intellectual disability, 88
  treatment
    algorithms, 94
    general guidance, 92
    NICE guidance, 92
    recommended duration, 94
developmental disorders
  comparison with cognitive disorders, 1
  definition, 1, 51
  grading, 1
Diabetes Remission Clinical Trial (DiRECT), 41
Diagnostic and Statistical Manual (DSM)
  ADHD, 199
  anxiety, 74
  bipolar disorders, 102
  children and adolescents, 299
  dementia, 254
  depression, 87, 89
  intellectual disability, 2, 51
  mania, 104
  paraphilic disorders, 169
  personality disorders, 155, 157
  PTSD, 62, 64
  schizophrenia, 118
  substance use disorders, 169, 180
Diagnostic Assessment for the Severely Handicapped-II (DASH II), 103
Diagnostic Criteria for psychiatric disorders for use in adults with learning disabilities DC-LD (2001), 75
Diagnostic Manual – intellectual disability DM-ID (2007), 75
diagnostic overshadowing, 2, 76, 89, 105, 225, 300, 331
Dialectical Behaviour Therapy (DBT), personality disorders, 158, 159
DisDAT (Distress Assessment Tool), 270, 276, 281
disorders of intellectual development, definition, 1
disulfiram, alcohol use disorder, 185, 192
Down syndrome
  accelerated ageing, 322
  ADHD, 199, 204
  as cause of intellectual disability, 2
  case studies, 228–9, 333
  dementia, 255–6, 258, 262, 333
  differential diagnosis, 255–6
  older people, 322, 333
  premature menopause, 311
  prevalence of ADHD, 199
  risk factor for autism, 210
  sleep disorders, 225
Dravet syndrome, 246
dysphagia
  age of onset, 276
  associated risks, 285
  clinical presentation, 275
  contributing medications, 280
  expert group consensus statements, 292–3
  prevalence, 32, 276, see also eating and drinking difficulties

eating and drinking difficulties, 275–94
  administration of medication via PEG tubes, 291–2
  aspiration pneumonia, 275–6, 282, 285
  associated conditions and syndromes, 277
  case studies, 280, 285, 289
  choking, 276, 282–3
  clinical presentation, 275–6
  contributing medications, 280
  definition, 275
  differential diagnosis, 276
  eating and drinking with acknowledged risk (EDAR), 285–6
  expert group consensus statements, 292–3
  feeding tubes, 289–92
  IDDSI Framework, 283
  management, 281
  nutrition and hydration support algorithm, 284
  positive behaviour support strategies, 282
  posture and positioning, 282
  prevalence, 275, 276
  referral to MDT, 280
  reflux, 276, 281, 287
  resources, 293–4
  salivation management, 282, 286–8
  symptoms and possible causes, 278–9
  texture modification, 282
  thickeners, 283
  weight algorithm, 284
  see also dysphagia; salivation management
Ehlers–Danlos syndrome, 63
electrocardiography (ECG), 106, 124
electroconvulsive therapy (ECT), 302
electroencephalography (EEG), 227, 233
emotional regulation, 63
end-of-life care, NICE guidance, 270–1
England
  medication reduction programmes, 13

  public campaign to stop overuse of medication in intellectual disability, 6
  see also STOMP and STAMP programmes
epilepsy, 238–52
  and ADHD, 201
  antiseizure medications, 17, 247
  autism, 209
  case studies, 89, 97, 242, 248, 250, 289, 317, 333
  catamenial epilepsy, 311
  classification of seizures, 239
  correlation with intellectual disability, 238, 240
  definition, 238
  developmental and epileptic encephalopathies, 240
  diagnosis, 240–1
  diagnostic criteria, 238
  different types, 239
  differential diagnosis, 240–2
  duration of treatment, 248–9
  expert group consensus statements, 250–1
  good prescribing practice, 244
  ILAE classification framework, 239
  management, 108
  medication treatment prescribing principles, 247
  treatment guidelines, 244
  mood stabilisers, 103
  mortality, 238–9
  NICE guidelines, 243, 244
  non-medication management, 244
  older people, 333
  overview of management, 242–4
  polypharmacy, 238
  presentation in intellectual disability, 241
  prevalence, 2, 15, 31, 238–9
  resources, 251–2
  seizure diary, 241, 249
  sleep disorders, 223, 225, 233
  specific guidance for management in intellectual disability, 245–6

  sudden unexpected death in epilepsy (SUDEP), 239, 243, 249, 250
  treatment guidelines, 242–6
  see also antiseizure medications (ASM)
Equality Act (2010), 31
eye movement desensitisation and reprocessing therapy (EMDR), 65

feeding tubes, 289–92
5-P formulation model, 53
fluoxetine
  autism, 216
  bipolar disorder, 108
Fragile X syndrome
  as cause of intellectual disability, 2
  challenging behaviour, 63
  prevalence of ADHD, 200
  risk factor for autism, 210
  self-injurious behaviour, 133
  sleep disorders, 225
fronto-temporal dementia, 258

GABA agonists, anxiety disorders, 78
gender reassignment treatments, 302
genetic causes of intellectual disability, 2
genetic syndromes
  associated with risk of autism, 210
  poor sleep patterns, 225
  prevalence of ADHD, 199
  sleep disorders, 224
Gillick competency, 300
Glasgow Antipsychotic Side-effect Scale (GASS), 56
Glasgow Anxiety Scale for people with an intellectual disability (GAS-ID), 83
Glasgow Depression Scale for People with a Learning Disability (GDS-LD), 89

Health and Care of People with Learning Disabilities (NHS Digital 2022), 14

Health of the Nation Outcome Scale (HoNOS), 56
health outcomes in intellectual disability, 2
HELP framework (Health, Environment, Lived experience, Psychiatric problems), 53
heroin dependence, medication treatments, 194
heroin use, prevalence in intellectual disability, 184
hyoscine, 288
hyperacusis, 61
hypnotics, monitoring recommendations, 35
hypoxia at birth, as cause of intellectual disability, 2

Independent Mental Capacity Advocate (IMCA), 8
Insomnia Severity Index, 226
insomnia, case study, 228–9, 233, 234
Integrated Theory of Sexual Offending (ITSO), 170
intellectual disability (ID), 1–9
and evidence-based practice, 4
causes, 2–3
definitions, 1, 51
diagnostic criteria, 2
health outcomes, 2
prevalence, 51
psychiatric disorders and challenging behaviour, 2–3
retrospective diagnosis, 51
International Classification of Diseases (ICD)
ADHD, 200
anxiety, 74
autism, 209
bipolar disorder, 102
children and adolescents, 299
dementia, 254
intellectual disability, 2, 51
paraphilic disorders, 169
personality disorders, 155

premenstrual dysphoric disorder (PMDD), 310
PTSD, 62, 64
schizophrenia, 118
substance use disorders, 180
International Dysphagia Diet Standardisation Initiative (IDDSI, 2019), 283
intoxication, definition, 181

Jacobsen syndrome, sleep disorders, 225

Karolinska Sleepiness Scale, 226

lamotrigine, 108
Learning Disability Mortality Review (LeDeR), 31, 44, 276, 321
Lennox Gastaut syndrome, 246
Lesch–Nyhan syndrome, 133
Lewy body dementia, 258
Liberty Protection Safeguards, 282
life expectancy in intellectual disability, 2, 321
lifestyle-associated diseases, prevalence in intellectual disability, 2
lithium, 106
Liverpool University Neuroleptic Side Effect Rating Scale (LUNSERs), 56

Makaton signing, 7
Maudsley Prescribing Guidelines in Psychiatry, 327
medication, potential problems in intellectual disability, 192
menopause, 311
menstrual cycle, 311–12, 313–16
Mental Capacity Act (2005), 281
mental capacity, and consent to treatment, 5
Mental Health Act (2017), 281, 302
mental health conditions, 51–8

assessment, 53
challenging behaviour, 52
diagnostic assessment, 53
prescribing, 54–6
psychotropic medications, 56–7
self-assessment for clinicians, 57
prevalence
in intellectual disability, 51
population based rates, 52
resources, 58
symptom clusters, 55
Mentalisation Based Treatments (MBT), personality disorders, 158
methadone, 187
methylphenidate, ADHD, 203–4
mindfulness, intervention for obesity, 42
mood stabilisers
antiseizure medications, 103
APA recommendations, 158
bipolar disorder, 105, 108
monitoring recommendations, 34
overprescribing, 148
paraphilic disorders, 173
personality disorders, 158
with comorbid illness, 110–11
withdrawal of, 110
Moss Psychiatric Assessment Schedules (MPAS), 127
multi-disciplinary team (MDT)
deprescribing of psychotropic medication, 23
eating and drinking difficulties, 281
epilepsy, 243
psychosis, 121
myography, 227

NACHBID trial, 136
naltrexone
alcohol misuse, 185, 192
opioid dependence, 187
self-injurious behaviour, 141
National Institute for Health and Care Excellence (NICE)
ADHD, 34, 206

National Institute (cont.)
  alcohol use disorders, 185
  anxiety disorders, 77, 79
  autism, 211–12
    antipsychotics, 218
  bipolar disorders, 108, 110, 112
  challenging behaviour, 20, 141–7, 148
  childhood mental health problems, 301
  depression, 92
  end-of-life care, 270–1
  epilepsy, 243, 244
  obesity, 40, 41
  personality disorders, 158
  psychosis, 120
  psychotropic medications
    monitoring, 41
    prescribing of, 21
  PTSD, 65
  schizophrenia, 120
  self-injurious behaviour, 145
National Prescribing Observatory for Mental Health Audits, 57
neurodevelopmental conditions, see attention deficit and hyperactivity disorder (ADHD); autism spectrum disorder (ASD)
neurofibromatosis, risk factor for autism, 210
nidotherapy, personality disorders, 159

obesity, NICE guidelines, 40, 41
oculography, 227
offending behaviour, 52, 160, 161, 181
off-licence prescribing
  antiseizure medications, 249
  psychotropic medications, 4
olanzapine
  bipolar disorder, 105, 106, 108
  epilepsy, 245
  schizophrenia, 126
older people, 321–35
  anticholinergic burden score, 326

case study, 333
Down syndrome, 322, 333
expert group consensus statements, 334
frailty and accelerated ageing, 322
key issues related to prescribing in intellectual disability, 322–5
leading causes of death, 321
life expectancy in intellectual disability, 321
medication considerations, 325–30
non-medication approaches, 331–2
pharmacokinetic and pharmacodynamic changes, 322–4
physical health conditions, 321
polypharmacy, 324–5
practical considerations, 330–1
prescribing considerations, 327–30
psychotropic medications, 325, 327
resources, 334–5
support strategies, 332

paraphilic disorders
  aetiology, 170
  assessment, 174
  'counterfeit deviance' theory, 170
  definition, 169–70
  differential diagnosis, 170–1
  duration of treatment, 175
  expert group consensus statements, 175
  medication treatments, 173, 174
  non-medication treatments, 173–4
  prevalence, 171
  resources, 175–7
  treatment algorithm, 175–6
  treatment guidelines, 174–5
  treatments in general population, 171–3

treatments in intellectual disability, 173
see also sexual offending
Parent version of the Young Mania Rating Scale (P-YMRS), 104
perimenopause, 311
personality disorders, 155–65
  antisocial personality disorder, 155, 157–8, 300
  APA guidelines, 158
  assessment, 161
  borderline personality disorder, 155, 157–8
  case study, 156–7, 164
  causes, 156
  cluster system, 155
  comorbid mental illnesses, 159
  definition, 155–6
  differential diagnosis, 156
  duration of treatment, 163
  expert group consensus statements, 164
  medication treatments, 160–1, 162–3
  NICE guidelines, 158
  non-medication treatments, 159–60, 161
  prevalence, 157
  resources, 165
  risk factors, 156
  symptom domains, 162
  treatments in general population, 158
  treatments in intellectual disability, 159–64
  unrecognised complex PTSD, 65
pharmacodynamics, definition, 5
pharmacogenomics, 5
pharmacokinetics, definition, 5
physical health conditions, 31–47
  annual health check, 31
  constipation, 44–6
  expert group consensus statements, 47
  monitoring recommendations, 32–40
  prevalence, 31

reasonable
    adjustments, 31–2
resources, 47
weight gain and obesity
    bariatric surgery, 44
    behavioural
        approaches, 41
    changing
        medication, 42–3
    definitions and
        categories, 40–1
    general principles, 41
    lifestyle changes, 41
    management
        algorithm, 45
    medication for
        management of
        obesity, 43–4
    obesogenic risk of
        antipsychotics and
        antidepressants, 42
    prevalence, 40
    psychotropic medications
        and, 41
pica, 132, 276, 304
Picture Exchange
    Communication
    System (PECS), 7
polycystic ovary syndrome
    (PCOS), 310
polypharmacy, 5
polysomnography, 227, 233
positive behaviour
    support (PBS)
    ADHD, 204
    autism, 212–13
    case studies, 23, 194
    challenging behaviour, 54
    childhood mental health
        problems, 304
    definition, 54, 212
    resources, 147
post-traumatic stress disorder
    (PTSD)
    autism, 62
    case study, 66–7
    NICE recommendations, 65
    overlap with other
        psychiatric
        disorders, 64
    prevalence, 61, 64
    trauma, 61–2
Prader–Willi syndrome (PWS)
    challenging behaviour,
        63
    risk factor for autism, 210

self-injurious behaviour
    and, 133
sleep disorders, 225
transcutaneous vagus nerve
    stimulation, 63
pregabalin, use in anxiety
    disorders, 77
premature birth, as cause of
    intellectual
    disability, 2
premenstrual disorders,
    309–10, 313
prescribing medication
    overview, 4–5
    and metabolism, 5
    collaborative decision-
        making, 7
    communication issues, 6–7
    concerns about overuse, 6
    consent to treatment, 5, 8–9
    mental capacity/
        incapacity, 7–8
    person-centred approach, 9
    pharmacogenomics, 5
    polypharmacy, 5
    practice, 6
    psychotropic medications,
        see psychotropic
        medications,
        prescribing of
    prescribing practice, potential
        impact on people
        with intellectual
        disability, 2
propranolol, 66
Psychiatric Assessment
    Schedule for Adults
    with Developmental
    Disabilities Checklist
    (PAS-ADD
    Checklist), 104
psychosis
    cognitive behaviour
        therapy, 121
    late adolescent onset, 297
    NICE guidelines, 120
    prevalence, 120
    suitability of bariatric
        surgery, 44,
    see also schizophrenia
psychosocial interventions
    autism, 211
    NICE recommendations, 212
    schizophrenia, 124–5
    sleep disorders, 234
    substance misuse, 188, 194

psychotropic medications
    autism, 4, 211, 217
    challenging behaviour,
        negative
        consequences, 61
    epilepsy, 238
    ethical considerations, 299
    gradual withdrawal, 218
    health problems associated
        with, 31
    importance of regular
        review, 6
    long-term physical health
        consequences, 13
    monitoring
        NICE guidelines, 41
        RCPsych standards, 57
    monitoring
        recommendations,
        32–40
        ADHD medications, 34
        antidementia
            medications, 35
        antidepressants, 32
        antipsychotics, 33, 35–6
        anxiolytics, 35
        hypnotics, 35
        mood stabilisers, 34
        specific tests and
            monitoring for
            serious mental health
            illness, 36–40
    older people, 325, 327
    personality disorders,
        158, 163
    prescribing
        overview, 13
        deprescribing in
            challenging
            behaviour
            guidance, 21
        practical example,
            23
        relapse and
            recurrence, 26
        withdrawal
            problems, 24
        expert group consensus
            statements, 27
        for challenging behaviour,
            3, 6, 54
        good practice, 148–9
        medication review
            programmes, 17–18
        effectiveness, 18–19
        USA example, 18

psychotropic (cont.)
  withdrawal of antipsychotic medications, 19
  NICE NG11 standards, 21
  off-licence, 4
  overprescribing, 6, 20, 23–4, 148
  prevalence, 13–15
  RCPsych principles, 21
  RCPsych recommendations, 57
  resources, 27–8
  reviews of clinical practice in England, 13
  standards, 57
  STOMP and STAMP programmes, *see* STOMP and STAMP programmes
  surveys, 90
  relationship with obesity, 41
  self-assessment tool for clinicians, 57
  standards and recommendations, 56–7
  Winterbourne View report, 20
pulse oximetry, 227

quetiapine, bipolar disorder, 106, 108

rapid cycling bipolar disorder, 103, 108–9
reflux, 276, 281, 287
relapse prevention therapy, for treatment of sexual offenders, 171
REPOS (Rotterdam Elderly Pain Observation Scale), 270
restraint, 61
Rett syndrome
  self-injurious behaviour, 133
  sleep disorders, 225
risperidone
  anxiety disorders, 79
  autism, 4, 216, 218
  bipolar disorders, 105
  PTSD, 66
  RCT, 304
  schizophrenia, 122
Rubinstein–Taybi syndrome, sleep disorders, 225

salivation management
  botulinum toxin injections, 289
  definition of salivation and saliva control, 286
  difficulty in, 287
  medication treatments, 287–8
  evidence base, 288
  prevalence of issues with, 286
  role of saliva, 286–7
  surgical relocation of salivary duct, 289
Sanfilippo syndrome, sleep disorders, 225
schema therapy, personality disorders, 159
schizophrenia, 118–28
  assessment, 124
  case studies, 126
  causes of, 118
  definition, 118
  diagnostic tools, 120
  differential diagnosis, 119–20
  duration of treatment, 125
  expert group consensus statements, 127
  medication treatments, 122–3, 124, 125
  NICE guidelines, 120
  non-medication treatments, 121, 124
  prevalence in intellectual disability, 120
  resources, 127–8
  treatment guidelines and algorithm, 124–5
  treatment in general population, 120
  treatment in intellectual disability, 121–3
seizures
  definition, 238
  seizure diary, 241, 249
selective serotonin reuptake inhibitors (SSRIs)
  anxiety disorders, 77
  autism, 214, 216
  childhood mental health problems, 303, 304
  paraphilic disorders, 172
  PTSD, 66
  withdrawal of, 24
self-harm
  autism, 209, 218

definition, 133
self-injurious behaviour, 131–52
  behavioural interventions, 135
  case studies, 134–5, 305
  causes of, 133
  clinical features, 144–5
  clinical subtypes, 133
  definition, 132–3
  differentiation from self-harm, 133
  expert group consensus statements, 150–1
  medication treatment, evidence base, 138–41
  NICE guidance, 145
  prevalence, 133
  psychological therapies, 135
  resources, 151–2
  risk factors, 133
  symptom of mental illness/disorder, 55
  treatment, 144–5
  treatment algorithm, 146
serotonin–noradrenaline reuptake inhibitors (SNRIs), 77, 81, 83, 326
sertraline, anxiety disorders, 77, 79
Sex Offender Treatment Programme (SOTP), 173
sexual abuse
  prevalence in adults with intellectual disability, 171
  risk factor for personality disorders, 156
sexual offending
  aetiology, 170
  association with intellectual disability, 171
  paraphilias and, 169
  treatment of sexual offenders, 171–3
  see also paraphilic disorders
sleep disorders, 223–36
  antidepressants, 232
  antihistamines, 232
  antipsychotics, 233
  behaviour disturbances, 235
  behaviour strategies, 230
  breathing disorders, 225, 233
  case studies, 228–9, 233, 234

causes of sleep
difficulties, 224
circadian rhythm sleep-wake
disorders, 233
definition, 223
diagnosis, 225–7
further investigations, 227
sleep diary, 228
sleep history, 226–7
differential diagnosis, 224–5
expert group consensus
statements, 235
hypnotics, 232, 234
insomnia, 223, 224, 227,
231, 232
insomnia, CBT, 229
International Classification
of Sleep Disorders,
categories, 223
long-term management,
234
medication treatments, 230
melatonin, 230, 231–2, 234
movement disorders, 233
narcolepsy, 233
non-medication
treatments, 231
obstructive sleep apnoea,
225, 227, 233
potential consequences, 225
prescribing strategies, 231
prevalence, 223–4
resources, 235–6
screening tools, 226
sleep hygiene, 230, 231
treatment in intellectual
disability, 229–31
withdrawal of
medication, 234
Smith–Magenis syndrome,
305
case studies, 305
physical health
treatments, 305
prevalence of ADHD, 200
self-injurious behaviour
and, 133
sleep disorders, 225
sodium valproate
bipolar disorder, 106, 107
development of PCOS,
311, 312
epilepsy, 247
monitoring
requirements, 107
paraphilic disorders, 173

risks of exposure during
pregnancy, 24,
106, 247
speech and language therapy
(SLT), eating and
drinking difficulties,
282, 283–7, 289
STOMP and STAMP
programmes
case studies, 23–4
guidance, 21–2
influence on prescribing,
81, 94
initiation and effects, 13,
14–15
pledges, 20
prescribing for children and
adolescents, 303, 305
STOP-Bang
Questionnaire, 226
Stopping Over-Medication of
People with
a Learning Disability,
see under STOMP and
STAMP programmes
Substance Use and Misuse in
intellectual disability
Questionnaire
(SumID-Q), 182
substance use disorders,
180–96
aetiology, 181
alcohol, 185, 191–2
assessment, 190
cannabis, 186, 193
case studies, 184, 194–5
classes of substance, 180
clinical presentation in
intellectual disability,
182–3
cocaine, 187
definition, 180–1
diagnostic tools, 182
differential diagnosis, 181–2
expert group consensus
statements, 195
intoxication, 181
medication treatments, 187,
188–94
non-medication treatments,
188–90, 191–4
opioids, 187, 194
prevalence, 183–4
recommendations for
addiction service
providers, 194

resources, 196
risk factors for substance
misuse, 181
tobacco, 186, 192–3
treatment in general
population, 185–7
treatment in intellectual
disability, 188–94
sudden unexpected death in
epilepsy (SUDEP),
239, 243, 249, 250
suicidality
autism, 209
mentalisation based
treatments, 158
substance use disorders, 182
Supporting Treatment and
Appropriate
Medication use in
Paediatrics, see under
STOMP and STAMP
programmes
Systematic Tool to Reduce
Inappropriate
Prescribing
(STRIP), 19

Talking Mats, 7
The Healthcare Intelligence
Network (THIN), 14
therapeutic interventions,
HELP framework, 53
thiamine, alcohol-related
disorders, 185, 191
tobacco use
medication treatments,
186, 193
NICE
recommendations,
186
non-medication treatments,
192–3
prevalence in intellectual
disability, 183
transcutaneous vagus nerve
stimulation, Prader–
Willi Syndrome, 63
trauma, 61–9
and autism, 66
case study, 66–7
challenging behaviour, 63–4
consequences of unresolved
trauma, 62
everyday traumas, 61
expert group consensus
statements, 68

trauma (cont.)
  meaning of, 62
  mental health, 61–2
  personality disorders, 156
  psychiatric diagnoses, 64–5
  PTSD, 61–2
  resources, 69
  treatment, 65–6
  two-phased approach, 61
tuberous sclerosis
  risk factor for autism, 210
  sleep disorders, 225

valproate, *see* sodium valproate
vascular dementia, 258
velocardiofacial syndrome, prevalence of ADHD, 200
venlafaxine, 66, 93, 333
vitamin D deficiency, risk factor for autism, 210

Whorlton Hall, 61
Williams syndrome
  prevalence of ADHD, 200
  risk factor for autism, 210
  sleep disorders, 225
Winterbourne View, 13, 20, 61
women's health issues, 309–18
  adolescence and puberty, 311
  case study, 317
  catamenial epilepsy, 311
  childbearing years, 310
  contraception, 310
  expert group consensus statements, 317–18
  hormone replacement therapy, 311
  issues specific to intellectual disability, 311–12
  menstrual cycle, 311–12, 313–16
  medication management, 314–16
  perimenopausal issues, 311
  polycystic ovary syndrome, 310
  premenstrual disorders, 309–10
  resources, 318
  screening services, access to, 309